Recent Results
in Cancer Research

86

Fortschritte der Krebsforschung
Progrès dans les recherches sur le cancer

Editor in Chief: P. Rentchnick, Genève
Co-editor: H. J. Senn, St. Gallen

Vascular Perfusion in Cancer Therapy

Edited by
K. Schwemmle and K. Aigner

With 136 Figures and 79 Tables

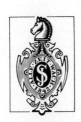

Springer-Verlag
Berlin Heidelberg New York Tokyo 1983

Professor Dr. Konrad Schwemmle
Dr. Karl Aigner

Allgemeinchirurgische Klinik des Zentrums für Chirurgie,
Justus-Liebig-Universität, Klinikstrasse 29, 6300 Giessen, FRG

Sponsored by the Swiss League against Cancer

ISBN 3-540-12346-6 Springer-Verlag Berlin Heidelberg New York Tokyo
ISBN 0-387-12346-6 Springer-Verlag New York Heidelberg Berlin Tokyo

Library of Congress Cataloging in Publication Data. Main entry under title: Vascular perfusion
in cancer therapy. (Recent results in cancer research — Fortschritte der Krebsforschung;
v. 86) Bibliography: p. Includes index. 1. Cancer-Chemotherapy-Addresses, essays, lectures.
2. Perfusion (Physiology)-Addresses, essays, lectures. 3. Thermotherapy-Addresses, essays,
lectures. I. Schwemmle, K. (Konrad), 1934– . II. Aigner, K. (Karl), 1947– . III. Series:
Recent results in cancer research; v. 86. RC261.R35 vol. 86 616.99'4s [616.99'406]
83-10211 [RC271.C5]

© Springer-Verlag Berlin Heidelberg 1983
Printed in Germany.

Typesetting and printing: v. Starck'sche Druckereigesellschaft m.b.H., Wiesbaden
Binding: J. Schäffer OHG, Grünstadt
2125/3140—5 4 3 2 1 0

Contents

Contents

List of Contributors*

---

* Addresses given at beginning of each contribution
1 Page on which contribution begins

Selective Embolization and Organ Perfusion with Cytostatics

Pharmacokinetics of Intra-Arterial Chemotherapy[*]

F. O. Stephens

Department of Surgery, Sydney Hospital, University of Sidney, Sydney, N.S.W., 2000, Australia

Introduction

Since the advent in 1944 of the use of a war-gas product, nitrogen mustard, in clinical medicine for treatment of lymphomas, a wide range of chemical agents with tumoricidal properties have been developed. These agents are especially toxic to cells in the process of division, normal as well as neoplastic. Although a great deal of research has been done to discover agents more specifically selective in destroying neoplastic cells, present studies and management methods are most often designed to determine the drug combinations, timing and ways of administration which result in a maximal antineoplastic effect with minimal disturbance to normal tissues and cells.

Treatment programs using anticancer drugs are designed to capitalise on exploitable differences between cancer cells and normal cells. This may include not only the differences in cellular kinetics and drug pharmacology but also anatomical and physiological features of the cancer cell population. Because cancer cells divide constantly, there are proportionately more of them sensitive to most anticancer drugs at any given time. Cancer cells are also slow dividers, and are therefore longer exposed to drugs which predominantly affect cells in the division process (Hall 1970). Efforts are made to select cytotoxic agents and combinations of agents with a known affinity for the type of cancer cell being treated. Sometimes all or the bulk of cancer cells to be eradicated are supplied with blood by one major artery. This can be cannulated, allowing the cytotoxic agents to be delivered selectively and in higher concentrations to the region containing the tumour. To date, such localization has not been widely exploited.

In the most common use of cytotoxic agents to eradicate, control or palliate widespread or systemic malignancy known to be present the chemotherapeutic agents are most appropriately given systemically, either by mouth or by intramuscular or intravenous injection.

The second use is as adjuvant chemotherapy, i.e., to eradicate occult systemic disease which may or may not be present after a primary cancer has been removed. Here again the agents are best given systemically.

---

[*] The work of the Sydney Hospital Oncology Service is supported by the New Sourth Wales State Cancer Council and by many friends and colleagues associated with Sydney Hospital — this is gratefully acknowledged. My thanks are also due to Mr. John Stewart and Mr. Bill Hsu of the Sydney Hospital Hallstrom Institute for mathematical and computer help, and for preparing the graphs

A third use is to reduce advanced or aggressive localised cancer in patients in whom distant metastases are unlikely. The objective is to improve the prospects for cure by planned subsequent standard local treatment, usually radiotherapy and/or surgery. This may be called "reducing" or "basal" chemotherapy (Stephens 1976, 1978). When the tumour to be treated is contained in a region supplied by one regional artery there would seem to be an advantage in delivering the agents directly into the regional artery supplying the tumour. This technique is most commonly appropriate in treating advanced or aggressive neoplasms of the head and neck or of the limbs. Although it has also been used in dealing with advanced localised tumours which recurred after treatment by radiotherapy with or without surgery, results with recurrent tumours in general have been poor (Nervi et al. 1970; Stephens 1970; Morrow et al. 1977; Jussawalla and Shetty 1978; Swenerton et al. 1979).

Recently, reducing or basal chemotherapy has begun to be used as well in patients in whom there is also a significant risk of systemic spread, which may already be present. This may apply to breast carcinoma (especially when the local tumour is advanced), to sarcoma in limbs or to carcinoma of the stomach (Stephens et al. 1979, 1980a, b). In this situation it may be appropriate to use both basal chemotherapy given by regional arterial infusion preceding definitive local treatment and adjuvant chemotherapy following definitive local treatment.

Regional chemotherapy by i.a. infusion is most appropriate in the "basal" or "reducing" situations described above. The cytotoxic agents are thus delivered in a greater concentration to the region embracing an advanced or aggressive tumour so that the tumour may be reduced to proportions which are more readily eradicated by definitive radiotherapy and/or surgery. Regional chemotherapy may also be used by infusing the hepatic artery in situations where systemic metastatic disease appears to be confined to the liver.

This paper outlines the pharmacokinetic and clinical principles concerned in the use of regional i.a. infusion of anticancer agents.

Pharmacokinetic Factors

Figure 1 illustrates the circulatory system. If 100% of the agent or combination of agents used is infused through a small artery with relatively small blood flow supplying a small percentage of body tissues, the initial concentration of agent flowing to the region will be greater than if a large artery supplying a large proportion of blood to tissues is infused. Therefore, the smaller the blood flow through the artery infused, the greater will be the initial concentration of agents in the regional tissues. In clinical practice the smallest appropriate regional artery is selected for infusion.

The more rapidly the agents are detoxified or excreted after they have entered the systemic venous circulation, the greater will be the relative effect of the initial circulation through the arterial tumor vascular bed. If, for example, all of an agent passing through liver and kidneys were eliminated, there would be a very rapid fall off in plasma concentration during subsequent circulation to both tumour and nontumour tissues. Conversely, with slow drug elimination a higher concentration of agents during subsequent circulation to both tumour and nontumour tissues would be maintained, although only a fraction of the initial high concentration would remain in the region of the artery originally infused. Some data on the methods and rates of elimination of the commonly used agents are available in clinical practice.

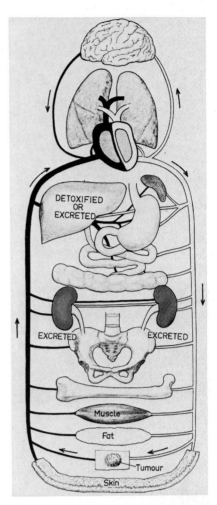

Fig. 1. The circulation. Note the relatively small artery which supplies the region containing a localised tumour; this is often the case. Delivery of anticancer agents into the artery of supply results in a significantly greater concentration of the agent in the region of the tumour than would systemic administration

A third factor is the amount of an agent infused which enters the tissues and tissue fluid but re-enters the venous and lymphatic circulation chemically unchanged. Whilst knowledge about this factor is limited, it seems that it would not greatly affect the end result, other than by allowing more time for a portion of the agent to act chemically on susceptible cells, and also resulting in a delay in detoxification and excretion of the agent.

The important factor which is largely unknown is the amount of agent which functions in a chemically active fashion against the tumour cells and normal cells. As there is no evidence that these agents are catalysts, they are presumably altered in the active metabolic process.

Figures 2 and 3 illustrate these four factors, comparing i.a. with i.v. infusion principles. The relative size of the vessel infused is usually known.

The proportion of agent detoxified or eliminated by liver and/or kidneys is also largely known. Of the agents most commonly infused (bleomycin, adriamycin, fluorouracil (5-FU) and methotrexate), bleomycin would seem to be the most slowly eliminated. About one-third of the amount is eliminated on each passage through the renal circulation. As a slow elimination is least favourable for i.a. infusion, it is assumed in Figs. 4—7 that the rate

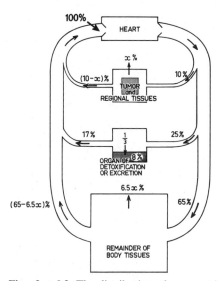

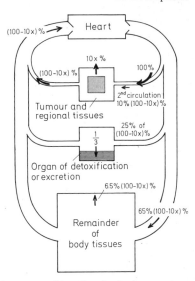

Figs. 2 and 3. The distribution of an agent in the region of a tumour and in other body tissues after intravenous (Fig. 2, *left*) or intra-arterial (Fig. 3, *right*) administration. If 100% of the agent is infused intravenously, and an artery carrying 10% of the blood supplies the region of the tumour and x% of the agent passing through the tumour circulation is biologically active against the tumour, then it is likely that if 100% of the agent is infused into the artery supplying the tumour, 10x% of the agent will be active against the tumour during the first circulation. After the initial circulation, distribution of the agents in the two models will be similar and the advantage of the high concentration of the first circulation will depend upon the rate of excretion or detoxification of the agent infused

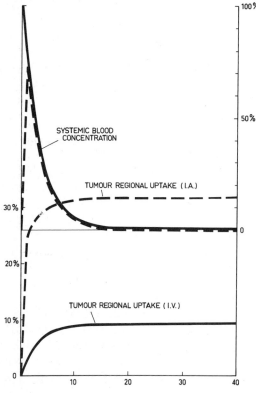

Fig. 4. Difference in concentration of the agent in regional tissue after i.a. administration (*broken lines*) as compared with after i.v. administration (*continuous lines*), assuming that one part in four of the agent passing through the tumour circulation is biologically active against the tumour cells (x = ¼). The upper scale indicates the difference in systemic blood concentration, which is minimal. Even though the regional uptake is some 3 times greater after i.a. administration, in absolute values this is unlikely to be sufficient to make a significant difference in systemic blood concentration. The abscissa indicates the time scale, measured by the number of circulations. In the clinical situation the slopes of the curves will be similar to those shown here but the time scale will be more protracted, as some of the agent will move temporarily into the tissue fluid and subsequently return unchanged into the circulation, resulting in delayed detoxification or excretion

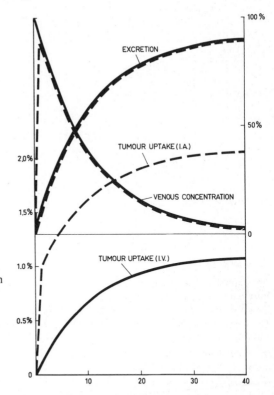

Fig. 5. Concentration of agent in regional tissue, venous concentration, and excretion of agent are compared for i.a. and i.v. infusion, assuming the tumor cell uptake is one part in 100 ($x = \frac{1}{100}$) of the agent passing through the regional circulation. Abscissa values as in Fig. 4. In each comparison *broken line* represents i.a. infusion and *continuous line* i.v. infusion

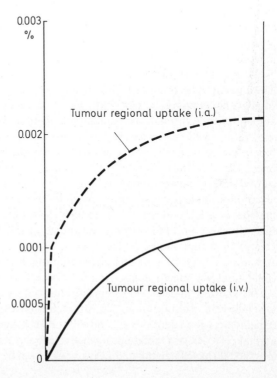

Fig. 6. Same comparison of regional uptake of agent as in Figs. 4 and 5, but with the assumption that only one part in 100,000 of the agent passing through the tumour circulation is biologically active

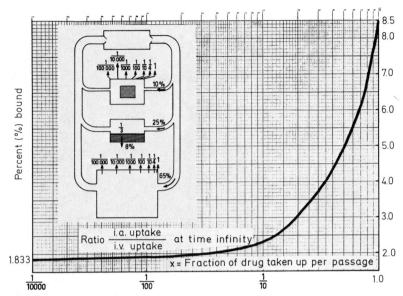

Fig. 7. The relative advantage of i.a. over i.v. uptake in regional tissues, assuming the same conditions as in Figs. 4–6, but with a range of biologically active agents against tumour cells (and normal cells) varying from 100% to only one part in 10,000 of the agent infused being biologically active on each circulation. *Inset* compares with Figs. 2 and 3

of elimination of the agents compared is as for bleomycin. The rate of elimination of adriamycin is about twice as rapid as that of bleomycin (60% cleared on each passage through the liver (Chen and Gross 1980). Methotrexate is eliminated (by the kidneys) twice as rapidly as bleomycin (MIMS Annual 1980) and up to 50% of 5-FU is extracted on each passage through the liver (Chen and Gross 1980). The regional advantage of i.a. over i.v. administration would therefore be significantly greater for adriamycin, methotrexate and 5-FU than that shown in the figures.

The amount of agent entering regional tissues on initial and subsequent passes through the capillary circulation is largely unknown. However, it is likely to be a fixed proportion of the amount passing through the capillary circulation. When i.a. infusion is used, the amount should therefore be greater by a factor which is in inverse proportion to the percentage of blood flow through the artery infused, during the initial circulation only. For example, if one external carotid artery is infused, the factor would be about 25 times, as an external carotid artery carries about 4% or V_{25} of the arterial circulation. In Figs. 4–7, the assumption made is that an artery carrying 10% of arterial circulation is infused, i.e., about the size of a femoral artery, whereas in fact most arteries infused are smaller than the femoral artery and the regional advantage of i.a. over i.v. infusion would therefore be greater than that shown in the figures.

As stated, a proportion of each agent entering the tissues returns unchanged to the venous circulation, serving to delay eventual tissue excretion. For example, Ensminger et al. (1978) showed hepatic vein concentration of carmustine (BCNU) to be greater than systemic vein concentration V_2 h after infusion of BCNU into the hepatic artery. The remainder of the agent is metabolised in its biochemical activity against tumour cells and normal cells. As this metabolically active proportion is not known, values ranging from V_4 to 1/100,000 have been taken for Figs. 4–6. It will be seen that the greater the metabolically active proportion in the tumour and regional tissues on each passage through the circulation, the greater the advantage of i.a. as opposed to i.v. infusion.

Although it is known that the cytotoxic agents used have a greater affinity for tumour cells than for cells of most normal tissues (Lee et al. 1980), it is assumed in Figs. 4–6 that there is no difference in sensitivity to the agents between tumour and normal cells. This, too, will therefore underestimate the true advantage of regional arterial infusion in being concentrated in tumour cells and in avoiding systemic toxicity in tissues outside the region infused.

It will be seen from Fig. 6 that in a model in which an artery with 10% of blood flow is infused and the agent used is excreted at about the rate of bleomycin excretion, there is an anticipated twofold increase (1.8 times) in the amount of drug available to the tumour, even if as little as 1 part per 100,000 is taken up in cellular activity and even if the tumour cells have no greater uptake of the drug than other tissues. If 25% of the drug flowing through is taken up by cells (Fig. 4) the advantage with i.a. will be at the very least 3.5 times better than with i.v. delivery. On the other hand, venous concentration and excretion (and consequently systemic toxicity) will be virtually the same for i.a. and i.v. methods of infusion. The proportion of cytotoxic agents taken up by cells in regional tissues is significantly greater when delivered regionally by i.a. infusion than by the i.v. route, but in absolute quantities the amount taken up regionally is not so great as to make a significant difference in the amount reaching the systemic circulation. Figure 7 is a composite graph showing that the relative advantage of i.a. over i.v. delivery in the fraction of drug biochemically taken up by regional cells ranges from all to as low as 1 part per 10,000.

Review of the Literature

How, then, do these theoretic calculations compare with results of studies already published? Lee et al. (1980) showed that i.a. infusion of adriamycin resulted in a higher tissue metabolism than did i.v. infusion. Whilst there was a higher initial plasma concentration of adriamycin recorded following i.v. administration, this was short-lived. However, they found a significantly increased concentration of adriamycin metabolites in plasma following i.a. administration, indicating that a greater proportion had been biochemically active. They also showed selective adriamycin uptake as follows:

Tumour and liver > Lymphnodes > Muscles and bone marrow > Fat > Skin.

Anderson et al. (1970) showed a greater concentration of methotrexate in a leiomyo-sarcoma after a single i.a. (common iliac) bolus injection than after a single i.v. injection of an equal dose.

Didolkar et al. (1978) compared isolation perfusion, i.a. infusion and i.v. infusion of adriamycin. Because the high tissue levels reached with isolation perfusion were not reached with i.a. infusion, they concluded that i.a. infusion was not effective. However, their own tables of biopsies of tissues taken 1 h after infusion show that there was a greater proportion of adriamycin in skin and muscle of the limb infused than in the opposite limb and a considerably greater concentration in blood from the femoral vein of the side infused.

Chen and Gross (1980) used sophisticated mathematics to pharmacokinetically compare theoretical tissue uptake of agents after i.a. and i.v. infusion. They concluded that the pharmacokinetic model "confirms the general belief that intra-arterial infusion produces an increase in local tissue levels and a reduction in systemic drug availability". They also noted that the increase in local drug concentration depends largely on the blood-flow rate of the infused artery and the rate of drug elimination of the rest of the body; "A low arterial blood-flow rate and a high drug-elimination rate will ensure a high local drug level". In the model they studied Chen and Gross calculated that for i.a. infusion of an artery carrying 100 ml blood/min (i.e., about 8% of circulation) there would be advantges of 2.1 times for adriamycin, 2.5 times for bleomycin, 4.17 times for methotrexate, 7.07 times for melphalan, and 22.67 times for 5-FU. Having made these calculations, they went on to make observations and to study clinical reports. They made two statements about adriamycin:

1. "If the region to receive infusion is the liver no improvement in tumor kill is expected, but there should be a reduction in systemic toxicity".
2. „If an organ other than the liver receives the infusion there should be an increase in the regional drug level and hence the tumor regression, but no reduction in systemic toxicity".

They analysed a paper by Bern et al. (1978) and wrote that "the only study that actually compared i.a. infusion versus i.v. bolus injection of adriamycin reported no significant difference in either antitumor effect or toxicity for both groups".

They accepted this comparison of only four i.a.-infusion versus four i.v.-bolus-treated patients, with two in each group having good responses, as indicating that their pharmacokinetic study was in error. They stated, "There are several possible reasons for this discrepancy between theoretic predictions and the clinical results", and then went on to give explanations.

This dismissal of all their theoretical evidence on the basis of totally inadequate clinical findings seems an extraordinary interpretation of the situation.

They also wrote that the theoretical evidence of increased benefit of i.a. infusion of both bleomycin and methotrexate was not borne out by the clinical evidence, again quoting a small number of inadequate clinical studies, but stated that for 5-FU the clinical evidence supported the theoretical advantage.

An examination of MEDLARS has revealed papers in English from 32 independent centers, covering i.a. infusion methods other than via the hepatic artery which have been used clinically over the past decade. This review cannot claim to be exhaustive, but in 27 of the 32 papers the authors concluded that i.a. chemotherapy was advantageous; in two others no conclusion was reached, and in only three papers was no advantage seen from the use of i.a. infusion. These statistics are quite different from those of a decade or two earlier when i.a. infusion techniques were used largely in patients with recurrent tumours in avascular tissues after failed radiotherapy and/or surgery; in most such cases only single agents were used. In the majority of these papers of a decade or more ago, including a report by the writer (Stephens 1970), the conclusion reached was that chemotherapy used in patients with advanced localised tumours was largely ineffective, and the use of the i.a. route of delivery seemed to offer no particular advantage. It has since been appreciated that carcinoma which recurs in scar tissue after surgery or radiotherapy is poorly vascularised, and agents which depend upon blood flow to get to the tumour site are not likely to be as effective in such situations as they are when used before blood supply has been impaired by previous surgery or radiotherapy (Nervi et al. 1970; Stephens 1970; Jussawalla and Shelty 1978). In the case of hepatic artery infusion for primary or secondary liver malignancy, reports from 18 centres were discovered, with 15 indicating favourable results, two undecided and one finding no advantage.

An experimental model has been designed by a group working with rats, at the Netherlands Cancer Institute, Amsterdam (Schouwenberg et al. 1980). A squamous carcinoma was implanted in front of each ear of the rats and tumour responses to i.a. infusions of bleomycin, methotrexate and 5-FU were compared. The agents were given by 7-day continuous infusion into the external carotid artery on one side. The tumour on the opposite side was regarded as a systemic chemotherapy control.

The tumour used did not respond to methotrexate, no matter how it had been administered, but the response of the tumours on the side of regional infusion which was 3.75 times greater in the case of bleomycin and 3 times greater in the case of 5-FU than that of the tumour on the opposite side. In other words, 3.75 times more bleomycin or 3 times more 5-FU was required to achieve the same effect systemically as was achieved by regional i.a. infusion.

These workers also found that the greatest antitumour effect was achieved by intermittent i.a. administration of combinations of the agents infused.

Clinical Observations

Disulphine blue is a dye with a molecular weight similar to those of many of the agents used; in fact, its mol. wt. of 567 is greater than the mol. wt. of 5-FU (130), BCNU (214), mitomycin C (335), methotrexate (454) and adriamycin (544), but less than those of actinomycin D (1,255) and bleomycin (1,400). It is therefore of some interest to observe the distribution of disulphine blue after an i.a. bolus injection, and the delay before the concentration in the regional tissues becomes so dispersed that it is no longer obvious. Observations in our patients have shown that 3–4 h after i.a. injection the dye remains in the regional tissues in an obviously greater concentration than on the opposite side. This supports other evidence that particles of this molecular weight are unlikely to pass through the capillary circulation on the initial circuit without a significant proportion passing into regional tissues as well.

There is also consistent clinical evidence of a greater effect, albeit toxic, of agents in the distribution of an infused artery (Stephens et al. 1980c). After infusion of an external

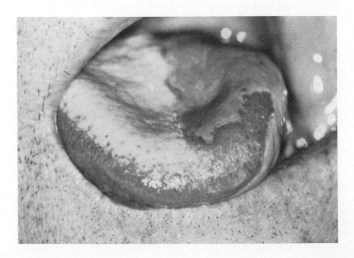

Fig. 8. Ulceration and mucositis on the left side of the tongue during infusion of the left external carotid, with an overgrowth of fungal organisms on the right side of the tongue. The changes in the tongue are invariably different on either side of the midline

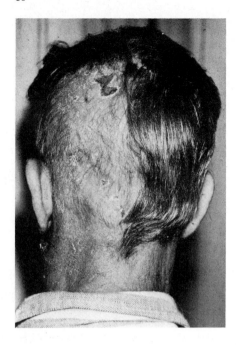

Fig. 9. Skin changes and loss of hair on the left side during infusion of the left external carotid artery. The changes are consistently different on either side of the midline, with evidence of a greater reaction on the side corresponding to the infused artery

carotid artery there is invariably more obvious stomatitis and mucositis with pain and discomfort on the side infused than on the opposite side (Fig. 8). There is also more hair loss on the side infused (Fig. 9). After infusion of an arm or leg with bleomycin there is often evidence of red patches and blistering of the skin of the fingers on the side infused bot not on the opposite side.

Again, indium bleomycin injected into an infused femoral artery resulted in increased radioactivity (and presumably increased bleomycin) in the region of the infused artery for at least 24 h (Stephens et al. 1980c).

At least one agent (cyclophosphamide) is not activated until it has been modified by passage through the liver. There would seem, therefore, to be no advantage in using the i.a. route of administration, as cyclophosphamide itself does not act by direct effect on tumour cells as other agents in common use appear to.

Conclusion

Evidence is accumulating that in treating large or aggressive localised malignant tumours best results may be achieved by first reducing the size, extent and viability of the tumours with "basal" or "reducing" chemotherapy and then capitalising on the reduced tumour size by radiotherapy and/or surgical exicision which are better able to eradicate residual disease (von Essen et al. 1968; Koyama et al. 1975; Auersperg et al. 1978; Mavligit et al. 1981; Stephens et al. 1981a, b). Pharmacokinetic studies supported by clinical evidence of increased regional toxicity suggest that basal chemotherapy has an increased regional effect if the chemotherapeutic agents are infused directly into a regional artery supplying the tumour, rather than into the systemic circulation. Using similar doses of cytotoxic agents, the regional effect will be increased by i.a. regional infusion but systemic side effects may be similar to i.v. administration. Alternatively, a reduced dose may be given i.a. to achieve the same local effect as the standard dose given i.v. with reduced risk of systemic side effects.

Although it is the distinct impression of members of the Sydney Hospital Surgical Oncology Service that clinical results achieved in reduction of tumour size are more impressive after regional (i.a.) than after systemic (i.v.) chemotherapy, and systemic side effects are distinctly reduced, adequate randomised clinical trials have not been carried out either in the Sydney Hospital Service or elsewhere. The main disadvantages of using regional chemotherapy are the increased regional toxicity in the distribution of the artery infused, the small risk of complications of the infusion system, and especially the need for hospitalisation for a month or so while the i.a. infusion is administered.

Therefore, properly controlled randomised clinical trials should be conducted to compare clinical results of i.a. and i.v. chemotherapy administration. As no one centre is likely to have a sufficient number of patients with large and aggressive tumours to justify such a randomised trial, it would seem mandatory that co-operative studies be carried out, involving multicentric groups.

Summary

Advanced or aggressive, but localised, malignancies can often be reduced to more curable proportions by the use of "basal chemotherapy", that is, using chemotherapy as the first mode of treatment, prior to definitive radiotherapy and/or surgical excision. In using anticancer agents, drug combinations, timing and methods of administration are employed which exploit differences between cancer cells and normal tissues and cells. One exploitable difference which is often overlooked is the fact that localised tumour is often supplied with blood by one artery; this can be cannulated so that the agents used can be delivered selectively in high concentration to the region containing the tumour. The advantage in delivering drugs regionally by intra-arterial infusion depends upon the size of the artery infused, the rate of excretion or detoxification of the agents used, the amount of the agent infused entering the tissues – especially from the first circulation, and especially the amount of agent entering the tissues which is biologically active against tumour cells. Taking all these factors into account, mathematical calculations indicated that under the worst possible circumstances infusion of anticancer agents intra-arterially should be at least 1.8 times more effective regionally than intravenous administration. In most situations and with most agents used the advantage would be significantly greater than this. These calculations are supported by evidence in the literature and by observations of a greater regional effect, albeit toxic, of intra-arterial administration of the agents. These effects include more pronounced loss of hair in the region of distribution of the artery infused, and increased skin and mucosal ulceration in the distribution of the artery infused.

The disadvantage of using intra-arterial infusion delivery is the need for hospitalisation. Therefore, properly controlled, randomised clinical trials should be conducted to compare clinical results of intra-arterial and intravenous chemotherapy administration.

References

Anderson LL, Collins GJ, Ojima Y, Sullivan RD (1970) A study of the distribution of Methotrexate in human tissues and tumors. Cancer Res 30: 1344–1348

Auersperg M, Furlan L, Marolt F, Jereb B (1978) Intra-arterial chemotherapy and radiotherapy in locally advanced cancer of the oral cavity and oropharynx. Int J Radiat Oncol Biol Phys 4: 273–277

Bern MM, McDermott W, Cady B, Oberfield RA, Trey C, Clouse ME, Tullis JL, Parker LM (1978) Intraarterial hepatic infusion and intravenous adriamycin for treatment of hepatocellular carcinoma. Cancer 42: 399–405

Chen HG, Gross JF (1980) Intra-arterial infusion of anticancer drugs: theoretic aspects of drug delivery and review of responses. Cancer Treat Rep 64: 31–40

Didolkar MS, Kanter PM, Baffi RR, Schwart HS, Lopez R, Baez N (1978) Comparison of regional versus systemic chemotherapy with adriamycin. Ann Surg 187: 332–336

Ensminger WD, Thompson M, Come S, Egan EM (1978) Hepatic arterial BCNU: a pilot clinical pharmacologic study in patients with liver tumors. Cancer Treat Rep 62: 1509–1512

Hall TC (1970) Clinical oncology for medical students and physicians. In: Rubin P (ed) The American Cancer Society, p 61

Jussawalla DJ, Shetty PA (1978) Experiences with intra-arterial chemotherapy for head and neck cancer. J Surg Oncol 10: 33–35

Koyama H, Wada T, Takahashi Y, Iwanaga T, Aoki Y, Wada A, Terazawa T, Kosaki G (1975) Intra-arterial infusion chemotherapy as a preoperative treatment of locally advanced breast cancer. Cancer 36: 1603–1612

Lee YN, Chan KK, Harris PA, Cohen JL (1980) Distribution of adriamycin in cancer patients. Cancer 45: 2231–2239

Mavligit GM, Benjamin R, Patt YZ, Jaffe N, Chuang V, Wallace S, Murray J, Ayala A, Johnston S, Hersh EM, Calvo DB (1981) Intraarterial cis-platinum for patients with inoperable skeletal tumors. Cancer 48: 1–4

MIMS Annual (1980) IMS Publishing, Division of Intercontinental Medical Statistics (Australia), Artarmon, NSW, Australia

Morrow CP, Di Saia PJ, Mangan CF, Lagasse LD (1977) Continuous pelvic arterial infusion with bleomycin for squamous carcinoma of the cervix recurrent after irradiation therapy. Cancer Treat Rep 61: 1403–1405

Nervi G, Arcangelli G, Casale C, Cortese M, Guadagni A, Le Pera V (1970) A reappraisal of intra-arterial chemotherapy. Cancer 26: 577–582

Schouwenburg PF, Van Putten LM, Snow GB (1980) External carotid artery infusion with single- and multiple-drug regimens in the rat. Cancer 45: 2258–2264

Stephens FO (1970) Intra-arterial infusion of chemotherapeutic agents Methotrexate and "Epodyl" in patients with advanced localized carcinomata recurrent after radiotherapy. Aust NZ J Surg 39: 371–379

Stephens FO (1976) CRAB care and cancer chemotherapy. Med J Aust 2: 41–46

Stephens FO (1978) CRAB chemotherapy. Am J Surg 135: 375–378

Stephens FO, Harker GJS, Dickinson RTJ, Roberts BA (1979) Preoperative basal chemotherapy in the management of cancer of the stomach: a preliminary report. Aust NZ J Surg 49: 331–335

Stephens FO, Crea P, Harker GJS, Roberts BA, Hambly CK (1980a) Intra-arterial chemotherapy as basal treatment in advanced and fungating primary breast cancer. Lancet 2: 435–438

Stephens FO, Crea P, Harker GJS, Lonergan DM (1980b) Intraarterial infusion chemotherapy in salvage of limbs with advanced neoplasms. Aust NZ J Surg 50: 387–392

Stephens FO, Harker GJS, Crea P (1980c) The intraarterial infusion of chemotherapeutic agents as "basal" treatment of cancer: evidence of increased drug activity in regionally infused tissues. Aust NZ J Surg 50: 597–602

Stephens FO, Harker GJS, Hambly CK (1981a) Treatment of advanced cancer of the lower lip – the use of intra-arterial or intravenous chemotherapy as basal treatment. Cancer 48: 1309–1314

Stephens FO, Kalnins IK, Harker GJS, Crea P, Smith ER (1981b) Intra-arterial infusion chemotherapy in the treatment of advanced squamous carcinoma of the tongue and floor of the mouth. Surg Gynecol Obstet 152: 816–818

Swenerton KD, Evers JA, White GW, Boyes DA (1979) Intermittent pelvic infusion with vincristine, bleomycin and mitomycin C for advanced recurrent carcinoma of the cervix. Cancer Treat Rep 63: 1379–1381

von Essen CF, Joseph LBM, Simon GT, Singh AD, Singh SP (1968) Sequential chemotherapy and radiation therapy of buccal mucosa carcinoma in South India. AJR 102: 530–540

Infusion Chemotherapy in Inoperable Pancreatic Carcinoma

S. Bengmark and Å. Andrén-Sandberg

Department of Surgery, University of Lund, 221 85 Lund, Sweden

One of the most common cancers in Europe and North America is that originating in the exocrine pancreas. In Sweden it constitutes 4% of all cancers and approximately 6% of all deaths from cancer. The incidence in Sweden has increased more than 100% during the last 15 years. In the United States today, pancreatic cancer is exceeded only by bronchial, colorectal, and mammary cancer as a cause of death. The increase in number of cases is only higher for bronchial cancer − a similar development can be expected in Sweden and the rest of Western Europe.

The results of treatment of pancreatic carcinoma today are discouraging. Several factors contribute to this: the long asymptomatic stage and the lack of tools to help in early detection of the disease. Most patients consult doctors for the first time when the disease is already too advanced. Moreover, even if early radical operation of the pancreatic carcinoma is tried, prognosis is still bad and only a minority of patients can be regarded as healed. There are good reasons, therefore, for finding new ways to treat this type of cancer.

Approximately 10%−15% of patients with pancreatic carcinoma receive radical surgery. In approximately 85% of cases the cancer is judged to be nonresectable. Treatment must then be restricted to decompression of the bile ducts and, if necessary, to restoration of gastrointestinal tract continuity. Median survival time for this group of patients is approximately 4 months. Thus, it is natural to try radiotherapy and chemotherapy in addition.

Until recently, radiotherapy was considered to have no effect on pancreatic carcinoma. However, with the development of megavolt treatment, reports have appeared showing that patients receiving high doses of radiotherapy have not only some relief of symptoms but also a longer survival time. Radiotherapy does not yet qualify as a routine tool in the treatment of such patients; still more studies are needed to convincingly demonstrate its efficiency.

Many reports in the literature deal with the effects of chemotherapy on pancreatic carcinoma. Common to all, however, is that the number of patients studied is too small to afford any definite conclusion. Most patients who are candidates for a phase II study of chemotherapy in pancreatic carcinoma have a very large tumor, but the results of the therapy can usually only be judged from its effect on peripheral metastases, which are most often of minor importance.

The drug most often tried in treatment of pancreatic cancer is 5-fluorouracil (5-FU). A review of the literature shows it to be effective in up to 67% of cases, mean 28%. On occasion other drugs such as streptozotocin and adriamycin have been tried in small groups with a somewhat higher response, but the scientific quality of these studies is not uncontroversial.

In the use of combination chemotherapy a somewhat higher response rate has been reported. Some studies claim 40% response with the combination of 5-FU, adriamycin, and mitomycin or of streptozotocin with mitomycin C. The price to be paid for these short remissions has been high, however, mainly in the form of general manifestations of toxicity. Thus, we are not yet convinced that any cytotoxic drug or combination of drugs is efficient enough, considering the cost-benefit aspect, to warrant routine use.

One way to decrease the general toxicity without decreasing the effect on the tumor is to administer the drug by regional intra-arterial infusion. The complex arterial anatomy of the pancreas, however, makes it less suitable for intra-arterial infusion than, for example, the liver. However, modern, super-selective angiography techniques make it quite possible. Waddell (1973) reported dramatic effects of 5-FU in combination with testolactone when given to patients with inoperable cancer. This led us to try 5-FU with and without testolactone in a randomized study conducted from 1974 to 1976. Cytologically verified pancreatic carcinoma was localized in the head of the pancreas in nine patients and in the body of the pancreas in ten patients. Of the 19 patients, nine had verified hepatic metastases. Laparotomy, gastroenterostomy, and biliary shunt were performed on all 19.

About 1 month after laparotomy all patients received a catheter through the brachial artery, with the tip localized in the vessel to the pancreatic tumor. The drug was administered over a period of 1 month using a Sigmamotor infusion pump. A dose of 10 mg 5-FU/kg body wt. per day was given, followed by oral administration of 50 mg 5-FU/kg body wt. Testolactone was given in doses of 50 mg 3 times a day. The effect of the treatment was measured angiographically with the use of the catheter introduced for the treatment. In no case was it possible to demonstrate any decrease of the tumors by angiography. However, some changes in the vascular architecture of the tumor were shown, indicating some effect. Some of the patients noticed a decrease in pain, but most important, the mean survival time compared with historical controls was not influenced by 5-FU, with or without testolactone.

The treatment was not without complications. In nine of 19 patients the angiography was done at the end of the treatment. Brachial artery thromboses were demonstrated, but none of the patients had any clinical symptoms, and this complication is probably of no significance. However, two patients had cerebral manifestations in connection with the withdrawal of the catheter, probably due to small arterial emboli. In some of the cases the complications were significant and this points to a potential risk; four of 14 patients demonstrated thrombi in the artery of the abdomen, the hepatic artery, the gastroduodenal artery, or the splenic artery. Whether this was due to the catheter, to an underlying disease, or to a combination of the two is not known. Only one of the patients developed abscesses despite the advanced stage of the disease and the long term of treatment.

It can be concluded that no methods are today available for intra-arterial cytostatic infusion of proven value in patients with inoperable pancreatic carcinoma. It is obvious that new paths should be tried. Infusion chemotherapy with other drugs and in other doses, possibly in combination with irradiation, may prove helpful.

Reference

Waddell WR (1973) Chemotherapy for carcinoma of the pancreas. Surgery 74: 420–429

Intra-Arterial Infusion in Tumors of the Pelvis

R. A. Oberfield

Section of Oncology, Lahey Clinic Medical Center, 41 Mall Road, Box 541, Burlington, MA 01805, USA

Tumors of the pelvis which are accessible to regional arterial infusion therapy are primarily of the bladder, the prostate, the cervix, the ovaries, soft tissues, and bone, and, in the case of recurrent malignancy, of the colorectal area. Among the estimated cancer statistics for 1982 in the United States (Silverberg 1982) are the following:

1. There were 37,000 new cases of *bladder cancer,* including 10,600 deaths; many of these patients had pain and hematuria. The 5-year survival rate for stages B2 and C of bladder cancer is 20%−43%; for stage D, about 10%.
2. There were 73,000 new cases of *prostate cancer,* including 23,300 deaths. This disease has about a 40% mortality, especially in patients with extracapsular extension; 5-year survival rate is 10%−25%.
3. There were 16,000 new cases of *cervical cancer,* including 7,100 deaths.
4. There were 18,000 new cases of *ovarian cancer,* including 11,400 deaths.

Hence, about 144,000 new cases of cancer of the pelvis were diagnosed, with 52,400 of these resulting in death. If we take into consideration the additional 60,000 patients presenting with colorectal tumors involving the pelvis, there is a large number of patients for whom local surgery, radiotherapy, or systemic chemotherapy is ineffective, and who may benefit from pelvic infusion therapy.

About 20 years ago our clinic started a program of chemotherapy using prolonged regional arterial infusion (Sullivan and Zurck 1965; Watkins et al. 1970; Sullivan 1962) of antimetabolites, in the hope of obtaining greater antitumor benefits. Our method (Sullivan 1962; Oberfield and Sullivan 1969; Oberfield et al. 1973; Oberfield 1975) was employed until about 1970; since then only a few patients have had infusion chemotherapy because of increased interest in systemic chemotherapy. However, a review of the literature of the past 10 years on regional chemotherapy shows that there have been sporadic attempts to use it, with interest increasing again in view of discouraging results with systemic treatment. It also revealed that our original treatment methods (Sullivan 1962, Oberfield 1975) had been the basis for studies during that period. Therefore, I will review our experience at the Lahey Clinic with arterial infusion chemotherapy of the pelvis, and then some of the work of other investigators in recent years, especially those series involving larger numbers of patients.

Surgical Methods

The pelvis and lower extremities take their blood supply from the internal hypogastric and external iliac arteries. The ovaries take their blood supply from the aorta and the superior and inferior gluteal arteries supply the buttocks, which is the basis for fluorescence. All nonresectable malignant tumors involving the pelvis are considered for hypogastric artery infusion. If, in addition to the pelvis the lower extremities are involved, the common iliac artery is catheterized. Palliation is the aim of treatment, except when it attempts to improve on existing treatment, such as radiotherapy and surgery, as adjuvant therapy.

Internal Iliac Artery Catheter Placement

Catheterization of both internal iliac arteries is always carried out because of the extensive collateral exchange. The extent of disease is determined on exploratory laparotomy. A

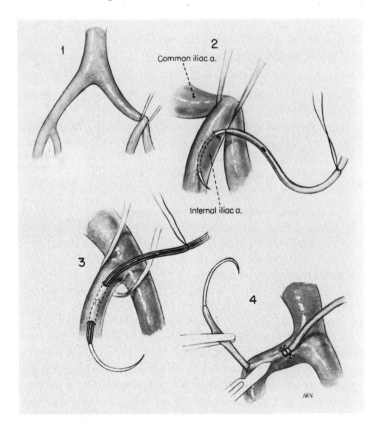

Fig. 1. Catheterization of internal iliac artery using swaged-needle technique. *1*, Countertraction is maintained by a nylon tape. *2*, A swaged-needle catheter is introduced 2−3 cm into the lumen of the internal iliac artery, to emerge well above the bifurcation of the internal iliac artery into dorsal and ventral trunks. *3*, As the needle catheter is advanced, a segment bearing a hole traverses the arterial lumen. Entry of blood into the catheter through this hole proves that the arterial lumen has actually been traversed so that the catheter tip will later come to lie within the vessel lumen. *4*, The catheter is secured and cut off cleanly with a scalpel [from Watkins E Jr, Sullivan RD (1964)]

swaged-needle catheter is inserted into each internal iliac artery (Fig. 1). The position is confirmed by demonstration of fluorescence over the medial aspect of the buttocks by the superior gluteal artery (Fig. 2).

Common Iliac Artery Catheter Placement

The surgical procedure for the common iliac artery is shown in Figs. 3–5. The Teflon catheter exiting from the skin area is attached to a portable chronometric infusion pump. Patients also have used a high-volume pump for drugs that cannot be dissolved in a small volume of fluid.

Fig. 2. Diagrams of areas of skin fluorescence characteristic of internal and common iliac arteries. The fluorescence is observed under ultraviolet light upon injection of these arteries with 5–10 ml of fluorescein dye [from Watkins E Jr, Sullivan RD (1964)]

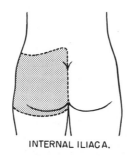

INTERNAL ILIAC A.

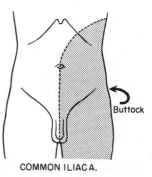

COMMON ILIAC A.

Buttock

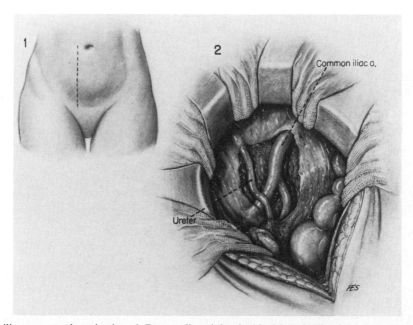

Common iliac a.

Ureter

Fig. 3. Common iliac artery catheterization. *1*, Paramedian abdominal incision. *2*, The right common iliac artery, its bifurcation, and the ureter are exposed

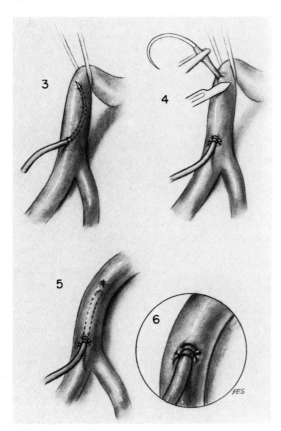

Fig. 4. Common iliac artery catheterization. *3,* A swaged-needle catheter is introduced upstream into the arterial lumen. The catheter is firmly secured with sutures at the point of entrance. *4,* The emerging portion of catheter is secured. If gentle traction is exerted upon the catheter before being severed, the cut end will retract into the lumen. Bleeding from this site is controlled with gauze pressure or a single arterial silk suture. *5* and *6,* Details of completed catheterization

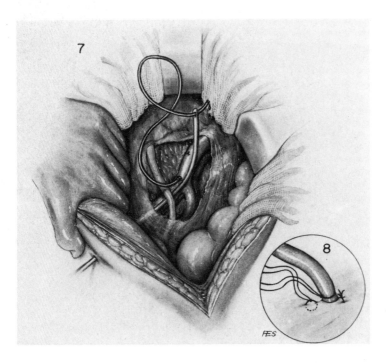

Fig. 5

Regional Chemotherapy Program

After placement, the catheter is attached to a chronometric infusion apparatus pump (Fig. 6). Infusions are continued for 1 month to 1 year, depending on the patency of the catheters and the cooperation of the patient in carrying out the infusion program. We have used predominantly methotrexate, floxuridine (FUDR), and fluorouracil (5-FU), as outlined in Table 1. Patients receiving chemotherapy are initially hospitalized; white blood cell counts are performed daily, hemoglobin and platelet counts, 3 times a week. Methotrexate and FUDR are administered through the pump − 50 mg a day and 0.1−0.3 mg/kg per day respectively, with citrovorum factor given in addition − 10 mg orally every 9 h or 6 mg intramuscularly every 6 h. After the onset of toxicity, manifested by bone marrow depression secondary to methotrexate, administration of the drug is discontinued, but administration of citrovorum factor is continued until abatement of toxicity. Patients receiving FUDR have local toxicity manifested by mucositis with erythema of the skin progressing to vesiculation, depending on the duration of the treatment. Systemic toxicity develops after the administration of large doses of methotrexate in the range of 350−500 mg after 7−10 days. A high-volume pump, in which large volumes of fluid are necessary, is used for patients who require drugs other than methotrexate.

Patients selected for treatment have been diagnosed on the basis of a tissue biopsy, have measurable disease which allows objective evaluation, and symptoms sufficiently progressive to justify treatment. They are aware of the problems of chemotherapy, and have a survival expectancy of at least 1 month, permitting completion of at least a single course of treatment.

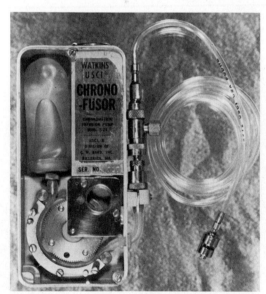

Fig. 6. The clock-driven chronometric infusion pump allows prolonged arterial chemotherapy infusion on an ambulatory basis

Fig. 5. Common iliac artery catheterization. *7*, Through a small stab incision, a catheter-passing instrument is passed retroperitoneally into the abdomen, and the catheter is directed underneath the ureter to an immobile skin area, such as the anterior superior iliac spine. *8*, Catheter is secured to the skin [from Watkins E Jr, Sullivan RD (1964)]

Table 1. Effective antimetabolites[a]

Drug	Dose	Route
Methotrexate	50 mg/24 h	Arterial infusion
Citrovorum factor	6 mg every 6 h	Intramuscular
(antidote)	10 mg every 8 h	Oral
Methotrexate	5 mg/24 h	Arterial infusion
Fluorouracil (5-FU)	$5.0-7.5$ mg $\cdot$ kg^{-1} $\cdot$ 24 h^{-1}	Arterial infusion
Floxuridine (FUDR)	$0.1-0.3$ mg $\cdot$ kg^{-1} $\cdot$ 24 h^{-1}	Arterial infusion

[a] Revised from Oberfield et al. 1973

Results

Of 55 patients who were catheterized at the Lahey Clinic, 52 received an adequate course of treatment, and objective response was obtained in 16 cases (31.5%). Several cases have been selected for review (Sullivan and Watkins 1963).

Case 1, Epidermoid Carcinoma of the Cervix. The patient was a 35-year-old woman with epidermoid cancer of the cervix, diagnosed by biopsy in January 1960. The cervix was covered by a fungating mass, and the tumor extended to the vaginal walls (Fig. 7a). The uterus was fixed by masses extending to the pelvic walls. Bilateral hypogastric artery catheters were inserted, and the patient received an i.a. dose of 25 mg methotrexate per side every 24 h and 6 mg citrovorum factor i.m. every 6 h. Over a 25-day period the patient

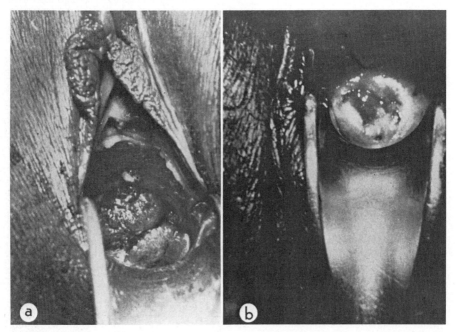

Fig. 7a, b. Epidermoid carcinoma of cervix. **a** Before therapy. Note extensive fungating lesion extending to the vaginal wall. **b** After therapy. Complete tumor regression has apparently occurred [from Sullivan RD, Watkins E Jr (1963)]

was given 12 days of therapy. There was progressive decrease in visible tumor, and by the 29th day after initiation of treatment there was no clinical evidence of residual cancer (Fig. 7b). The patient remained clinically well, and had experienced normal menstrual periods for 25 months when lost to follow-up.

Case 2, Epidermoid Carcinoma of the Bladder. The patient was a 56-year-old man with inoperable epidermoid carcinoma of the bladder diagnosed in October 1960. For several months before receiving arterial infusion therapy he had noted constant dysuria and hematuria. Intravenous pyelography showed a small bladder with a filling defect on the left side (Fig. 8a); the left kidney was not visualized. The patient was given methotrexate for 11 days, infused into both hypogastric arteries in the same dose as that used for case 1. Hematuria ceased by the 6th day of therapy, and the patient became asymptomatic. Cystoscopy after treatment showed that the bladder tumor had regressed by approximately 90%, and several urethral lesions had completely disappeared. Intravenous pyelography showed good concentration of the contrast material on the left side, with a moderate degree of hydronephrosis (Fig. 8b). In addition, there was improvement in the filling defect on the left side of the bladder. The patient was asymptomatic for three months when hematuria recurred. He refused further therapy.

Arterial Infusion of Melanoma Involving the Pelvis

We have previously reported our results with arterial infusion chemotherapy for melanoma (Oberfield and Sullivan 1969). Six patients received adequate courses of infusion involving the pelvis and inguinal region. Of five patients with tumor involving the inguinal region,

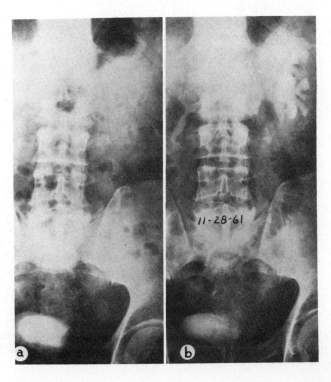

Fig. 8a, b. Epidermoid carcinoma of bladder. **a** Before therapy. Intravenous pyelogram showing nonfunction of the left kidney and a filling defect on the left side of the bladder. **b** After therapy. Note improved function of the left kidney and the decrease in size of the filling defect of the bladder [from Sullivan RD, Watkins E Jr (1963)]

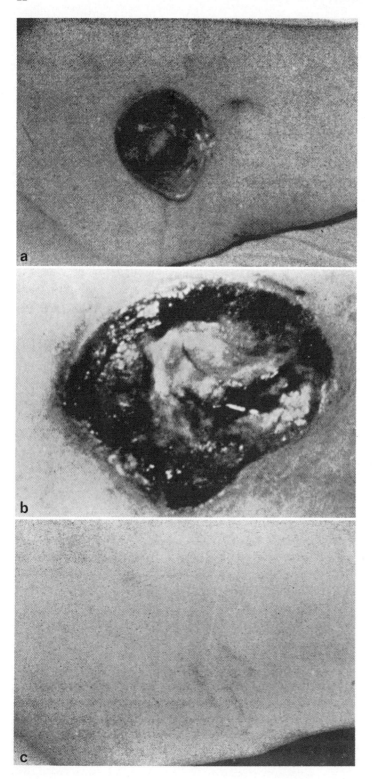

four had objective response, as did the one patient whose disease involved the pelvis. The common iliac artery was used for infusion. Complications included leakage of infusate in two patients; bleeding at catheter site, two patients; pulmonary embolism, two patients; mycotic aneurysm, two patients; and septicemia, two patients.

Case 3, Melanoma of Pelvis and Lower Extremity IM (Oberfield and Sullivan 1969). The patient was a 54-year-old woman who noted a mass on her right leg in 1962. Shortly thereafter a second mass was noted on her right thigh. Both leasions increased in size during the next 2 months, and the patient was seen at the Lahey Clinic in April, 1962.

Examination revealed a mass 10 cm in diameter that was thickened and reddened, with black discoloration and necrosis over the medial portion of the right thigh (Fig. 9a and b). A smaller mass over the posterior part of the right thigh at the midthigh level and a palpable mass in the right inguinal area were also noted. On April 17, biopsy of the right inguinal mass and the thigh lesions confirmed melanoma.

On April 23 an abdominal exploration was made to determine the extent of disease. Lymph nodes along the right iliac artery to the aortic bifurcation were involved, and biopsy showed melanoma. Palpable nodes were present at the level of the left renal artery and periaortic chain. These nodes were enlarged, soft, and necrotic. On the same day, a Teflon catheter was inserted directly into the right common iliac artery, and infusion therapy begun. Methotrexate, 50 mg per 24-h infusion, was given, along with 10 mg citrovorum factor taken orally every 8 h. The patient received two courses of methotrexate, the first for 7 days and the second for 8 days. After the first course, the tumor had decreased by 80%, and on June 2 no tumor was palpable. The catheter was removed on June 5 and the patient was discharged from the hospital. Follow-up examinations in May, 1967 (Fig. 9c) and 6 years after treatment revealed no evidence of tumor.

Review of the Literature

Arterial Infusion for Cancer of the Cervix

Smith et al. (1972) treated 26 patients using either methotrexate with citrovorum factor, or 5-FU, in combination with radiotherapy (Table 2). Fluorouracil and radiotherapy were better tolerated than methotrexate and radiotherapy. Control of cancer was obtained in 46% of their patients. Morrow et al. (1977) administered bleomycin using percutaneous catheters via the femoral artery in 20 patients, with partial remission in two. Swenerton et al. (1979) used vincristine, bleomycin, and mitomycin C via percutaneous infusion of the femoral artery in 20 patients. However, the toxicity was considerable in both series (Morrow et al. 1977; Swenerton et al. 1979) (Table 3), consisting of pulmonary fibrosis (probably due to bleomycin), renal failure, septic emboli, intravaginal fistula, bone marrow depression, or septicemia. Toxicity is high when percutaneous catheters are used in such high-risk patients.

Fig. 9a—c. Appearance of lesion on April 5, 1962, before infusion of drug into left common iliac artery. Distant view (**a**) and close-up (**b**). On May 1, 1967, 6 years after treatment, only residual scar (**c**) is present [from Oberfield RA, Sullivan RD (1969)]

Table 2. Arterial infusion for cancer of cervix

Study, year	No. of patients	Treatment	Response (n)
Smith et al. 1972	26	Methotrexate plus citrovorum factor, or 5-FU, and radiation	? ↓ recurrence
Morrow et al. (GOG)[a] 1977	20	Bleomycin	Partial remission (2)
Swenerton et al. 1979	20	Vincristine, bleomycin, mitomycin C	Partial remission (3)

[a] Gynecology Group, Philadelphia

Table 3. Incidence of toxicity in 20 patients with cervical cancer who received drugs via percutaneous i. a. infusion[a]

Type of toxicity	No. of episodes
Pulmonary fibrosis, pneumonitis	7
Renal failure	4
Septic emboli	3
Enterovaginal fistula	3
Bone marrow depression	3
Oral ulcer	2
Septicemia	1

[a] Adapted from Morrow et al. (1977) and Swenerton et al. (1979)

Table 4. Arterial infusion for bladder cancer

Study, year	No. of patients	Treatment	Response (%)
Nevin et al. 1974	30	5-FU, bleomycin, adriamycin, radiation	75.0
Ogata et al. 1973	33	Mitomycin C, surgery	51.5
Wallace et al. 1982	18	cis-Platinum + 5-FU − i.a. Adriamycin + mitomycin − i.v.	50.0

Arterial Infusion for Cancer of the Bladder

Nevin et al. (1974) treated 30 patients with 5-FU, bleomycin, adriamycin, and radiotherapy, occasionally giving adriamycin and bleomycin together, with 75% response (Table 4). Ogata et al. (1973) treated 33 patients using mitomycin C and surgery with a 51.5% response rate. Wallace et al. (1982), using cis-platinum and 5-FU i.a. together with adriamycin and mitomycin C i.v., had a 50% response rate.

Commentary

What will be the status of pelvic arterial infusion chemotherapy in the future? I think we should continue to explore this method of treatment in view of the limited results achieved with systemic chemotherapeutic agents, such as *cis*-platinum, adriamycin, and mitomycin C in such locally advanced cancers. Until we have more effective methods of treatment, regional infusion chemotherapy can be used to advantage for pelvic tumors, but it should be performed only in well-equipped institutions, and a well-motivated and well-trained team of physicians and nurses is mandatory to avoid excessive morbidity.

References

Morrow CP, DiSaia PJ, Mangan CF, Lagassé LD (1977) Continuous pelvic arterial infusion with bleomycin for squamous carcinoma of the cervix recurrent after irradiation therapy. Cancer Treat Rep 61: 1403–1405

Nevin JE III, Melnick I, Baggerly JT, Easley CA Jr, Landes R (1974) Advanced carcinoma of bladder: treatment using hypogastric artery infusion with 5-fluorouracil, either as a single agent or in combination with bleomycin or adriamycin and supervoltage radiation. J Urol 112: 752–758

Oberfield RA (1975) Current status of regional arterial infusion chemotherapy. Med Clin North Am 59: 411–424

Oberfield RA, Sullivan RD (1969) Prolonged and continuous regional arterial infusion chemotherapy in patients with melanoma. JAMA 209: 75–79

Oberfield RA, Cady B, Booth JC (1973) Regional arterial chemotherapy for advanced carcinoma of the head and neck: a ten-year review. Cancer 32: 82–88

Ogata J, Migita N, Nakamura T (1973) Treatment of carcinoma of the bladder by infusion of the anticancer agent (mitomycin C) via the internal iliac artery. J Urol 110: 667–670

Silverberg E (1982) Cancer statistics 1982. Cancer 32: 15–31

Smith JP, Randall GE, Castro JR, Lindberg RD (1972) Hypogastric artery infusion and radiation therapy for advanced squamous cell carcinoma of the cervix. AJR 114: 110–115

Sullivan RD (1962) Continuous arterial infusion cancer chemotherapy. Surg Clin North Am 42: 365–388

Sullivan RD, Watkins E Jr (1963) Effects of the prolonged intravenous and intra-arterial infusion of cancer chemotherapeutic compounds. AJR 89: 590–597

Sullivan RD, Zurek WZ (1965) Chemotherapy for liver cancer by protracted ambulatory infusion. JAMA 194: 481–486

Swenerton KD, Evers JA, White GW, Boyes DA (1979) Intermittent pelvic infusion with vincristine, bleomycin, and mitomycin C for advanced recurrent carcinoma of the cervix. Cancer Treat Rep 63: 1379–1381

Wallace S, Chuang VP, Samuels M, Johnson D (1982) Transcatheter intraarterial infusion of chemotherapy in advanced bladder cancer. Cancer 49: 640–645

Watkins E Jr, Sullivan RD (1964) Cancer chemotherapy by prolonged arterial infusion. Surg Gynecol Obstet 118: 1–19

Watkins E Jr, Khazei AM, Nahra KS (1970) Surgical basis for arterial infusion chemotherapy of disseminated carcinoma of the liver. Surg Gynecol Obstet 130: 581–605

The Use of Nitrogen Mustard in the Treatment of Intractable Pelvic Pain

J. C. Lathrop and R. E. Frates

Rhode Island Hospital, Brown University, 110 Lockwood Street, Providence, RI 02903, USA

The standard treatment for patients experiencing severe, unrelenting pain secondary to malignant disease in the pelvis has been oral or intramuscular administration of analgesic therapy. This results in a cyclic recurrence of pain prior to each succeeding dose of narcotic. The medication, as well as an attendant to administer it, must always be available. Addiction to the drug is common. The patient is usually very depressed, partly as a result of the pain, which provides a constant reminder of the presence of a probably fatal condition.

For many years systemic chemotherapy has been used to control the growth of pelvic malignancies (Parker and Shingleton 1962). Chemotherapeutic agents are used primarily when surgery or radiation therapy is considered to be inappropriate. The pain associated with such lesions gradually diminishes as the tumor volume is reduced. In some patients the pain is so severe that an initial attempt to control this symptom is warranted, prior to an effort to directly affect tumor growth. Many patients are better able to tolerate chemotherapy if the associated pain has been controlled.

Previous experience with abdominal and pelvic perfusion of nitrogen mustard in an attempt to control pelvic malignancies produced prolonged pain relief in many patients (Lathrop et al. 1963). Since the technique was so complex and difficult, and available in only a few centers, however, its use could not be justified as a reasonable method for the palliation of pelvic pain in patients with advanced malignancy. Percutaneous retrograde catheterization of the femoral artery, because of its simplicity, offered a reasonable method of placing a therapeutic dose of nitrogen mustard into the pelvic circulation.

The use of intra-arterial chemotherapy in the treatment of malignant diseases was introduced in 1950 by Klopp et al. In the following years a variety of techniques for arterial perfusion and infusion were recorded, employing many different chemotherapeutic agents, alone or in combination. Many patients were observed to have considerable pain relief in addition to reduction of tumor volume (Bateman et al. 1966; Cavanagh et al. 1965; Laufe et al. 1966; Masterson and Nelson 1965; Ross and Shingleton 1964).

Riebeling (1962) was the first to specifically address the problem of pain relief. He injected a single large dose of nitrogen mustard into the aorta and followed this promptly with radiation therapy. Of nine patients so treated, seven had very satisfactory relief of pain. Ross and Shingleton (1964) observed a pain-remission rate of about 70% in a small series of patients using this technique. At Lyon, Colon and Mayer (1965) reported a very large series of 101 patients receiving intra-arterial injections of 20–30 mg nitrogen mustard. They observed pain reduction of at least 50% in 55% of their patients.

Recent Results in Cancer Research, Vol. 86
© Springer-Verlag Berlin · Heidelberg 1983

The present study was undertaken to evaluate the ability of intra-arterial nitrogen mustard to control intractable pelvic pain secondary to malignant disease. The goals of the study were threefold: pain reduction by at least 50%; significant pain relief for 2 or more weeks; improvement in physical performance.

Materials and Methods

From January 1963 to January 1982 a series of 73 patients with intractable pelvic or lower-extremity pain, secondary to a pelvic malignancy, was studied at Rhode Island Hospital. The use of pelvic irradiation for pain relief was precluded for 62 patients who had previously received the maximum. Nine patients with primary colon lesions had received no prior radiation therapy. All patients were experiencing severe pain, requiring frequent large doses of analgesics (usually morphine), and were being considered for intrathecal alcohol injection or spinal cordotomy. For nearly all patients, physical function was severely impaired by pain.

In the early years of the study, patients were given general anesthesia and percutaneous retrograde catheterization of the femoral artery was carried out. Utilizing radiologic control, the catheter tip was positioned just above the aortic bifurcation and below the renal arteries. Pneumatic tourniquets previously placed about both thighs were inflated to a pressure of 550 mm Hg. Nitrogen mustard, in a dose of 0.4 mg/kg body wt., was then placed in a solution and promptly injected as a bolus into the catheter. After 10 min the tourniquets were deflated and the catheter removed. The patient was returned to his or her room with instructions not to flex the thigh for 6 h. In most instances the patient had recovered from the procedure by the next day.

Pneumatic tourniquets on the thigh prevented a significant excape of drug to the lower extremities, thus protecting the bone marrow of the leg and permitting a greater concentration of medication in the pelvis. As the activity of nitrogen mustard is rapidly dissipated once it is placed in solution, it was not necessary to occlude extremity circulation for a period longer than 10 min (Calabresi and Parks 1970).

Since 1973 the method of administration has been modified. Following insertion of the catheter into the aorta, pelvic angiography is carried out and the vasculature studied. With this technique better localization of the pelvic tumor, especially of its blood supply, is made. Selective insertion of the catheter into the appropriate hypogastric artery or its smaller branches can then be done, permitting the injection of a higher concentration of nitrogen mustard into the tumor mass. In addition, the necessity for pneumatic tourniquets about the thigh is eliminated. The maximum total dose of nitrogen mustard remains at 0.4 mg/kg body wt., but each side should receive no more than 0.2 mg/kg.

Results

A total of 83 arterial infusions with nitrogen mustard were performed on 73 patients, of whom eight had two infusions and one received three. Table 1 indicates the primary origin of the various malignancies encountered.

Subjective evaluation by the patient was used to provide a rough estimation of pain reduction (Table 2). The patients were divided into two groups, those having intra-aortic therapy and those in whom selective arterial infusion was accomplished. Eleven patients

Table 1. Site of origin of malignancies

Site	Number of malignancies		
	Intra-Aortic	Selective	Total
Cervix	28	18	46
Uterus	3	4	7
Ovary	9	1	10
Colon	12	4	16
Urethra	1	0	1
Clitoris	1	0	1
Lung	0	1	1
Vulva	0	1	1
Total	54	29	83

Table 2. Patient evaluation of pain relief

Level of relief	Number of patients (%)	
	Intra-aortic	Selective
Excellent ($\geq$ 75%)	35 (65)	17 (59)
Good (50%$-$75%)	7 (13)	7 (24)
Poor ($<$ 50%)	8 (15)	3 (10)
None	4 (7)	2 (7)
Total	54	29

Table 3. Minimum duration of pain relief

	Number of patients (%)	
	Intra-aortic	Selective
None	4	2
Less than 2 weeks	10	7
$^{1}/_{2}$$-$1 month	14	7
1$-$2 months	9	8
2$-$6 months	12	3
6$-$12 months	2	1
12+ months	3	1
Total	54	29

noted some relief, but only of a minor degree. These patients are identified separately from those with no response at all for purposes of comparison and grading of response. Maximum relief of pain occurred within the first 24 h following treatment. Pain reduction or relief was sustained by the largest segment of patients for periods of 2$-$8 weeks, with many reporting a considerably longer period (Table 3); 16 noted a short period of relief but had complete recurrence of pain in less than 2 weeks.

NO. OF PATIENTS

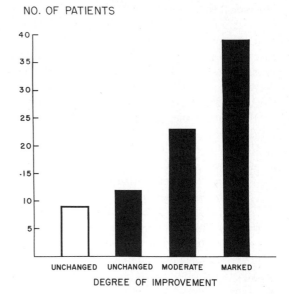

Fig. 1. Relative degree of physical performance improvement following nitrogen mustard injection. *White bar* indicates patients (*n* = 9) whose improvement was prevented by other than pelvic pain

Pain relief obtained by intra-aortic infusion was compared to that achieved by selective arterial infusion. There was no apparent difference in the degree of pain relief or its minimum duration of time (Tables 2 and 3).

Physical performance was evaluated before and after treatment on a graded scale; improvement was then tabulated (Fig. 1).

In eight patients whose pain clearly originated unilaterally it was possible to selectively inject the nitrogen mustard on the affected side. This permitted reduction of the total dose by at least 50%, resulting in a greatly decreased risk of generalized toxicity, while allowing a greater concentration of medication at the tumor site than could have been achieved by an intra-aortic infusion.

Of nine patients who had repeat infusions, seven received them because of their excellent response to the first infusion. In the two remaining, infusions were carried out in selected vessels in an effort to improve the poor result of the previous intra-aortic injection; each noted slight improvement. No increase in complications or toxicity was noted in patients receiving repeat infusions. Many patients were in a preterminal condition (not expected to survive for more than 3 months) at the time of initial treatment and died before their pain recurred to an extent that would indicate a repeat infusion. A small number of patients underwent spinal cordotomy after pain recurrence in lieu of repeat infusion. Additional patients were able to satisfactorily control any residual or recurrent pain with oral analgesics.

Toxicity produced by this procedure was relatively mild. Leukocyte counts reached a nadir at about 10 days after infusion and rarely dipped below 1500/mm^3. About half of the patients experienced nausea and vomiting lasting for approximately 6 h after infusion.

The complications of this procedure may be quite severe. Following a pelvic perfusion with 60 mg nitrogen mustard, Sholes (1960) described a patient who experienced motor and sensory damage to the lumbosacral plexus and severe leg pain. Parker and Shingleton (1962) observed sciatic paralysis in two patients following perfusion with high doses of nitrogen mustard. Colon and Mayer (1965) reported five cases of necrosis of portions of the abdominal wall, with skin grafting required for one patient; hemorrhage and thromboses occurred in ten patients, and four deaths resulted from the procedure.

In our series complications were uncommon. Among six patients experiencing marked relief from primary pain, a new pain of less severity was produced in the thigh; in one instance this was associated with a drug rash. In this case, leg discomfort and paresthesias decreased over the following ten months and the original pain did not recur. An embolus lodged in the great toe of one patient, but this contributed little to her morbidity. In another patient the guide wire inadvertently perforated the external iliac artery and the catheter was passed to an extravascular position in the pelvis. Upon verification of its position by injection of radio-opaque material, the catheter was promptly withdrawn with no untoward effects.

Two patients experienced major complications. Sciatic paralysis with buttock ulceration and necrosis developed in one, apparently as a result of excessive concentration of drug in the superior gluteal artery at the time of a second hypogastric artery infusion. Partial recovery of function was observed 2 months after treatment. Another patient suffered acute hemorrhage from the groin puncture site and required transfusions. This resulted from excessive leg motion following catheter removal. There were no deaths in this series of patients attributable to either the procedure or the drug.

The direct effect of nitrogen mustard in reducing the size of the masses was not routinely evaluated, since most of the tumors were felt to be drug-resistant. One patient with an ovarian malignancy was observed to have marked reduction in tumor size after each of two infusions.

Discussion

Quantitation of pain relief is very difficult because of the subjective nature of pain. Since several patients had been receiving narcotics for pain for considerable periods and were approaching addiction, the reduction of the pain medicine requirement was of only limited value as a parameter for measuring success.

The mechanism of pain relief is not clear. According to Woodhall et al. (1962), when nitrogen mustard was placed directly on the sciatic nerve, axis cylinder swelling, intrafascicular hemorrhage, and endoneural thickening resulted; nerve conduction was severely affected. Mahaley and Woodhall (1962) studied two patients histologically following nitrogen mustard perfusion. One had leg numbness associated with minimal histologic changes at amputation 14 days following perfusion. The other experienced nearly complete anesthesia and paralysis after infusion with 60 mg nitrogen mustard. The myelin and axis cylinders showed marked structural changes at autopsy 7 days later.

Several patients were evaluated by unprejudiced neurologists prior to and following nitrogen mustard infusion in this study. Except for paralysis or paresthesias in two patients, and relief of pain, no alterations could be found in the neurologic examination. This suggests that the neurologic effects may have been dose related.

The nonmyelinated pain-transmitting nerve fibers could have been affected by the lesser doses and, as the relative dose increased, dysfunction could have occurred in the myelinated nerves. More information regarding this phenomenon might be obtained by studying the conduction of impulses along nerve fibers under the influence of varying drug concentrations.

Six patients obtained no pain relief following nitrogen mustard infusion. Of these, three had compression fractures of the vertebra secondary to metastatic disease. The remaining three patients had massive tumor volume, suggesting that it was not possible to perfuse a sufficient amount of involved nerve tissue to significantly reduce the pain.

Pain relief of less than 2 weeks' duration was experienced by 17 patients. One who experienced little relief was found to have a drug addiction rather than residual tumor. Two patients were known to have lumbosacral spine metastases and only the peripheral component of their pain responded to treatment. Eleven patients had tumor present above the pelvis. In these patients the sensory nerves related to the suprapelvic disease were not able to be adequately perfused with nitrogen mustard and they experienced only a minor degree of relief. One patient experienced excellent pain relief, but died 12 days after treatment. Two patients had previously undergone hypogastric artery ligation which severely limited the ability of the drug to gain access to the sensory nerves responsible for the pain. Fischer et al. (1966) have suggested that the degree of vascularity of the tumor is crucial to the success of chemotherapeutic pain relief. In the angiographic studies performed in this series, those patients demonstrating major pelvic vascular obstruction experienced much less pain relief and for a shorter duration of time.

The advantages of selective arterial infusion are substantial. The drug may be concentrated in the pelvis by avoidance of dissemination into the external iliac artery. The risk of thrombophlebitis is considerably reduced since it is not necessary to apply pneumatic tourniquets to the thighs. Eight patients in this series had pain limited to one side of the pelvis. In these subjects it was possible to give one-half of the full dose (0.2 mg/kg) but deliver it all unilaterally to the site of pain origin, which nearly completely eliminated the risk of systemic toxicity. Five patients received a fraction of the dose in other selected vessels, as well as in the hypogastric arteries. This was done when angiography indicated that other accessible vessels appeared to be directly supplying the tumor.

Conclusions

A substantial degree of pain relief may be anticipated in patients experiencing pelvic and lower extremity pain through treatment by arterial infusion with nitrogen mustard. Advantages of the procedure include low toxicity, an acceptable morbidity and complication rate, and the relative availability and ease of performance of the procedure. Pain in the entire pelvis may be alleviated, contrasting with results obtained by unilateral cordotomy. Patients experiencing satisfactory relief may expect a similar result should they require a second infusion. An outstanding point is the freedom from the cyclic return of pain and associated depression that is characteristic of pain control by oral or intramuscular analgesic therapy.

Individuals with some element of pain arising from disease situated above the pelvic circulation may expect less satisfactory pain relief, as this area cannot be perfused with a significant amount of nitrogen mustard by this method. Patients having vascular obstruction from either tumor mass or prior hypogastric artery ligation may anticipate at most only modest pain relief from this procedure. The treatment will not relieve pain arising from compressed fractures of the vertebrae.

Nitrogen mustard infusion is recommended as the next step in the attempt to control intractable pelvic and lower-extremity pain resulting from malignancy, after the failure of oral or intramuscular analgesics. It may also be used in the attempt to control pain temporarily in anticipation of the use of systemic chemotherapy designed to produce tumor regression. Intrathecal alcohol injections and spinal cordotomy should be reserved for those patients experiencing inadequate relief with nitrogen mustard infusion.

Summary

Substantial relief of discomfort may be anticipated by most patients suffering from pelvic and lower-extremity pain who are treated by arterial infusion of nitrogen mustard. Seventy-three patients with intractable pain secondary to malignancy arising in the pelvis received 83 percutaneous pelvic arterial infusions of this drug. Sixty infusions (72%) resulted in marked relief from pain for periods averaging 6–8 weeks. Advantages of the procedure are low toxicity, relative simplicity and availability of technique, and an acceptable rate of complications with minimal morbidity. Patients experiencing satisfactory results may expect significant relief from a second infusion for recurrent pain. The most rewarding result is the freedom from the cyclic return of pain characterized by oral and intramuscular analgesic therapy. Little or no relief can be expected in patients with pain caused by compression fractures of the vertebrae, or where the tumor burden is so great that adequate perfusion of the involved nerves is not possible.

One should consider this procedure for controlling pain before resorting to the more dangerous and potentially disabling techniques of spinal cordotomy or intrathecal alcohol injection.

References

Bateman JR, Hazen JG, Stolinsky DC, Steinfeld JL (1966) Advanced carcinoma of the cervix treated by intra-arterial methotrexate. Am J Obstet Gynecol 96: 181–187

Calabresi P, Parks RW Jr (1970) Alkylating agents, antimetabolites, hormones, and other antiproliferative agents. In: Goodman LS, Gilman A (eds) The pharmacological basis of therapeutics, 4th edn. MacMillan, New York, p 1354

Cavanagh D, Martin DS, Ferguson JH (1965) Closed pelvic perfusion in advanced gynecologic cancer. South Med J 58: 549–557

Colon J, Mayer M (1965) Resultats de la chimiotherapie intraarterielle dans le traitment des algies dues aux cancers pelviens. Marseille Chir 17: 147–159

Fischer G, Colon J, Mayer M, Dargent M (1966) Interer de l'arteriographie au cours de la chimiotherapie intra-arterielle des cancers. Ann Radiol (Paris) 9: 367–376

Klopp CT, Alford TC, Bateman J, Berry GN, Winship T (1950) Fractionated intra-arterial cancer chemotherapy with methyl bis-amine hydrochloride; a preliminary report. Ann Surg 132: 811–832

Lathrop JC, Leone LA, Soderberg CH Jr, Colbert MP, Vargas LL (1963) Perfusion chemotherapy for gynecological malignancy. Trans New Engl Obstet Gynecol Soc 17: 47–56

Laufe LE, Blockstein RS, Parisi FZ, Lowy AD Jr (1966) Infusion through inferior gluteal artery for pelvic cancer. Obstet Gynecol 28: 650–659

Mahaley MS Jr, Woodhall B (1962) The effect of anticancer agents on nervous tissue. Cancer Chemother Rep 16: 543–544

Masterson JG, Nelson JH Jr (1965) The role of chemotherapy in the treatment of gynecologic malignancy. Am J Obstet Gynecol 93: 1102–1108

Parker R, Shingleton W (1962) Chemotherapy in genital cancer: systemic therapy and regional perfusion. Am J Obstet Gynecol 83: 981–1003

Riebeling M (1962) Massive intra-aortic injections of nitrogen mustard (Dichloren), 5-fluorouracil, Nitromin, and Endoxan prior to roentgen irradiation for advanced tumors of the uterus. Radiology 79: 132–133

Ross RA, Shingleton HM (1964) Treating carcinoma of the cervix as a disease. Am J Obstet Gynecol 88: 307–313

Sholes DM Jr (1960) Pelvic perfusion with nitrogen mustard for cancer: a neurological complication. Am J Obstet Gynecol 80: 481–484

Woodhall B, Mahaley S Jr, Boone S, Huneycutt H (1962) The effect of chemotherapeutic agents upon peripheral nerves. J Surg Res 2: 373–381

Intra-Arterial Perfusion Therapy with 5-Fluorouracil in Patients with Metastatic Colorectal Carcinoma and Intractable Pelvic Pain

J.-H. Beyer[1], H. W. von Heyden[1], H.-H. Bartsch[1], M. Klee[1], G. A. Nagel[1], R. Schuster[2], and H. J. von Romatowski[2]

1 Abteilung für Hämatologie/Onkologie, Medizinische Universitätsklinik, Robert-Koch-Strasse 40, 3400 Göttingen, FRG
2 Abteilung für Radiologie, Medizinische Universitätsklinik, Robert-Koch-Strasse 40, 3400 Göttingen, FRG

Introduction

Patients with colorectal carcinoma frequently exhibit pelvic and/or perineal pain due to metastatic invasion of the lumbosacral plexus. The pain cannot be alleviated in some of these patients even by combinations of analgesics, systemic cytotoxic chemotherapy, or local irradiation. The patients are often confined to bed and are dependent on morphine derivatives. Prior to attempting irreversible neurosurgical procedures, such as rhizotomy or chordotomy, it is justifiable to try local intra-arterial perfusion therapy with cytotoxic drugs.

In 1979 we started a phase II trial with 5-fluorouracil (5-FU) pelvic perfusion in patients resistant to prior systemic 5-FU therapy, to determine whether high local doses of 5-FU could overcome such resistance.

Patients and Methods

The study comprised 18 patients with histologically verified colorectal carcinoma, in relapse after prior surgery, and intractable pelvic or perineal pain. None of them responded to combinations of analgesics. 17 of 18 patients had previously been treated unsuccessfully with 5-FU chemotherapy, radiotherapy, or the combination of both. Angiography and computer tomography of the pelvis were performed before and after the perfusion therapy to verify tumor size and the correct sites for catheters.

One 7-French side-winder catheter was placed in each internal iliac artery. Alternatively, one 7-French pigtail catheter was located in the aortic bifurcation. The catheters were sutured to the skin and during perfusion the patients were confined to bed. After cessation of treatment the correct placement of the catheters and tumor size were confirmed by angiography, and the catheters were then removed.

A dose of 15−30 mg 5-FU/kg body wt. per day was administered for 1−5 days through a perfusion pump. Heparinization was performed with 800 IU heparin i.v./h continuously when using one catheter, with 400 IU heparin i.v./h continuously through each catheter when using two.

The effect of the treatment was correlated to the subsequent amount of analgesic required. We divided the results into four groups:

1. No effect.
2. Absolute pain relief.
3. 50% less analgesics required as compared with pretreatment.
4. Use of analgesics is 50%−100% of pretreatment requirement.

Some patients received a second perfusion following successful treatment, and one received a third.

Results

Profiles of the 18 patients treated are given in Table 1. The results of treatment including dosage and number of treatments are demonstrated in Table 2. In all cases but one where there was excellent pain relief, no tumor regression was demonstrable after cessation of perfusion therapy.

In general the side effects of this treatment were minimal: two patients suffered from diarrhea for a short time; one demonstrated a minimal leukopenia of $3,800/mm^3$; nine of ten who were perfused with 30 mg 5-FU/kg/day for 5 days showed redness and swelling of the skin over the perfusion region, which later turned light brown with subsequent hyperpigmentation.

Severe side effects were seen in one female patient: GJ, 69 years old, was perfused with 30 mg 5-FU/kg/day for 5 days to treat local recurrent tumor and perineal pain. On days 2, 7, and 8 following cessation of therapy arterial embolizations of the left leg occurred, despite sufficient heparinization. Three embolectomies were performed successfully. The histological examination of these emboli showed arteriosclerotic, not thrombotic material. On the 9th day a new embolism occurred, requiring leg amputation; 3 weeks later the patient died of septicemia following pneumonia and renal failure. The histology of the leg again revealed arteriosclerotic material in the arteries.

Discussion

As shown by this study, patients with intractable pain in the pelvic and perineal regions, caused by locally recurrent and/or metastatic colorectal carcinoma, and which is unresponsive to combinations of analgesics, systemic cytostatic chemotherapy and/or radiotherapy, can be treated successfully using intra-arterial perfusion therapy with 5-FU. The quality of life can be enhanced for such patients (Beyer et al. 1980; Häfstrom et al. 1979). They are not confined to bed or dependent on analgesics and can live normal lives.

The analgesic effect of this therapy cannot be explained by reduction in tumor size. With the exception of one patient, no tumor remissions could be demonstrated where there was considerable or complete pain relief after 5-FU perfusion. One possible explanation may be that 5-FU has an effect on nerve-plain receptors (Cavanagh et al. 1975; Stevens et al. 1960).

Our results concerning therapeutic and side effects are comparable to those of other investigators (Ariel 1957; Cavanagh et al. 1975; Fischerman et al. 1974; Häfstrom et al. 1979; Klopp et al. 1950; Krakoff and Sullivan 1958; Lathrop and Frates 1980; Stevens et al. 1960; Tully et al. 1979). However, some side effects described by other authors, such as

Table 1. Perfusion therapy of the pelvis with 5-FU in 18 patients with colorectal carcinoma and intractable pain

Sex	n	Age range in years	Age (years), mean value	Pretreatment			
				Chemo-therapy	Radio-therapy	Chemo- and Radiotherapy	None
Male	7	51−71	63.3	5	2	0	0
Female	11	47−69	60.3	2	4	4	1

Table 2. Results of treatment for 18 patients

Result	Patient			Pain relief in weeks	5-FU i.a. (mg/kg/day)
	Name	Age	Sex		
No effect	JG	63	M	0	20 × 2
	PR	47	F	0	30 × 1
Absolute pain relief	HP	64	M	3	15 × 1
	AF	71	M	9[b]	15 × 2
	MM	54	F	6	15 × 3
	AS	59	F	8[b]	20 × 2
	EH	57	F	3	30 × 1
	EH*	57	F	16[a]	30 × 1
	SM	51	F	28	30 × 5
	BK	63	F	16[a]	30 × 5
	DE	68	F	28[b]	30 × 5
	KA	62	M	32	30 × 5
	ML	65	F	4	30 × 5
	ML*	65	F	4	30 × 5
Less than 50% of pretreatment amount of analgesics required	AF	71	M	6	15 × 2
	AS	59	F	3	20 × 2
	VA	66	M	4	30 × 2
	DE	68	F	8	30 × 5
	WF	51	M	10	30 × 5
	KE	69	F	4	30 × 5
	GJ	69	F	5	30 × 5
	KCh	61	F	4	30 × 5
More than 50% of pretreatment amount of analgesics required	MF	68	M	6	30 × 5

[a] Patients EH and ML experienced complete pain relief after each of two consecutive therapies
[b] Complete pain relief after the second perfusion

thrombosis, bleeding, displacement of catheters, and local or general infections, were not seen in our series.

One patient was lost owing to arteriosclerotic embolism. Therefore, patients with severe arteriosclerosis are considered a high risk for this procedure.

Summary

In a phase-II trial, 18 patients with intractable pelvic and perineal pain caused by local recurrent and/or metastatic colorectal carcinoma resistant to combinations of analgesics, systemic cytostatic chemotherapy and/or radiation were treated with intra-arterial perfusion therapy using 15–30 mg 5-FU/kg body wt./day for 1-5 days. Of 18 patients, ten achieved complete pain relief for 3–32 weeks (mean, 15.7 weeks); after the perfusion therapy eight used less than 50% of the amount of analgesics required before treatment; one patient had only a minor response; two patients were treated unsuccessfully. Side effects were mild and controllable. One patient died subsequent to arterial embolism in the leg where the catheter was placed; pelvic perfusion therefore appears risky in patients with severe arteriosclerosis.

References

Ariel IM (1957) Treatment of inoperable cancer by intra-arterial administration of mechlorethamine. Arch Surg 74: 516–524

Beyer J-H, Heyden HW, Klee M, Nagel GA, Schiller U, Bornikoel K, Schuster R (1980) Intraarterielle Perfusionstherapie des kleinen Beckens mit 5-Fluorouracil bei therapieresistenten Schmerzen des metastasierenden Kolonkarzinoms. Verh Dtsch Ges Inn Med 86: 470–772

Cavanagh D, Hovadhanakul P, Comas MR (1975) Regional chemotherapy – A comparison of pelvic perfusion and intra-arterial infusion in patients with advanced gynecologic cancer. Am J Obstet Gynecol 123: 435–441

Fischerman K, Briand P, Olsen J, Nielsen OV (1974) Intra-arterial combined cancer chemotherapy in technically inoperable carcinoma of the anus and rectum. Acta Chir Scand 140: 416–421

Hafström L, Jönsson P-E, Landberg T, Owman T, Sundkvist K (1979) Intraarterial infusion chemotherapy (5-fluorouracil) in patients with inextirpable or locally recurrent rectal cancer. Am J Surg 137: 757–762

Klopp CT, Alford TC, Bateman J, Berry GN, Winship T (1950) Fractionated intra-arterial cancer; chemotherapy with methyl bis amine hydrochloride. A preliminary report. Ann Surg 132: 811–832

Krakoff IH, Sullivan RD (1958) Intra-arterial nitrogen mustard in the treatment of pelvic cancer. Ann Int Med 48: 839–850

Lathrop JC, Frates RE (1980) Arterial infusion of nitrogen mustard in the treatment of intractable pelvic pain of malignant origin. Cancer 45: 432–438

Stevens GM, Thomas SF, Wilbur BC (1960) Intra-aortic nitrogen mustard for the palliation of advanced pelvic cancer. Radiology 75: 948–953

Tully JL, Lew MA, Connor M, D'Orsi CJ (1979) Clostridial sepsis following hepatic arterial infusion chemotherapy. Am J Med 67: 707–710

Palliative Therapy of Pelvic Tumors by Intra-Arterial Infusion of Cytotoxic Drugs

M. E. Heim, S. Eberwein, and M. Georgi

Onkologisches Zentrum, Klinikum der Stadt Mannheim, Fakultät für Klinische Medizin Mannheim der Universität Heidelberg, Postfach 23, 6800 Mannheim, FRG

The treatment of patients with inoperable pelvic tumors is a major problem of clinical oncology. In most cases, colorectal or bladder carcinomas cause intractable pain in the pelvic region requiring high-dose analgesic treatment and sometimes even nerve blocks or neurosurgery. There is no curative systemic treatment for these cancers, but palliative therapy can improve the quality of life of symptomatic patients. The best results in the treatment of colorectal cancers were obtained by combination chemotherapy using 5-fluorouracil with nitrosourea derivatives (Queißer and Heim 1981), while adriamycin is the most active single drug for the treatment of bladder cancers. Because of their short half-life and high systemic clearance rate these cytotoxic drugs seem especially suited for local cancer chemotherapy (Chen and Gross 1980).

We treated 20 patients with inoperable malignant pelvic tumors using intra-arterial cytotoxic chemotherapy. Patients were selected on the basis of the following criteria:

1. Histologically proven inoperable primary or metastatic tumor.
2. Vascularization of the tumor by branches of the internal iliac arteries.
3. Performance status $\geq$ 50% on Karnofsky index.
4. No bone marrow depression, cardiac, hepatic or renal dysfunction.
5. Intractable tumor-related pain; intractable bleeding from urinary bladder or rectum.

All patients had intractable pelvic pain, and one had intraluminal bleeding; eight patients had been pretreated by radiation therapy, and one had had prior 5-fluorouracil monochemotherapy (Table 1); 13 patients had inoperable colorectal pelvic tumors, five had advanced urinary bladder cancer, and two had carcinoma of the prostate.

Table 1. Patients treated by intra-arterial chemotherapy

Site of primary tumor	No. of patients	Age	Female	Male	Pretreatment	
					RT	CT
Colorectum	13	49−73	5	8	6	1
Urinary bladder	5	51−83	1	4	2	−
Prostatic	2	50, 51	−	2	−	−

RT, radiation therapy; CT, chemotherapy

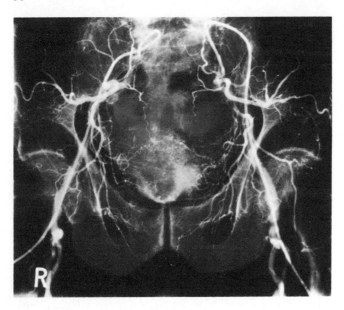

Fig. 1. Pretreatment arteriography of both internal iliac arteries in a patient with bladder carcinoma

Table 2. Results of intra-arterial chemotherapy

Type of tumor (n)	Objective partial tumor regression	Stable disease	Subjective improvement (pain relief)
Colorectal (13)	2	3	11
Bladder (5)	1	2	2
Prostate (2)	2	–	2

Catheters were placed percutaneously into both internal iliac arteries and the position of the catheter tip was determined by arteriography before each course of drug infusion (Fig. 1). Before each cycle the tumor extension was measured by CAT scanning. Biochemical parameters and tumor markers, as well as the amount of analgesic drugs required for pain relief, were documented throughout therapy.

Colorectal tumors were treated with 24-h infusions of 10 mg 5-fluorouracil (5-FU) per kg body wt. via one internal iliac artery for 5 days, and with 30-min infusions of 40 mg carmustine (BCNU)/m² via the other internal iliac artery for the same period. This cycle was repeated after 6 weeks, and response to treatment was evaluated after 12 weeks. Patients with advanced bladder or prostate cancer received 20–30 mg adriamycin/m² for 3 days. The cycle was repeated 4 weeks later, and evaluation followed after 8 weeks; the intra-arterial chemotherapy was continued in patients who demonstrated improvement or partial remission.

We observed subjective improvement with a decrease in analgesic drug consumption in 15 of 20 patients. In one case urinary bladder hemorrhage stopped dramatically after intra-arterial adriamycin infusion (Table 2). Objective partial tumor regression was observed in 5 of 20 patients, i.e., the two cases of prostate cancer one case of bladder cancer, and two of colorectal cancer. The objective tumor response in colorectal cancers was, as expected, very low.

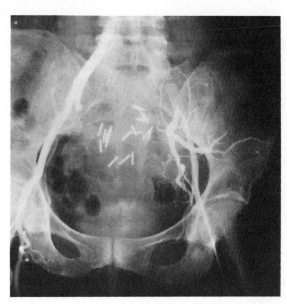

Fig. 2. Thrombosis of right internal iliac artery as complication of intra-arterial chemotherapy in a patient with inoperable rectal carcinoma

Table 3. Side effects of intra-arterial chemotherapy in 20 patients studied

Carcinoma (n)	Cytotoxic agent	Side effect	No. affected
Colorectal (13)	5-FU and BCNU	Local cutaneous inflammation	3
		Thrombosis of internal iliac artery	1
		Local suprapubic paresthesias	1
		Loss of appetite	5
		Nausea	2
Bladder and prostate (7)	Adriamycin	Alopecia	7
		Nausea	3
		Loss of appetite	2
		Leukopenia ($< 2,000/\mu l$)	2
		Local cutaneous inflammation	1

The frequency of side effects was tolerable (Table 3): four patients experienced local cutaneous inflammation, one patient had paresthesias, and another a complete internal iliac artery thrombosis (Fig. 2). All patients receiving adriamycin developed alopecia; gastrointestinal and bone-marrow toxicity were low.

In conclusion we can state that intra-arterial chemotherapy is very effective in reducing pain in patients with pelvic tumors. The objective tumor response is comparable to the results in systemic chemotherapy of colorectal cancer (Queißer and Heim 1981), the five bladder and two prostate cancers comprise too small a group for us to draw any conclusions. In a prospective randomized study Grage et al. (1979) compared systemic and intra-arterial chemotherapy in patients with hepatic metastases from colorectal cancer. While there was no significant difference in terms of response rate and survival, the intra-arterial infusion arm was associated with a greater incidence of side effects. To compare intravenous and intra-arterial chemotherapy in pelvic colorectal carcinoma, we have started a controlled randomized trial with 5-FU and BCNU combination therapy at our institution. Apart from objective response criteria, we are monitoring subjective improvement by measuring the amount of analgesic drugs needed for pain relief. This study should answer the question of whether there is an advantage to local intra-arterial chemotherapy in inoperable pelvic colorectal carcinomas.

References

Chen H-S, Gross JF (1980) Intraarterial infusion of anticancer drugs: theoretic aspects of drug delivery and review of responses. Cancer Treat Rep 64: 31–40

Grage TB, Vassilopoulos PP, Shingleton WW, Jubert AV, Elias EG, Aust JB, Moss SE (1979) Results of a prospective randomized study of hepatic artery infusion with 5-fluorouracil versus intravenous 5-fluorouracil in patients with hepatic metastases from colorectal cancer: A Central Oncology Group study. Surgery 86: 550–555

Queißer W, Heim ME (1981) Chemotherapy in alimentary tract malignomas. Hepatogastroenterology 5: 276–283

Catheter Embolization in the Central Nervous System and the Gastrointestinal Tract

F. W. Schumacher, J. Hunold, and S. Bayindir

Medizinisches Zentrum für Radiologie, Klinikum der Justus Liebig-Universität Giessen, Klinikstrasse 29, 6300 Giessen, FRG

Therapeutic transarterial embolization has been known for 20 years. The first experience with embolization to produce an occlusion to treat intracerebral arteriovenous malformation was reported by Luessenhop in 1960.

The development of sophisticated techniques for selective blood vessel catheterization and the production of differentiated materials for selective occlusion have made catheter embolization possible for a variety of diseases (Berenstein and Kricheff 1979; Chuang and Wallace 1980).

In the central nervous system primary vascular malformations can be treated curatively. Preconditions are an exact angiographic study of the frequently very complex blood supply and an evaluation of the risk of unintentional embolization in the normal vessels.

Spontaneous or post-traumatic arteriovenous fistulas are supplied by the internal carotid artery. For example, the cavernous sinus fistulas can be occluded by placing a detachable balloon inside the fistula, using a technique reported by Serbinenko (1974). In cooperation with the center for Neurosurgery we have performed occlusions of post-traumatic arterio venous fistulas, following a technique reported by Debrun et al. (1978). After the balloon is placed inside the fistula it is filled with contrast medium or silicon, and can be detached by sliding forth the outer part of the coaxial catheter system.

Embolization of hypervascular tumors supplied by the internal carotid or vertebral artery, using occlusion agents such as Gelfoam or BCA, of course carries the risk of ischemic cerebral damage.

Primary craniofacial angiomatous tumors can be curatively treated without greatly endangering or disturbing the patient. Additional vessels, however, which can take over the blood supply after embolization of the main vessel require angiographic controls and frequent reembolization.

Hypervascularized carcinoma in the craniofacial area can be treated palliatively or preoperatively. Glomus tumors very often have shunts with the internal carotid or vertebral artery; frequently a permanent occlusion cannot be achieved, and unintentional embolization of intercerebral vessels has been reported (Kvam et al. 1980; Ahn et al. 1980).

Most retromedullary spinal hemangiomas that are fed by the posterior spinal artery can be treated by embolization; therefore this method, performed with Ethibloc or Gelfoam or dura chips can be regarded as first choice treatment. Djindjan et al. (1973) reported that embolization of intramedullary spinal angiomas fed by the anterior spinal artery may be possible and helpful in some selected cases. Hypervascularized bone tumors with compression of the spine can be treated in a similar fashion.

Embolization in the gastrointestinal tract can be performed in those parts that are fed by the celiac trunk, as sufficient collaterals prevent extensive gut-wall necrosis. Therefore a number of reports have been published dealing with embolization in this area. Embolization is usually performed after angiographic localization of the side of hemorrhage in duodenal ulcers, gastric ulcers, or hemorrhage caused by other diseases. Vogel et al. (1981) reported that embolization was successful in 85% of cases, selective vasopressin infusion in only 60%.

In 1979 a patient with a hypervascularized tumor in the head of pancreas was treated by embolization of the gastroduodenal artery. Gelfoam was used as an occluding agent, and a temporary cessation of the hemorrhage was achieved. A second embolization with Ethibloc was performed in this patient in 1980, as the angiographic study had shown that some parts of the gastroduodenal artery were still perfused. Because of multiple collaterals from adjacent vessels, complete occlusion of all vessels was not possible; however, the patient is still alive 2 years later, as occasional minor hemorrhage can be handled by transfusions.

Material that blocks smaller caliber arteries is used to occlude the inferior mesenteric artery for rectosigmoidal hemorrhage. Occlusions in the periphery would lead to ischemic necrosis. Only a few reports about embolization of the inferior mesenteric artery are in the literature (Goldberger and Bookstein 1977; Bookstein et al. 1978; Mitty et al. 1979; Chuang et al. 1979; Vogel and Bücheler 1981). A 66-year-old patient with severe radiation-induced colitis was successfully treated by embolization of branches of the inferior mesenteric artery. In a second session, embolization of both internal iliac arteries was performed and the neccessity for blood transfusion was drastically reduced. An angiographic study showed that branches of the inferior mesenteric artery remained closed for 10 months. In another patient the hemorrhage was also drastically reduced. In a third patient hemorrhaging was very severe; the embolization stopped the bleeding but the patient died shortly after the procedure because of untreatable shock.

In conclusion, curative embolization of vessels is possible in selected cases. In the central nervous system and the craniofacial region especially, angiomas can be treated favorably. In many cases hypervascularized tumors can be treated palliatively. Embolization seems to be especially suited in the treatment of acute hemorrhage caused by neoplasm.

References

Ahn HS, Kerber CW, Deeb ZL (1980) Extra- to intracranial arterial anastomoses in therapeutic embolization: recognition and role. AJNR 1: 71

Berenstein A, Kricheff JJ (1979) Catheter and material selection for transarterial embolization: Technical considerations. Radiology 132: 619

Bookstein Jj, Naderi MJ, Walter JF (1978) Transcatheter embolization for lower gastrointestinal bleeding. Radiology 127: 345

Chuang VP, Wallace S (1980) Current status of transcatheter management of neoplasms. Cardiovasc Intervent Radiol 3: 256

Chuang VP, Wallace S, Zornoza J, Davis LJ (1979) Transcatheter arterial occlusion in the management of retrosigmoidal bleeding. Radiology 133: 605

Debrun G, Lacour P, Caron JP, Hurth M, Comoy J, Keravel J (1978) Detachable balloon and calibrated-leak balloon techniques in the treatment of cerebral vascular lesions.l J Neurosurg 49: 635

Djindjan R, Cophignong J, Rey A, Theron J, Merland JJ, Houdart R (1973) Superselective arteriographic embolization by the femoral route in neuroradiology. Neuroradiology 6: 132

Goldberger LE, Bookstein JJ (1977) Transcatheter embolization for treatment of diverticular hemorrhage. Radiology 122:613

Kvam DA, Michelsen WJ, Quest DO (1980) Intracerebral hemorrhage as a complication of artificial embolization. Neurosurgery 7:491

Luessenhop AJ, Spence WT (1960) Artificial embolization of cerebral arteries: report of use in a case of arteriovenous malformation. JAMA 172:1153

Mitty HA, Efremedia S, Keller RJ (1979) Colonic stricture after transcatheter embolization for civerticular bleeding. AJR 133:519

Serbinenko FA (1974) Balloon catheterization and occlusion of major central vessels. J Neurosurg 41:125

Vogel H, Bücheler E (1981) Transkatheter, Verschluß der A. mes. inferior. Röntgenblätter 34:223

Vogel H, Betz J, Bücheler E (1981) Komplikationen des transkatheteralen Verschlusses von Abdominalarterien. Röntgenblätter 34:342

Percutaneous Embolization of Urological Tumors

J. Hunold, F. W. Schumacher, and S. Bayindir

Medizinisches Zentrum für Radiologie, Klinikum der Justus Liebig-Universität Giessen, Klinikstrasse 29, 6300 Giessen, FRG

When the world-famous fictional detective Sherlock Holmes had to solve a crime, he asked himself the seven "W" questions. With incomparable penetration he was able to solve the problem and have the criminal convicted.

Medicine and criminology have many parallels. The problem we are engaged in is percutaneous embolization of urological tumors. We will try to answer three questions:

1. Why? The question of indication.
2. How? The question of technique.
3. With what? The question of embolization material.

The embolization of renal tumors can be done either preoperatively or as a palliative measure. Preoperative embolization facilitates the subsequent operative procedure, in that:

1. Blood loss is reduced to a minimum.
2. Demarcation of the renal tumor in normal renal parenchyma is clear.
3. Ligation of the V. renalis before the A. renalis is possible, which keeps the lymphogenous and hematogenous distribution of tumor cells to a minimum.

We use palliative tumor embolization for patients with untreatable tumors, to stop the tumor bleeding, to reduce the pain, and to reduce tumor cell mass.

Habigkhorst et al. (1977) suggest that embolization can replace short- and long-term preradiation of tractable tumors.

Evidently it is not possible to stimulate immunological resistance by embolization in order to destroy metastases or to extend survival time (Kjaer 1976a; Wallace et al. 1981). The purpose of embolization of the pelvic vessels is to control intractable bleeding caused by trauma, operation, radiation, or tumors of the pelvic organs. The most important indications for embolization are the bleeding caused by tumors of the bladder or invading growth of tumors of the uterus, prostate, and colon.

Embolization of the renal artery is done by the Seldinger technique. We use curved catheters, Charrière 7 or 8, as do many investigators. Others prefer balloon catheters; they do not anticipate a reflux of embolization material. We use balloon catheters only for preoperative blockade by nephrectomy, or for intraoperative renal perfusion.

The embolization of pelvic vessels is also done with curved catheters in a crossed technique via the femoral arteries. If this is impossible because of arteriosclerosis the ipsilateral way or the left axillary artery can be tried.

Recent Results in Cancer Research, Vol. 86
© Springer-Verlag Berlin · Heidelberg 1983

Since Brooks (1931) used autologous muscle for his first embolization in 1930, many other methods have been developed, including even thrombosis induced by anionic direct current (Sawyer et al. 1961; Setlarik and Deckert 1981). The embolization can be arranged in different ways; for example:

1. Localization of embolization, central, peripheral, or capillary.
2. Duration of embolization, varying or constant.
3. Character of embolization material, autologous, nonautologous, or liquids.

Our own experience from November, 1974 to March, 1982 is based on 139 embolizations of the renal artery and 43 embolizations of pelvic vessels.

From November, 1974 to December, 1976 our method was to occlude the renal artery with autologous muscle. We evaluated the results with 38 patients, 19 men and 19 women. In 30 cases the embolization was done preoperatively, in eight it was done palliatively. The median survival time was 60 months for the preoperative group and 10 months for the palliative group.

During the years following we revised the embolization method for the following reasons:

1. A second operation is necessary to get the muscle; several times we saw healing per secundam.
2. During reangiography following palliative embolization we often found recanalization. For example, it was necessary to do three embolizations over 12 months in one patient who suffered from a intractable renal tumor with metastases.
3. Histopathology of kidneys removed 2–7 days after embolization always showed ischemic infarction of the normal parenchyma. However, total infarction of the tumor was rare.

We now use balloon catheters, as do other examiners (Dotter et al. 1975), for short-therm central embolization of the urogenital tract. For a medium-term peripheral embolization we use Gelfoam and for a permanent capillary embolization we use Ethibloc.

References

Brooks B (1931) Discussion of paper by L. Noland and A. S. Taylor. Trans South Surg Assoc 43: 176–177

Dotter CT, Goldmann ML, Roesch J (1975) Instant selective arterial occlusion with 1-isobutyl-2-cyanoacrylate. Radiology 114: 227–230

Habigkhorst LV, Kreutz W, Eilers H (1977) Katheterembolisation der Nierenarterie, eine Alternative zur präoperativen Radiotherapie bei Nierentumoren? Radiologe 17: 509–513

Kjaer M (1976a) Effect of leucocyte washings on cellular immunity to human renal carcinoma. Eur J Cancer 12: 783–792

Kjaer M (1976b) Prognostic value of tumor-directed, cell-mediated hypersensitivity detected by means of the leucocyte migration technique in patients with renal carcinoma. Eur J Cancer 12: 889–898

Sawyer PN, Dennis G, Wesolowski SA (1961) Bioelectrical hemostasis in incontrol able bleeding states. Am Surg 153: 556

Sedlarik K, Deckert F (1981) Die Elektrothrombose – eine Alternative zur Gefäßembolisation mit Partikeln. Fortschr Geb Röntgenstr Nuklearmed Ergänzungsband 134,6: 643–648

Wallace S, Chuang VP, Swanson D (1981) Embolization of renal carcinoma. Radiology 138: 563–570

Chemoembolization:
A New Treatment for Malignant Tumors and Metastases

K.-H. Schultheis

Medizinisches Zentrum für Chirurgie, Klinikum der Justus Liebig-Universität Giessen,
6300 Giessen, FRG

In the treatment of malignant tumors and metastases surgical procedures are preferred. In some cases, however, inoperability presents problems.

Liver metastases are operable as long as (a) the physiological age of the patient is under 70, (b) only solitary, unilateral metastases are found, (c) no hepatomegaly is present, and (d) the alkaline phosphatase is within the normal range (Pettavel and Morgenthaler 1978).

In other cases the only option is palliative measures. Among these are (Madding and Kennedy 1972; Bergmark and Fredlund 1978; Lee 1978; Wallace and Chuang 1982):

1. Ligation of the hepatic artery.
2. Intra-arterial chemotherapy.
3. Dearterialization of the liver and intra-arterial chemotherapy.
4. Isolated liver perfusion (Aigner, personal communication).
5. Embolization of the hepatic artery.

All of these therapeutic approaches are based on certain facts. First, the liver has a double circulation system, allowing the hepatic artery to be ligated without danger. Second, liver tumors and metastases have arterial blood supply. After ligation of the hepatic artery, however, the tumor receives a new supply of blood from collateral vessels. Thus, Bengmark proposes total dearterialization of the liver by ligation of possible collateral vessels (Bengmark and Fredlund 1978). This total dearterialization of the tumors is also possible by peripheral embolization.

A new therapeutic method could be "chemoembolization." For this purpose the embolizing agent must fulfill two conditions: It must induce long-lasting peripheral closure of the vessels, and release a cytostatic agent over a long period of time. Kato et al. (1981) reported on the first steps in this direction with ethylcellulose mitomycin capsoles. They achieved the necessary closure of vessels with gelatin sponge. However, the effect of embolization lasted for only a short period, and the release of the single cytostatic agent (mitomycin) took place too quickly.

Not being aware of these problems, we mixed the embolizing agent Ethibloc, which guarantees a long-lasting peripheral closure of the vessels, with different cytostatic agents and examined the bioaviability of the agents. We were able to prove that a gradual release took place over a long period of time (Schultheis et al. 1981; Schultheis 1982).

Ethibloc is an excellent substance for the chemoembolization of arterial tumor vessels, the advantages of which are several. It effects a safe, long-lasting interruption of the nutritional blood supply. At the same time, the tumor is attacked by the locally released cytostatic agent. There are various indications for chemoembolization. For example, preoperative embolization can reduce the tumor, or it can be applied postoperatively after long infusion of cytostatic agents, or after isolated perfusion, via the still-inserted catheter.

Successful embolization of urological, gynecological, gastroenterological, and bronchial tumors, as well as of tumors of the head and neck, shows that super-selective embolization is practicable in all vascularized tumors using the modern catheter technique.

Summing up, we can say that the chemoembolization of malignant tumors and metastases is a new method of palliative treatment for tumors of various localizations. The best palliative measure is the one which offers minimal therapeutic risk combined with maximal quality of life. Our current experiments with animals will show how far this new method of therapy it successful.

References

Bengmark S, Fredlund PE (1978) Temporary dearterialization combined with intra-arterial infusion of oncolytic drugs inthe treatment of liver tumors. Prog Clin Cancer 7: 207−216

Kato T, Nemoto R, Hisashi M, Takahashi M (1981) Arterial chemoembolization with Mitomycin C microcapsules in the treatment of primary or secondary carcinoma of the kidney, liver, bone and intrapelvic organs. Cancer 48: 674−680

Lee YT (1978) Nonsystemic treatment of metastatic tumors of the liver − review. Med Pediatr Oncol 4: 185−203

Madding GF, Kennedy PA (1972) Hepatic artery ligation. Surg Clin North Am 52: 719−728

Pettavel J, Morgenthaler F (1978) Protracted arterial chemotherapy of liver tumors. Prog Clin Cancer 7: 217

Schultheis KH, Schulz A, Schiefer HG (1981) Schnellhärtende Aminosäurenlösung als mögliche Chemotherapeutika-Trägersubstanz zur Behandlung der chronischen Osteomyelitis. Unfallchirurgie 7: 324−333

Schultheis KH, Henneking K, Rehm KE, Ecke H, Schiefer HG, Breithaupt H (1982) Untersuchungen über die Freisetzungskinetik verschiedener Chemotherapeutika aus einer viskösen, im feuchten Milieu schnell aushärtenden Aminosäurenlösung und ihre mögliche klinische Anwendung. Langenbecks Arch Chir [Suppl] 199−205

Wallace S, Chuang VP (1982) The radiologic diagnosis and management of hepatic metastases. Radiologe 22: 56−64

Discussion

Cannulas for infusing gastric cancer are placed into the coeliac axis. The injection of disulphine blue dye which can be seen through a gastroscope indicates the correct position of the catheter.

Chemoembolization may serve as a kind of arterial occlusion combined with chemotherapy.

As soon as we have an exact, standardized intra-arterial treatment regimen, and know what amount of drug via which vessel can be given in what period of time, additional concepts such as radiotherapy can be discussed.

A trial should be performed, comparing intra-arterial with intravenous treatment. Some individual patients who had previously received systemic chemotherapy have served as their own control, comparing response when the same drug was given intra-arterially; however, this is not an argument against controlled studies.

There might be an advantage to intra-arterial administration, especially with those drugs that have a short half-life, such as 5-FU.

Prolonged and Continuous Percutaneous Intra-Arterial Hepatic Infusion Chemotherapy in Advanced Metastatic Liver Adenocarcinoma from Colorectal Primary

R. A. Oberfield

Section of Oncology, Lahey Clinic Medical Center, 41 Mall Road, Box 541, Burlington, MA 01805, USA

In the United States in 1982 123,000 new cases of colorectal cancer were estimated, with 57,000 deaths anticipated. At least 30,000 of these deaths will be caused by liver metastases, the only metastases present in 15,000 of these patients. In the cases where tumors are limited to the liver and supplied by one major artery, the hepatic artery, regional infusion chemotherapy would be desirable. Systemic chemotherapy with fluorouracil (5-FU) has had only about a 20% response rate for about 3–5 months without any increase in survival (Silverberg 1982). Radiotherapy has also been limited, and surgery is not suitable for bilateral disease. Over the past 10–15 years we have reported our experience with surgical placement of the catheter, with increases in response and survival (Cady and Oberfield 1972, 1974; Oberfield 1974; Sullivan and Zurek 1965; Watkins et al. 1970).

In 1969 we began a program of percutaneous infusion at the Lahey Clinic. The program is continuing at the present time, but in this article I will report our experience with a study of 60 patients including follow-up data on all of them (Oberfield et al. 1979).

The rationale for this method is that prolonged, continuous exposure of tumor cells to an antimetabolite is required for effective antimetabolic activity to develop in the tumor cell population. Cancer cells are vulnerable to an antimetabolite during deoxyribonucleic acid (DNA) synthesis, and prolonged exposure of the tumor to the antimetabolite would affect most of the vulnerable cells of the tumor population as they enter this phase. This exposure should exceed the doubling time of the tumor. In regional arterial infusion, a chronometric infusion pump continuously propels the drug through a small arterial catheter attached to it. Infusion is conducted around the clock for periods of weeks or months, with high concentrations of antimetabolites being delivered to the tumor site. This produces increased regional concentration of the drug with minimal systemic concentration, thereby limiting systemic toxicity.

Materials and Methods

Sixty patients with advanced liver adenocarcinoma metastatic from colorectal primary were referred to the Lahey Clinic for percutaneous hepatic arterial infusion chemotherapy. The first patient received treatment in December, 1969, and the last patient entered the study in July, 1976. Follow-up studies were completed for this report as of September, 1976, with five patients still alive. Four patients had died by March 13, 1977, and one patient died in

Recent Results in Cancer Research, Vol. 86
© Springer-Verlag Berlin · Heidelberg 1983

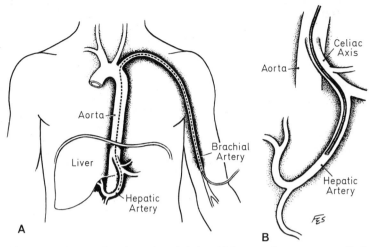

Fig. 1. A Passage of catheter into left brachial artery in upper arm. Catheter is then passed into descending aorta to common hepatic artery. **B** Enlarged view of catheter in common hepatic artery

November, 1977. Separate follow-up analysis to March 1977 did not alter results. All patients referred to the Lahey Clinic had histologic documentation of metastatic liver adenocarcinoma from the colorectal region with symptomatic evidence of disease progression – weight loss, right upper quadrant pain, malaise, fatigue, and clinical deterioration – combined with objective progression of disease as manifested by increase in liver size and worsening of results on liver enzyme tests, and shown on liver scans. Before catheterization, patients underwent baseline studies – blood chemistry profiles, liver scanning, and abdominal echography. The carcinoembryonic antigen test was performed occasionally.

All patients underwent percutaneous placement of an arterial catheter, using methods reported in detail elsewhere (Clouse et al. 1977). A preshaped, thin-walled, catheter was inserted into the brachial artery in the upper arm and passed into the thoracic aorta, the descending aorta, and the common hepatic artery (Fig. 1). For angiographic studies, the celiac and superior mesenteric arteries were injected separately with 35 ml of 60% meglumine sodium diatrizoate to outline the hepatic arteries. The hepatic artery was selectively catheterized and injected at 5 ml/s to delineate hepatic metastases. Patients whose right hepatic artery or entire hepatic arterial anatomy arose from the superior mesenteric artery were referred for surgical placement of the catheter, and were not included in the group of 60.

Catheter Care

The catheter was wrapped with nonallergenic tape to prevent sharp bends that predispose to cracking. An antibiotic ointment was applied at the arteriotomy site. The catheter was connected to a continuos infusion pump (Bowman, Brooklyn, NY; Sigma-Motor Middleport, NY; or, recently, Imed, Boston) by a long polyethylene tube that allowed the patient to ambulate at the bedside.

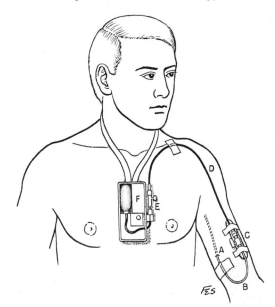

Fig. 2. Complete assembly for percutaneous hepatic artery infusion chemotherapy. *A*, exit site from the brachial artery; *B*, Teflon catheter; *C*, stopcock attachment connecting infusion Teflon catheter with vinyl tubing; *D*, vinyl tubing with male and female Luer-Loks; *E*, monoflow valve; *F*, chronometric infusion pump [Oberfield RA (1975)]

Chemotherapy

On the same day that the catheter was inserted patients started receiving 5-FU, 20 mg/kg body wt. daily by continuous arterial infusion for a total of 10 days, unless problems of toxicity prevented completion of treatment; the majority of patients were able to tolerate 10 days of chemotherapy. Angiography was performed to check the position of the catheter at the end of the infusion, although often the position was checked after the 5th day of infusion as well. If the catheter was still in good position, it was then attached to a portable chronometic infusion pump (the Watkins Chronofusor, U.S. Catheter and Instrument Corp., Glens Falls, NY), and if no toxicity was evident, patients began receiving 20 mg deoxyuridine (FUDR) per day by continuous infusion, at which point they were instructed in the use of the pump and discharged, receiving outpatient follow-up care (Fig. 2). During 5-FU infusion a leukocyte count was taken every other day, a hematocrit and platelet count twice a week, and liver enzyme tests weekly. Patients returned to the clinic for weekly evaluation at which time complete blood cell counts, platelet counts, and liver chemistries were performed. FUDR infusion was continued until the onset of toxic reactions, usually occurring within the first 5 weeks. A nonmedicated solution of distilled water was then infused until toxicity abated. Regional hepatic toxicity was manifested by an increase in the serum glutamic oxaloacetic acid and alkaline phosphatase, and occasionally in the bilirubin level. Systemic toxicity consisted in either a decrease in leukocyte count and platelets or gastrointestinal reactions (oral ulcers, diarrhea, vomiting). Catheter angiography was performed at 3- to 4-week intervals, and liver scans were made every 6 weeks. In some cases echograms were taken at 6-week intervals. Instruction in the use of the pump and catheter care was provided by a special oncology nursing team familiar with the problems of arterial infusion catheters and pumps (Carter 1977).

Early in the study we reported on 24 patients with colorectal cancer (Oberfield 1974). Other primary tumor sites were also treated, and our response rate with these cases was about 50%. The hepatic artery was used in 46% of cases, the celiac artery in 36%, and the splenic artery in 12%; the femoral artery and portal vein were rarely used. The median survival was 8.5 months. The celiac and hepatic artery infusions produced a 47% response rate, and splenic artery infusion resulted in a response rate of 10.6%.

Results

Of the 60 patients treated, 48 evaluable patients (80%) form the basis for analysis; 12 (20%) were eliminated because of inadequate treatment.

Patients Eliminated

Of the 12 patients eliminated, 10 had inadequate catheter time (median, 11 days); for the other two we had insufficient information for evaluation. Interestingly, two of the 12 (16.7%) had direct surgical placement of the catheter, one had a percutaneous infusion first and later had direct catheter infusion, three (25%) had terminal disease, and one developed infection that necessitated catheter removal after inadequate treatment time.

Objective Response

There was objective response in 36 (75%) of the 48 patients studied (Table 1): 15% (7 or 48) of patients had 100% response, 39% (19 of 48) had 50% response, 21% (10 of 48) had 25% response, and 25% (12 of 48) had no response. Median survival time from onset of treatment was 8.5 months, 6.9 months, and 4.7 months (100%, 50%, and 25% responders respectively) versus 3.6 months for nonresponders. The nonresponders had a median survival of 14.6 months from onset of diagnosis compared to 34.8 months for the 100% responders. Eight of the 12 nonresponders (66.7%) had poor infusion with clotting in the aorta and other complications, three (25%) had no catheter check after discharge, and five (42%) had direct surgical placement of the catheter for chemotherapy before having percutaneous infusion treatment.

Table 1. Objective response of 48 patients

Objective response (%)	No. of patients	(%)	Median survival from treatment (months)[a]	Patients without disease-free interval	
				Number	Percent
100	7	(15)	8.5	5/7	71.0
50	19	(39)	6.9	12/19	63.0
25	10	(21)	4.7	6/10	60.0
0	12	(25)	3.6	4/12	33.3

[a] $P = 0.103$ comparing all four groups. $P = 0.016$ comparing $\geq 50\%$ response with $< 50\%$ response (25% response and 0 response). No significant difference was noted between 0 response and 25% response

Significance of Disease-free Interval

Twenty-seven patients had no disease-free interval, and 21 had disease-free intervals greater than zero. In Table 1 the relationship of no disease-free interval to response is seen. In Table 2, comparisons between patients without disease-free intervals and patients with disease-free intervals greater than zero are given. The median survival from onset of treatment was generally less in those with no disease-free interval. In patients without disease-free intervals, 100% objective responders had a median survival of 7 months from treatment compared with 13.5 months survival of 100% responders with greater than zero disease-free interval; however, only two patients were in the latter category. In all categories of response, the median survival from diagnosis of disease to death was far longer for those with disease-free intervals greater than zero compared with those without disease-free interval. The long survival of eight nonresponders with a disease-free interval greater than zero is due to the fact that four of the eight were initially treated by direct surgical catheter infusion, with response. If we eliminate these four patients, survival from diagnosis decreases to 33 months. Patients without disease-free interval have an increased survival time from onset of metastases compared with patients with a disease-free interval greater than zero. The percentage of responses was slightly increased for patients without disease-free interval.

Table 2. Disease-free interval[a] and response

Objective response[b]	100%		50%		25%		None	
Disease-free interval	> 0	0	> 0	0	> 0	0	> 0	0
Number of patients	2 (10%)	5 (19%)	7 (33%)	12 (44%)	4 (19%)	6 (22%)	8 (38%)	4 (15%)
Treatment to death (months)	13.5	7	10.5	5	7	4.3	3.6	3.2
Metastases to death (months)	26.5	31	14.5	24	13	12.3	12	13.2
Primary diagnosis to death (months)	37.5	31	37.5	24	39	12.3	41	13.2

[a] $P > 0.10$ in all categories
[b] 100% response is complete disappearance of measurable lesions

Table 3. Relationship of sex to response and survival

Sex	Number	Median age (years)	Without disease-free interval	Objective response			Median survival from treatment, with > 50% regression (months)
				≥ 50%	25%	0%	
Male	31	58	22 (70%)	22 (71%)	5 (16%)	4 (13%)	8.9
Female	17	52	5 (30%)	4 (24%)	5 (30%)	8 (47%)	12.3

Analysis of the 21 patients with disease-free intervals greater than zero revealed that with increasing disease-free intervals, survival time from diagnosis until death increases, but no correlations seem to be significant in other categories, that is, infusion therapy to death, metastases to death, or catheter time in relation to increasing disease-free interval. Relationship of sex to response and survival is described in Table 3.

Relationship of Prior Treatment to Response

Radiation Therapy to Liver. Three patients received radiotherapy to the liver: one patient showed 50% response, one showed 25%, and one showed none. Survival from infusion therapy to death was 10.8 months in the 50% responder, who had had a long disease-free interval of 38 months, as compared with the 2.6-months survival of the nonresponder without a disease-free interval.

Primary Colorectal Resection Only. Of the eight patients who had primary resection without systemic chemotherapy, two were 100% responders, three were 50% responders, and three were 25% responders. In terms of the median, survival from treatment until death for these patients was 36.8 months, survival from metastases to death was 8.8 months, survival from treatment to death was 6.6 months, and the interval from diagnosis to metastases was 28 months; duration of catheter time was 5.6 months. Three patients had no disease-free interval.

Prior 5-FU Chemotherapy. Of the 18 patients who received 5-FU before arterial infusion chemotherapy, two received systemic chemotherapy orally and 16 intravenously. Sixteen of the 18 had primary resection in addition. Three of the 18 (17%) had responded to systemic 5-FU before arterial infusion therapy. Of 18 patients, 12 (68%) had a response of 50% or more regression to arterial infusion therapy, despite the fact that 83% of them had not responded to 5-FU systemically. Of the 15 patients (84%) without prior intravenous 5-FU response systemically and with no other treatment, two (13%) had a 25% response, and three (20%) had no response (Table 4).

Response in Relation to Catheter Treatment Time and Duration of Response

In Table 5, analysis is made in terms of response, showing catheter time and duration of response. Some patients, although they exhibited progression of disease, were continued on catheter treatment for another month or 2. Of 12 nonresponders, six had only percutaneous catheter placement, while six others had both direct and percutaneous

Table 4. Relationship of prior systemic 5-FU chemotherapy to intra-arterial responses

	No. of patients	Objective response			None
		100%	50%	25%	
Prior treatment	18	2 (11%)	10 (57%)	3 (17%)	3 (17%)
No prior treatment	15	2 (13%)	8 (54%)	2 (13%)	3 (20%)

Table 5. Response in relation to catheter treatment and duration of response

Treatment	No. of patients	Catheter time		Duration of response	
		Weeks	Months	Weeks	Months
A. Response (%)					
100	7	24.0	6.0	19	4.8
50	19	17.0	4.2	12	3.0
25	10	13.5	3.4	13	3.2
0	12	9.0	2.2	0	0
B. No response					
Percutaneous only	6	8.4	2.1	0	0
Direct and percutaneous	6	8.9	22	0	0
− Direct, then percutaneous	5	10.1	2.5	0	0
− Percutaneous, then direct	1	4.6	1.2	0	0

catheter placement (five had direct then percutaneous, and one had percutaneous then direct). Three patients who had percutaneous catheters first, with 50% objective response, later required direct placement of a catheter but showed no further response.

Relationship of Drug Dose to Response

Nonresponders received less 5-FU (< 9.8 g) and FUDR (< 150 mg) compared to responders (5-FU > 14 g; FUDR > 920 mg). Analysis was made correlating dose/kg body wt. but no significant difference was noted.

Relationship of Jaundice to Response

Of nonjaundiced patients, 52% had an objective response greater than 50%, with a median survival from treatment to death of 6.7 months. Of those with slight-to-moderate jaundice, 54% had an objective response greater than 50% with median survival from treatment to death of 4.8 months. Of those patients with severe jaundice, 56% had greater than 50% response, but the median survival from treatment to death was only 4.2 months.

Drug Toxicity

Local. During the initial 5-FU infusion, chemical hepatitis occurred in about 10% of patients. FUDR infusion resulted in local toxicity or chemical hepatitis in about 52%.

Systemic. Criteria for evaluation of toxicity were those of the Eastern Cooperative Oncology Group (Table 6).

Table 6. Toxicity criteria

	Degrees of toxicity				
	0	1	2	3	4
Oral stomatitis	0	Soreness	Ulcers, can eat	Ulcers, cannot eat	–
White blood cell count $\times$ 10^3	$\geq$ 4.5	3.0 – < 4.5	2.0 – < 3.0	1.0 – < 2.0	< 1.0
Platelet $\times$ 10^3	$\geq$ 130	90 – < 130	50 – < 90	25 – < 50	< 25
Gastrointestinal					
Nausea and vomiting	0	Nausea	Nausea and controlled vomiting	Vomiting intractable	–
Diarrhea	0	No dehydration	Dehydration	Severe, bloody	–

Oral. Of the 48 patients, 11 (23%) had 1+ oral toxicity. In this group, 36% had a 50% response, and 36% had no response. Duration of response was only 1 month – much less than in other groups.

Gastrointestinal. Of 41 patients (85%) with gastrointestinal toxicity, 21 had 1+ toxicity and 20 had 2+ toxicity. For 15 of this group toxicity was secondary to 5-FU (37%), and for 26 (63%), toxicity was secondary to FUDR. Five patients (10% of the total group) had no toxicity. In this group, one had 100% remission, three had 50% remission, and one had no response.

White Blood Cell Count. Eleven patients (23%) had toxicity. Eight had 1+ toxicity, two had 2+, and one had 3+. Ten of the 11 had toxicity from 5-FU, and one had 1+ toxicity from FUDR.

Platelet Count. Of the 10 patients (21%) with toxicity, nine had 1+ toxicity, and one had 3+ toxicity. Six of the 10 had toxicity from 5-FU, and the other four had 1+ toxicity from FUDR.

Complications Related to Arterial Catheter

Major and minor complications were recorded in this group of 48 patients (Table 7). Among major complications, complete or partial thrombosis of the common hepatic artery or the celiac artery occurred in 18.6% and 20.8% respectively, with no occlusions or thrombosis occurring in the brachial artery. Displacement of the catheter occurred in 33% of patients, with the total number of this complication occurring 43.8% of the time. Cracked catheters occurred in 25% of patients and were 31.3% of total complications. In Table 8 and 9 comparison is made between complete thrombosis and partial thrombosis in relation to survival factors and response. The median survival from treatment to death was 11.3 months in patients with partial occlusion compared to 6.9 months in patients having complete occlusion ($P = 0.20$); both groups are essentially comparable in terms of survival from onset of primary diagnosis (Table 8). Those patients with partial occlusion (Table 9) were all responders, as opposed to seven of nine patients (78%) with complete occlusion; a slightly higher percentage of 50%+ responders were in the partially occluded group (90% of patients with partial occlusion versus 67% in the complete occlusion group).

Table 7. Complications among 48 patients

	Total complications	
	Number	Percent
Major		
Complete thrombosis of common hepatic artery or celiac artery	9	18.8
Brachial artery thrombosis or occlusion	0	0
Partial thrombosis of common hepatic artery or celiac artery	10	20.8
Bleeding not controlled by pressure	3	6.3
Stenosis of common hepatic artery	1	2.1
Pseudoaneurysm of common hepatic artery	1	4.2
Catheter broken off in artery	1	2.1
Minor		
Displacement (occurred more than once in an individual patient)	21	43.8
Cracked catheter	15	31.1
Clotted catheter	7	14.6
Infection	2	4.2
Diminished pulse (or loss)	6	12.5
Bleeding controlled by pressure	3	6.3
Subintimal injection	3	6.3
Catheter pulled out by confused patient	1	2.1
Inability to reposition replace catheter	3	6.3
Inability to advance catheter through arch	0	0
Catheter kinked	4	8.3

Table 8. Arterial occlusion and survival (median values)

	Number	Primary diagnosis to death (months)	Metastases to death (months)	Treatment to death (months)
Complete occlusion	9	32.4	20.9	6.9[a]
Partial occlusion	10	36.5	17.9	11.3
No occlusion	29	20.5	14.5	4.1

[a] $P = 0.043$ comparing all three groups; $P = 0.05$ comparing occlusion (complete and partial) with no occlusion; $P = 0.20$ comparing complete occlusion with partial occlusion

Table 9. Arterial occlusion and response

	Number	Response			
		100%	50%	25%	None
Complete occlusion	9	1 (11%)	5 (56%)	1 (11%)	2 (22%)
Partial occlusion	10	4 (40%)	5 (50%)	1 (10%)	0
No occlusion	29	2 (7%)	9 (31%)	8 (27%)	10 (35%)

Arterial Occlusion vs Nonocclusion

In addition to the data relating to 19 patients with complete or partial occlusion, the data pertaining to the 29 patients without occlusion but with other complications (as noted in Table 7) were analyzed. Of these 29, 11 (38%) had 50%+ responses compared to 67% and 90% for complete and partial occlusion respectively (Table 9).

The duration of survival from treatment until death was only 4.1 months without occlusion compared with 11.3 months with partial occlusion and 6.9 months with complete occlusion (Table 8). If these 29 patients without occlusion are compared with the 19 patients with occlusion, the difference between the two groups does seem to be significant ($P = 0.05$).

Discussion

Table 10 reviews the experience of investigators who have reported experience with only percutaneous intra-arterial infusion, with sufficient numbers of patients to warrant meaningful data (Oberfield 1975; Misra et al. 1977; Patt et al. 1981; Shah et al. 1977). Other reports are available, but they cover small groups and do not add to the evaluation of this method of treatment. Catheter sites were not the same, and infusion programs varied. However, responses were within the same range, with median survivals also similar. For criteria of objective response investigators used reduction of liver size by at least 50% over 1–3 months, in addition to reduction of liver function tests. Systemic toxicity was similar, and complications from the catheter were similar to ours. Only one randomized study, that of the Central Oncology Group (Grage et al. 1979), was reported. Seventy-four patients were randomized into two treatment groups: one involved intra-arterial chemotherapy (direct surgical placement and percutaneously placed catheter) for 21 days, and the other had intravenous treatment as a loading course. Both groups of patients received weekly intravenous 5-FU after initial treatment. Of the 61 patients accepted for evaluation, responses were obtained in 34% of the arterial infusion patients versus 23% of the intravenously treated patients. Survivals were approximately the same in both groups – 53.5 weeks in the intra-arterially treated group and 43.2 weeks in the intravenously treated group. Durations of response were also about the same. Catheters were placed surgically in 12 patients, and percutaneously in 16. Survival curves for the two catheter treatments did not show a significant difference. Response rates in this study were much lower than those reported by others (Donegan et al. 1969; Labelle et al. 1968; Massey et al. 1971) and almost approximated those obtained from intravenous treatment. Again, both percutaneous and direct catheter groups were combined. Multiple institutions were involved, but the numbers were relatively too small to draw any definite conclusions.

Our study indicated that optimal responses can be obtained by a prolonged percutaneous infusion approach to colorectal cancer, using 5-FU and FUDR. Our response rates were similar, with 54% of patients having greater than 50% objective response, and a median survival from treatment of 8.5 months for 100% responders and 6.9 months for 50% responders. Of interest is the long survival from onset of metastases in our patients. As noted in Table 2, 100% responders with no disease-free interval had a survival from onset of metastases of 31 months, and 50% responders had a survival of 24 months. In our nonresponders, survival from onset of metastases was much longer than that previously reported in the literature (Jaffe et al. 1968), although many of our patients had received treatment.

Table 10. Percutaneous intra-arterial hepatic infusion treatment with fluorinated pyrimidines in metastatic liver adenocarcinoma from colorectal primary (Oberfield 1982)

Study, year	No. of patients	Percent colorectal primary	Percutaneous artery used	Intra-arterial infusion program	Response (%)	Median survival from intra-arterial treatment (months)
Massey et al. 1971	38	26	Femoral, 90%; axillary, 10%	5-FU, 15–30 mg/kg per 24 h, 4–21 days	42	10.8[a]
Ansfield et al. 1975	419	93	Brachial	5-FU, 20–30 mg/kg per 24 h, 4 days; 15 mg/kg per 24 h, 17 days; D/C intra-arterial; then IVP, 15 mg/kg per week; reinstitute intra-arterial treatment if progression	55	7.3
Petrek and Minton 1979	52	46	Femoral or axillary	5-FU, 1 g/day, 21 days	50	9.0
Oberfield et al. 1979	48	100	Brachial	5-FU, 20 mg/kg per 24 h, 10 days; FUDR, 20 mg/24 h until toxicity; resume FUDR after toxicity abates; prolonged treatment	54	7.7

[a] Mean

Complications from this technique have been reported for our group (Clouse et al. 1977), and the problem of whether occlusion has any influence on response is still unresolved. Increased responses with hepatic artery ligation have been reported (Balasegaram 1972; Fortner et al. 1976; Madding et al. 1970; Murray-Lyon et al. 1970). but overall survival has not been significantly prolonged, and morbidity due to the operative technique has increased.

The duration of survival from treatment and the duration of response with our percutaneous method were inferior to our previously reported experience involving direct surgical placement of catheter (Cady and Oberfield 1972, 1974; Oberfield 1972; Sullivan and Zurek 1965; Watkins et al. 1970). In 1965 (Sullivan and Zurek 1965) we reported response rates of 60%, and later (Cady and Oberfield 1972) of 67%, with median survival of 15 months in responders and 4.5 months in nonresponders. Our reviews (Cady and Oberfield 1974; Watkins et al. 1978) have also shown similar results with , again, a 67% response rate and median survival of 14 months contrasted with 8 months in those who had no response. Clinical improvement in our studies had occurred consistently in 71% of patients with survival of 16 months compared to a survival of nonresponders of 5 months ($P < 0.001$). The median survival of all responders was similar to that reported by Watkins et al. (1970, 1978). Since both direct surgical placement of catheter and the percutaneous catheter series have been performed in our institution by the same physicians, we believe our results are more valid than those obtained when data are pooled from several institutions with different techniques and different investigators. We believe that direct surgical placement of catheters is superior to percutaneous placement of catheters in terms of objective response, duration of response, and survival from treatment. No randomized study has ever been done, and a controlled study should be made comparing these two techniques. Percutaneous arterial infusion is not as adequate as the direct method because of the multiple complications and displacements of catheter that compromise good infusion with the former. Also, many of our patients selected for infusion chemotherapy by the percutaneous method are poor-risk patients who would not tolerate direct surgical placement of the catheter via laparotomy.

Conclusions

Our study has dealt only with patients who had colorectal adenocarcinoma with metastases to the liver. These patients were often too ill to be considered for direct surgical catheter placement or systemic chemotherapy, and many of the patients had already received intravenous 5-FU, which failed in about 83% of cases. Despite this, 68% of these patients achieved a response rate of about 50% or more with a median survival of 8 months. This method of treatment involved prolonged, ambulatory, percutaneous arterial infusion for periods often exceeding 2 years. Our results appear similar to Ansfield's data (Ansfield et al. 1971, 1975) with shorter treatment time, and prolonged treatment may not be needed for optimal antitumor effect. Direct surgical placement of the catheter in our previously reported experience has offered increased survival compared with our results with percutaneous catheter placement.

Disease-free intervals did not influence responses or survival except that patients without disease-free intervals had decreased survival. No relationship to age or sex was found. Prior treatment with radiotherapy did not influence treatment, although our series was small. Most of our nonresponders were patients who had had surgically placed catheters first and were then treated with percutaneous infusion. In addition, patients who failed to respond after percutaneous infusion did not generally benefit from a surgically placed catheter. Our data indicate that the effect of arterial occlusion on tumor growth may be a factor in enhanced response and survival, but patient population is too small to allow a definite conclusion. For the future, combined modalities should continue to be explored, employing radiotherapy, radioactive microspheres, isotopic immunoglobulins, drug combinations, hypothermia, hepatic artery ligation, and chemoembolization.

References

Ansfield FJ, Ramirez G, Skibba JL, Bryan GT, Davis HL Jr, Wirtanen GW (1971) Intrahepatic arterial infusion with 5-fluorouracil. Cancer 28: 1147–1151

Ansfield FJ, Ramirez G, Davis HL Jr, Wirtanen GW, Johnson RO, Bryan GT, Manalo FB, Borden EC, Davis TE, Esmaili ME (1975) Further clinical studies with intrahepatic arterial infusion with 5-fluorouracil. Cancer 36: 2413–2417

Balasegaram M (1972) Complete hepatic dearterialization for primary carcinoma of the liver: report of twenty-four patients. Am J Surg 124: 340–345

Cady B, Oberfield RA (1972) Infusion chemotherapy of liver metastases from large bowel cancer. Lahey Clin Found Bull 21: 89–95

Cady B, Oberfield RA (1974) Regional infusion chemotherapy of hepatic metastases from carcinoma of the colon. Am J Surg 127: 220–227

Carter J (1977) Role of the oncology nurse in regional infusion chemotherapy. AORN J 25: 662–668

Clouse ME, Ahmed R, Ryan RB, Oberfield RA, McCaffrey JA (1977) Complications of long term transbrachial hepatic arterial infusion chemotherapy. AJR 129: 779–803

Donegan WL, Harris HS, Spratt JS Jr (1969) Prolonged continuous hepatic infusion: results with fluorouracil for primary and metastatic cancer in the liver. Arch Surg 99: 149–157

Fortner JG, Kim DK, Barrett MK, Golbey RB (1976) Intrahepatic infusional chemotherapy using multiple agents for cancer in the liver. Proc Am Soc Clin Oncol 17: 293

Grage TB, Vassilopoulos PP, Shingleton WW, Jubert AV, Elias EG, Aust JB, Moss SE (1979) Results of a prospective randomized study of hepatic artery infusion with 5-fluorouracil versus intravenous 5-fluorouracil in patients with hepatic metastases from colorectal cancer: a Central Oncology Group study. Surgery 86: 550–555

Jaffe BM, Donegan WL, Watson F, Spratt JS (1968) Factors influencing survival in patients with untreated hepatic metastases. Surg Gynecol Obstet 127: 1–11

Labelle JJ, Lucas RJ, Eisenstein B, Reed MD, Vaitkevicius VK, Wilson GS (1968) Hepatic artery catheterization for chemotherapy. Arch Surg 96: 683–692

Madding GF, Kennedy PA, Sogemeier E (1970) Hepatic artery ligation for metastatic tumor in the liver. Am J Surg 120: 95–96

Massey WH, Fletcher WS, Judkins MP, Dennis DL (1971) Hepatic artery infusion for metastatic malignancy using percutaneously placed catheters. Am J Surg 121: 160–164

Misra NC, Jaiswal MS, Singh RV, Das B (1977) Intrahepatic arterial infusion of combination of mitomycin-C and 5-fluorouracil in treatment of primary and metastatic liver carcinoma. Cancer 39: 1425–1429

Murray-Lyon IM, Parsons VA, Blendis LM, Dawson JL, Rake MA, Laws JW, Williams R (1970) Treatment of secondary hepatic tumors by ligation of hepatic artery and infusion of cytotoxic drugs. Lancet 2: 172–175

Oberfield RA (1972) Practical aspects of investigation and treatment of colorectal cancer. Med Clin North Am 56: 665–675

Oberfield RA (1974) Prolonged and continuous percutaneous intra-arterial hepatic infusion chemotherapy in advanced liver cancer. Abstract. Proceedings XI International Cancer Congress, Florence, Italy, October 23, 1974, p 219

Oberfield RA (1975) Current status of regional arterial infusion chemotherapy. Med Clin North Am
    59: 411–424
Oberfield RA (1983) Intra-arterial hepatic infusion chemotherapy in metastatic liver cancer. Semin
    Oncol (in press)
Oberfield RA, McCaffrey JA, Polio J, Clouse ME, Hamilton T (1979) Prolonged and continuous
    percutaneous intra-arterial hepatic infusion chemotherapy in advanced metastatic liver adeno-
    carcinoma from colorectal primary. Cancer 44: 68–77
Patt YZ, Wallace S, Freireich EJ, Chuang VP, Hersh EM, Mavligit GM (1981) The palliative role of
    hepatic arterial infusion and arterial occlusion in colorectal carcinoma metastatic to liver. Lancet
    1: 349–350
Petrek JA, Minton JP (1979) Treatment of hepatic metastasis by percutaneous hepatic arterial
    infusion. Cancer 43: 2182–2188
Shah P, Baker LH, Vaitkevicius VK (1977) Preliminary experiences with intra-arterial adriamycin.
    Cancer Treat Rep 61: 1565–1567
Silverberg E (1982) Cancer statistics 1982. Cancer 32: 15–31
Sullivan RD, Zurek WZ (1965) Chemotherapy for liver cancer by protracted ambulatory infusion.
    JAMA 194: 481–486
Watkins E Jr, Khazei AM, Nahra KS (1970) Surgical basis for arterial infusion chemotherapy of
    disseminated carcinoma of the liver. Surg Gynecol Obstet 130: 581–605
Watkins E Jr, Oberfield RA, Cady B, Clouse ME (1978) Arterial infusion chemotherapy of diffuse
    hepatic malignancies. In: Ariel IM (ed) Progress in Clinical Cancer. Vol VII, Grune and Stratton
    New York pp 235–245

Arterial Infusion Chemotherapy for Hepatic Metastases*

J. Pettavel

Department of Surgery, University of Lausanne Medical School Center,
1003 Lausanne, Switzerland

In the treatment of primary and secondary liver cancer, the respective roles of surgery and chemotherapy are far from being established. Surgical treatment by itself is preferred for primary hepatic tumors, bulky solitary metastases, and smaller hepatic metastases limited to one lobe (Pettavel and Meyer 1979). In addition, the excision of one or even several metastases is generally preferable before instituting chemotherapy. The logical basis for arterial chemotherapy as treatment for liver metastases has been described elsewhere (Pettavel and Morgenthaler 1970). There is a considerable choice of methods, associated with different adjuvant means: mono- or polychemotherapy, continuous or intermittent injections, simultaneous or sequential chemotherapy. All these can be used alone or in association with some form of hepatic ischemia: complete liver dearterialization, ligation of one or all main liver arteries, temporary occlusion of the hepatic artery (Bengmark and Fredlund 1978), and eventually some form of arterial embolization.

I will limit my discussion to the long-term results of chemotherapy by arterial infusion, which I started to employ in 1965.

Material and Methods

Between 1965 and 1982 we infused 158 livers harboring primary or secondary malignancies for 3–24 months. We elected arterial infusion in 155 cases and portal infusions in three cases. Ligation of the proximal hepatic artery with distal infusion by chemotherapeutic agents was used in five cases. Ligation of a right or left hepatic artery, associated with infusion chemotherapy on the opposite side, was used four times. Major hepatic surgery was combined with arterial infusion seven times. Drugs infused include fluorouracil (1–3 g/day) until discrete oral mucosa toxicity; floxuridine (0.25 mg/kg per day) until completion of the treatment; mitomycin-C (10 mg/m², once every 4–6 weeks); rarely methotrexate with or without citrovorum factor rescue; rarely, adriamycin for hepatocarcinomas; dacarbazine and vincristine for melanomas.

Prior to instituting infusion, complete vascular perfusion of the liver was checked preoperatively by injection of fluorescein in the catheter. Additional arterial ligation or correction of the location of the tip of the catheter was often found to be necessary. Pre- and postoperative studies included the determination of CEA (Mach et al. 1978) and

---

* The advice of Jack Manpel, MD, is gratefully acknowledged

alkaline phosphatase levels. A hepatic angiogram is indispensable preoperatively to show the morphology of the hepatic arterial tree, since the so-called normal anatomy is found in only 45% of patients. Computed tomograms and/or ultrasonographic echograms of the liver are also routine pre- and postoperative examinations.

The origin of the primary cancer for the 158 patients who underwent hepatic infusion chemotherapy was as follows:

Origin	Number of cases
Colon and rectum	92
Stomach	9
Gall bladder and bile ducts	5
Breast	12
Hepatocarcinoma	12
Melanoma	12
Carcinoid tumor	5
Other	12

Classification of Liver Tumors in Stages

To accurately assess the results of the treatment of these tumors, one must bear in mind their evolution without therapy. This is especially valid for secondary tumors originating in the colon and/or rectum. Some authors, e.g., Pestana et al. (1964), Jaffe et al. (1968), Watkins et al. 1970, Nielsen et al. (1971), and more recently Wood et al. (1976), have presented several hundred cases with a mean survival time of 6−9 months and a median survival time of about 4,5 months. Nielsen et al. (1971), Cady and Oberfield (1974), Wood et al. (1976), and Pettavel and Morgenthaler (1976) were able to correlate the number and size of metastases with duration of survival. Lavin et al. (1980) insisted that initial performance status, weight loss, and prior chemotherapy status seem to be most prognostic for survival, and thus merit inclusion as stratification factors.

Our 1976 classification (Table 1; Pettavel and Morgenthaler 1978) includes three stages of evolution, and allows quite an accurate prognosis in each case. It has also been adopted by Patt et al. (1981).

Table 1. Lausanne classification of secondary liver malignancies originating in colon and/or rectum (1976); median survival of untreated cases ($n = 83$)

Stage	Liver enlargement	Elevated alkaline phosphatase	Median survival[a] (months)
1 ($n = 27$)	No	No	15.0
2 ($n = 26$)	One or the other		4.7
3 ($n = 30$)	Yes	Yes	1.4

[a] Mean survival for untreated cases = 4.5 months

Results

Operative Mortality

Our 30-day operative mortality was 4.7%. This is somewhat higher than was reported a few years ago (Pettavel and Morgenthaler 1978) because we have lately included some extremely high risk cases with the hope of improving their survival time.

Cancer Mortality

Our 30-day cancer mortality is 12%. It is sometimes difficult to evaluate where a given patient stands in relationship to the natural evolution of his disease. This is especially true of melanomas metastatic to the liver, where one feels that one is always too late, and of some breast carcinomas metastatic to the liver which have previously failed to respond to various systemic treatments.

Morbidity Secondary to Treatment

Morbidity due to toxicity is practically nil at the therapeutic dosage of fluorinated pyrimidines. However, certain cancer cells are not susceptible to chemotherapeutic agents at the level used with arterial infusions, in which case it is better to ligate the artery or to resort to embolization.

Arterial thrombosis due to the presence of the catheter is quite uncommon with standard Teflon or silicone catheters, especially if heparinized perfusates are used; on re-exploration we have found that obstruction of the hepatic artery is most often due to extension of the carcinoma into the hepatic pedicle.

Dislodgement of the catheter is rare if the arterial tree was entered through the gastroduodenal artery. However, ligation of the hepatic artery may produce necrosis and secondary dislodgement.

Gastroduodenal ulcerations may be seen especially after percutaneous placement of the catheter (Clouse et al. 1977). It is my opinion that the ulceration occurs secondary to the local action of the chemotherapeutic agent on the mucosa. We therefore place the catheter during laparotomy, and not percutaneously, in order to be able to ligate the many secondary arteries (e.g., the pyloric artery) that may lead the drug to the pyloroduodenal area instead of to the liver.

Iatrogenic liver abscesses as described by Jochimsen et al. (1978) are rare. We have only encountered this complication after ligation of a major artery.

Response

The response obtained by infusing liver metastases of miscellaneous origin has been reviewed elsewhere (Pettavel and Morgenthaler 1978). However, 72 of 78 patients infused for hepatic malignancies of colorectal origin constituted a comparatively homogeneous, well-staged group. Six of the 78 could not be evaluated; the 72 − who received chemoarterial infusions for more than 3 months − are analyzed in more detail. Of 55 who demonstrated objective response, 24 hat complete remission, 31 partial remission. The

Table 2. Results of chemoarterial infusion for > 3 months in 72 patients with secondary liver malignancies originating in colon and rectum

Result	No. of patients	Median survival (months)
Complete remission	24	19
Partial remission	31	9.7
No change, or progression	17	4.5

Table 3. Median survival times for 55 patients who received chemoarterial infusion for > 3 months for secondary liver malignancies originating in colon and rectum

Remission	Stage	No. of patients	Median survival (months)
Complete	2	6	26
	3	18	18
Partial	2	2	15.5
	3	29	9.5

remaining 17 showed either no change, or progression of the disease (see Tables 2 and 3 for further data).

Complete remission is defined as the return of the CEA level to normal and complete or almost complete disappearance of the lesions visualized by CT scanning or ultrasound for a minimum duration of 3 months. One must remember that large metastases do not always disappear completely and may be replaced by fibrous tissue, amorphous necrotic deposits, and ultimately by calcifications as has been discussed previously (Pettavel and Morgenthaler 1976). In partial remission, one of the mentioned objective parameters did not return to normal while the others did.

Remission of less than 3 months according to the criteria outlined above was considered "no change".

Discussion and Conclusion

The method of protracted arterial chemotherapy (hepatic arterial catheterization by laparotomy) appears to us to be the treatment of choice for hepatic metastases of colorectal origin and, to a lesser degree, for those of gastric and mammary origin. Melanomas merit a complementary study − in particular when they are of choroidal origin − as do carcinoid tumors.

With the method described, toxicity is remarkably infrequent. Operative mortality is equally low.

Surgical excision is indispensable for the treatment of a bulky hepatic tumor. In emergency situations, ligation of the hepatic artery perhaps temporarily at its point of origin should be considered, combined with terminal chemotherapeutic infusion into the distal artery. This method is not without risk, and some form of embolization may also be considered.

Should a hepatocellular tumor prove to be nonresectable due to its location, protracted arterial chemotherapeutic infusion could prolong the survival of the patient in comfort. In Table 3 survival is presented according to stage of disease; it is considerably longer in treated than in comparable untreated cases.

Arterial infusion should be instituted from the moment the diagnosis of metastases is made, for such lesions are much more sensitive to chemotherapy when they are still small and better vascularized. One may even wonder whether arterial or portal chemotherapy should not be used at the time of the initial operation in all cases of Dukes' C colorectal carcinoma, in order to destroy any infraclinical hepatic metastasis present.

References

Bengmark S, Fredlund PE (1978) Temporary dearterialization combined with intra-arterial infusion of oncolytic drugs in the treatment of liver tumors. In: Ariel IM (ed) Progress in clinical cancer VII. Grune and Stratton, New York, pp 207−216

Cady B, Oberfield RA (1974) Regional infusion chemotherapy of hepatic metastases from carcinoma of the colon. Am J Surg 127: 220−227

Clouse ME, Ahmed R, Ryan RB, Oberfield RA, McCaffrey JA (1977) Complications of long-term transbrachial hepatic arterial infusion chemotherapy. Am J Roentgenol 129: 799−803

Jaffe BM, Donegan WL, Watson F, Spratt JS Jr (1968) Factors influencing survival in patients with untreated hepatic metastases. Surg Gynecol Obstet 127: 1−11

Jochimsen PR, Zike WL, Shirazi SS, Pearlman NW (1978) Iatrogenic liver abscesses. Arch Surg 113: 141−144

Lavin P, Mittelman A, Douglass H Jr, Engstrom P, Klaasen D (1980) Survival and response to chemotherapy for advanced colorectal adenocarcinoma: an Eastern Cooperative Oncology Group report. Cancer 46: 1536−1543

Mach JP, Vienny H, Jaeger P, Haldemann B, Egeli R, Pettavel J (1978) Long-term follow-up of colo-rectal carcinoma patients by repeated CEA Radioimmunoassay. Cancer 42: 1439−1477

Nielsen J, Balslev I, Jensen HE (1971) Carcinoma of the colon with liver metastases. Acta Chir Scand 137: 463−465

Patt YZ, Chuang VP, Wallace S, Hersh EM, Freireich EJ, Mavligit GM (1981) The palliative role of hepatic arterial infusion and arterial occlusion in colorectal carcinoma metastatic to the liver. Lancet 349−351

Pestana C, Reitemeier JR, Moertel CG, Judd ES, Dockerty MB (1964) The natural history of carcinoma of the colon and rectum. Am J Surg 108: 826−829

Pettavel J, Meyer A (1979) Indication sélective à l'exérèse chirurgicale des métastases hépatiques. Schweiz Med Wochenschr 109: 794−796

Pettavel J, Morgenthaler F (1970) The treatment of hepatic metastases by long-term chemotherapeutic infusions. In: Saegesser F, Pettavel J (eds) Surgical oncology. Williams and Wilkins, Baltimore, pp 865−881

Pettavel J, Morgenthaler F (1976) Dix ans d'expérience de chimiothérapie artérielle des tumeurs primaires et secondaires du foie. Ann Gastroenterol Hepatol 12: 349−363

Pettavel J, Morgenthaler F (1978) Protracted arterial chemotherapy of liver tumors: An experience of 107 cases over a 12-year period. In: Ariel IM (ed) Progress in clinical cancer VII. Grune and Stratton, New York, pp 217−223

Watkins EJ, Khazei AM, Nahra KS (1970) Surgical basis for arterial infusion chemotherapy of disseminated carcinoma to the liver. Surg Gynec Obstet 130: 580−605

Wood CB, Gillis CR, Blumgart LH (1976) A retrospective study of the natural history of patients with liver metastases from colorectal cancer. Clin Oncol 2: 285−288

Transient Repeated Dearterialization Combined with Intra-Arterial Infusion of Oncolytic Drugs in the Treatment of Liver Tumors

S. Bengmark, A. Nobin, B. Jeppsson, and K.-G. Tranberg

Department of Surgery, University of Lund, 221 85 Lund, Sweden

After to the lymph nodes, the liver is the organ of the body which is most frequently the site of malignant growth. Using international data on cancer incidence, it can be calculated that there are roughly 200–250 thousand new cases of cancer diagnosed each year in the Federal Republic of Germany. Roughly 50,000 of these will sooner or later develop liver metastases. Approximately every 20th such patient will die of liver tumors.

The prognosis for patients with primary liver tumors is poor; in rare cases a patient may live for more than 6 months, but the median survival time after diagnosis is 2 months in Europe and the United States, and 1 month in Africa and Asia. Although the prognosis for liver metastases is generally better, for those with metastases from pancreatic or stomach cancer it is extremely bad. Occasionally such a patient will live for a year, but 75% die after 5 months. The best prognosis is for patients with metastases from colorectal cancer, 15%–20% of whom can live for more than a year; in rare cases a patient can live without treatment for more than 2 years.

We regard it as a challenge to find new tools to treat this huge group of patients.

Roughly 10% of patients with diagnosed hepatic malignancy can be resected. For the remaining 90% other types of treatment must be found. It has been known for a century that 70% of the hepatic portal venous blood can be diverted from the liver with survival of the patient. Von Haberer (1905) showed that ligation of the hepatic artery leads to death in cats, dogs, and rabbits, thereby demonstrating the importance of this vessel. Death following hepatic artery ligation was explained by Ellis and Dragstedt in 1938 who demonstrated that the liver harbors *Clostridium perfringens* or similar microorganisms. Under normal conditions these microorganisms are harmless but in a hypoxic situation, i.e., after ligation of the hepatic artery, they will grow and induce necrosis in the liver and sepsis, leading to the death of the animal. Markowitz et al. (1949) were able to show that treatment with penicillin for 7 days after hepatic artery ligation helped the animals survive. This observation later proved valuable for the human situation. In 1952 Markowitz suggested hepatic artery ligation as a tool for treating hepatic lacerations, aneurysms of the hepatic artery, arterioportal fistulas, and even hepatic malignancies.

In 1923 Segall showed that hepatic metastases receive the entire blood supply via the hepatic artery. This early study was based on three patients, but in 1937 Wright investigated 15 patients and in 1954 Breedis and Young reported on another 11. Finally, in 1965 Healey made a very extensive anatomical study of 45 patients. All these studies demonstrated that hepatic tumors are supplied totally by the hepatic artery. However, it has since been shown that this is not entirely true. Tumors weighing less than 30 mg usually

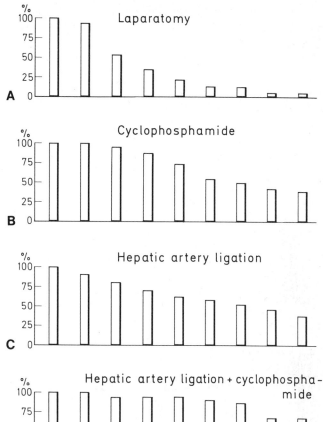

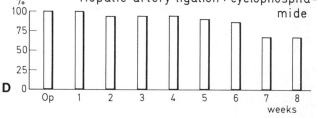

Fig. 1. Survival of rats with experimental methylcholanthrene-induced hepatic tumors after (**A**) laparotomy, (**B**) cyclophosphamide, (**C**) hepatic artery ligation, and (**D**) hepatic artery ligation combined with cyclophosphamide

have a double blood supply, as was clearly shown by Ackerman et al. (1969). For larger tumors a double blood supply is seen only in the extreme periphery of the tumor.

At the beginning of the 1960s laboratory experiments on animals were performed in Göteborg by Nilsson et al. (Nilsson et al. 1966); one of us (S. Bengmark) was working there at the time. Figure 1 shows the survival for rats with methylcholanthrene-induced hepatic tumors. Group A had no treatment except laparotomy. The animals in group B were treated with cyclophosphamide and those in group C with hepatic artery ligation; group D received a combination of ligation and medication. It is obvious that hepatic artery ligation quite a significant influence on survival, especially when combined with cyclophosphamide. These studies were encouraging.

In 1966 we were able to report on our first successful treatment with hepatic dearterialization (Almersjö et al. 1966). The patient had leiomyosarcoma in both liver lobes. Hepatic dearterialization was performed, where upon the tumors disappeared or decreased in size. After 6 weeks it was possible to perform another laparotomy; now resection and tumor enucleation were possible. In most of the tumors the pathologist was not able to demonstrate any surviving tumor cells. In one of the tumors living cells were found in the periphery of one tumor, obviously living saprophytically on surrounding hepatic parenchyma.

Fifteen years ago we were extremely optimistic regarding the future of the method. However, there proved to be several obstacles which we had not anticipated. It was not easy to obtain good results. As a matter of fact, when we collected data on a large series, no statistically significant influence could be demonstrated (Almersjö et al. 1976). The most important obstacle seemed to be the rearterialization occurring after single dearterialization. This occurred so rapidly that within days or a few weeks the surviving malignant cells were again being supplied with enough oxygen and nutrients to be able to continue to grow (Bengmark et al. 1969). This led us to try temporary dearterialization (Bengmark and Fredlund 1978; Jeppsson et al. 1979; Bengmark et al. 1981) in which all arterial connections to the liver except the hepatic artery are surgically divided. Slings are applied around the hepatic artery and is a catheter introduced into it through the gastroduodenal artery. Some days later the hepatic artery is occluded over a period of 9−16 h with the aid of the slings. In our opinion the advantages of temporary dearterialization are manifold. For one thing, the regeneration of arteries might not occur if the occlusion is as short as 16 h (Bengmark and Fredlund 1978). Another advantage is that the operative trauma and the trauma of the vascular exclusion of the liver do not coincide, which contributes to better survival. Finally, the hepatic artery can be used for infusion of oncolytic drugs, which is not possible when the hepatic artery is definitely ligated.

In 1981 we reported our first experience with temporary dearterialization (Dahl et al. 1981). Despite our efforts the complication frequency was quite high. Of 22 patients treated, three developed hepatic abscesses, two hepatic artery aneurysms, and another three catheter complications. In seven patients, or one-third of the group, the complications were so serious that some sort of reoperation had to be performed. For two patients the complications resulted in death.

Figure 2 shows the survival time for patients with colorectal cancer treated with temporary hepatic dearterialization. Although it is difficult to draw any definite conclusions regarding the value of temporary dearterialization, it is obvious that patients with extrahepatic growth do benefit a little from the treatment.

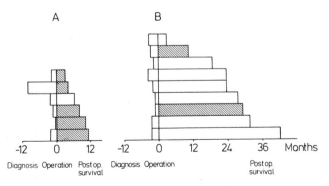

Fig. 2A, B. Survival times from diagnosis and from operation for 15 patients treated with transient liver dearterialization and regional fluorouracil infusion for colorectal carcinoma metastasizing to the liver. **A** With extrahepatic tumor growth; **B** without signs of extrahepatic tumor growth at operation *white fields* represent patients with less than 25% tumor involvement of the liver, *marked fields* patients with 25%−75% tumor involvement

Table 1. Diameter of metastases in 14 patients in whom an individual metastasis could be measured

Patient no.	Preoperative size	Size (cm) after dearterialization at					
		2 w	2 m	3 m	6 m	12 m	18 m
1	3			4	2.5		
3	10.5		10.5				
7	4.5				5	5	
8	4.5		4.5				
9	8	12					
10	5	5.5	8				
11	3	4					
12	3	3.5			2		2.5
13	8		6				
14	10	13	13				
15	6		8		3	2.5	
16	8	8					
17	8		6.5		8		
18	10.5					5	

Table 2. Liver size in centimeters measured from the caudal part of the right liver lobe to the dome of the right diaphragm

Patient no.	Preoperative size	Size after dearterialization at						Survival time
		2 w	2 m	3 m	6 m	12 m	18 m	
1	23		?	23	23	24		1 y 4m
2	?		22	24	21	25		2 y 3 m
3	26	?	28					11 m
4	25	25						3 m
5	> 35	> 35	> 35	> 35	> 35			10 m
6	?	24						8 m
7	27				28	28		1 y 7 m
8	21		23					2 y
9	26	33						4 m
10	21	?	> 35					5 m
11	23	29						4 m
12	24	26		22		23	21	alive 5 y
13	32		30					4 m
14	31	> 35	26					3m
15	18		19	16		17		3 y 6 m
16	29	27						1 m
17	28		26	26	23			11 m
18	25					23		2 y 8 m
19	?	?						6 m
20	26	29	23	23				2 y 5 m

?, caudal part of the right liver lobe for technical reasons could not be defined
> 35, liver was too big for the film size

S. Bengmark et al.

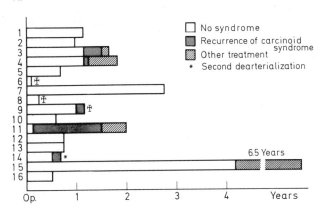

Fig. 3. Follow-up of 16 patients after temporary liver dearterialization, comparing symptomatic effects and survival times

Table 1 shows the diameter of the hepatic metastases in patients followed up for up to 18 months. In some cases a decrease in size could be observed. Most of the metastases, however, were stationary during longer or shorter periods.

Table 2 shows the influence of the size of the liver. In some cases a true decrease in the hepatomegaly could be observed. In most cases, however, hepatic size was stationary for a period of time. In conclusion, 13 of 16 patients with hepatic metastases from colorectal cancer seemed to show subjective and objective improvement lasting more than 2 months and a symptom-free period of more than 6 months.

Up to now temporary dearterialization has proven to be most successful in cases of metastatic carcinoid disease. In fact, this seems to be the only indication where we can today conclude that temporary dearterialization is effective (Bengmark et al. 1982a).

To date we have treated nine men and seven women, between 39 and 72 years of age. Figure 3 shows the survival time for these patients following temporary dearterialization. All patients survived the operation without complications. They were usually out of bed the day after operation. Temporary occlusion was performed 3–4 days later; however, in one patient it was postponed for 14 days due to postoperative carcinoid crisis. One patient developed a smaller hepatic abscess. Symptoms in connection with occlusion were mild, mainly some pain, fever, and tiredness. The hepatic enzymes in all patients except one were elevated after occlusion of the hepatic artery, but no clinical signs of hepatic insufficiency were noted. The hepatic enzyme values of all patients returned to normal within 6 weeks. To assure that complete occlusion was obtained, angiography was done during the procedure in five patients.

Three patients in our series have died, two 1 and 3 months postoperatively, of complications with hepatic abscess or leakage from intestinal anastomosis. These two patients had undergone intestinal resection in connection with preparation for hepatic dearterialization. The third patient died of carcinoid crisis after 14 months; the autopsy showed a duodenal cancer with hepatic metastases in lymph nodes, spleen, liver, and spine. The surviving 13 patients showed immediate relief from carcinoid symptoms after temporary dearterialization. 13 patients have been followed up for a minimum of 6 months, eight patients for 12 months, and five for more than 18 months. The symptom-free period extends as far as 42 months, the mean being 14 months.

Figure 4 compares the occurrence of carcinoid flush and diarrhea before and after the operation. The majority of patients had flush before the operation, but 3 and 6 months after, almost everyone was free from flush. Almost every patient had diarrhea before the operation, but occurrence was rare postoperatively. There were only a few cases of more

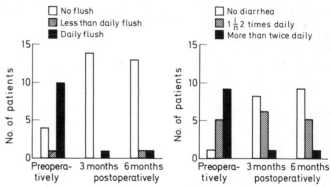

Fig. 4. The effect of temporary liver dearterialization on carcinoid flushing and diarrhea in 14 patients subjected to 15 dearterializations and followed up for at least 6 months

than two stools per day. Angiographic checking has shown regression and necrosis of the hepatic metastases in eight of the operated patients who survived more than 3 months. In four patients neither regression or progression could be demonstrated, and in two continuous progression was observed.

It is time to look to the future. Implantable pumps are being developed, which will be a great help in cytostatic treatment. We are also working with an implantable device for repeated hepatic artery occlusion. Experimental data from such studies will soon be published (Persson et al. 1982). Our group can look back on a 20-year period of various attempts to palliate patients with hepatic tumor growth; the way has not been easy, but today there is a small light of hope on the horizon (Bengmark et al. 1982b, c, d).

References

Ackerman NB, Lien WM, Kondi ES, Silverman NA (1969) The blood supply in experimental liver metastases. I. The distribution of hepatic artery and portal vein to "small" and "large" tumors. Surgery 66: 1067–1072

Almersjö O, Bengmark S, Engevik L, Hafström LO, Nilsson LAV (1966) Hepatic artery ligation as pretreatment for liver resection of metastatic cancer. Rev Surg 23: 377–380

Almersjö O, Bengmark S, Hafström LO, Leissner K-H (1976) of liver dearterialization combined with regional infusion of 5-fluorouracil for liver cancer. Acta Chir Scand 142: 131–138

Bengmark S, Fredlund PE (1978) Temporary dearterialization combined with intra-arterial infusion of oncolytic drugs in the treatment of liver tumors. In: Ariel IM (ed) Progress in clinical cancer, vol VII, pp 207–216

Bengmark S, Engevik L, Rosengren C (1969) Angiography of the regenerating human liver after extensive resections. Surgery 65: 590

Bengmark S, Dahl E, Fredlund PE (1981) Hepatic dearterialization and infusion treatment of liver tumors: In: Petersson HE (ed) Experimental tumour research. CRC Press, Boca Raton, Florida

Bengmark S, Ericsson M, Lunderqvist A, Mårtensson H, Nobin A, Saco M (1982a) Temporary liver dearterialization in patients with metastatic carcinoid disease. World J Surg 6: 46–53

Bengmark S, Hafström LO, Jeppsson B, Jönsson P-E, Nagasue N, Persson B, Sundqvist K, Szeleczky M, Tranberg K-G (1982b) Neuster Stand der Leberchirurgie. Zentralbl Chir 107: 689–696

Bengmark S, Hafström LO, Jeppsson B, Jönsson P-E, Rydén S, Sundqvist K (1982c) Metastatic disease in the liver from colorectal cancer: An appraisal of liver surgery. World J Surg 6: 61–65

Bengmark S, Hafström LO, Jeppsson B, Sundqvist K (1982d) Primary carcinoma of the liver: Improvement in sight? World J Surg 6: 54–60

Breedis C, Young G (1954) The blood supply of neoplasms in the liver. Am J Path 30: 969–985

Dahl E, Bengmark S, Fredlund PE, Tylén U (1981) Transient hepatic dearterialization followed by regional intraarterial 5-fluorouracil infusion as treatment for liver tumors. Ann Surg 193: 82–88

Ellis JC, Dragstedt LR (1938) Liver autolysis in vivo. Arch Surg 20: 8–16

Healey JE Jr (1965) Vascular patterns in human metastatic liver tumours. Surg Gynecol Obstet 120: 1187–1193

Jeppsson B, Dahl EP, Fredlund PE, Stenram U, Bengmark S (1979) Hepatic necrosis in the pig produced by transient arterial occlusion. Eur Surg Res 11: 243–253

Markowitz J (1952) The hepatic artery. Editorial. Surg Gynecol Obstet 95: 644–646

Markowitz J, Rappaport A, Scott AC (1949) Prevention of liver necrosis following ligation of hepatic artery. Proc Soc Exp Biol Med 70: 305

Nilsson LAV, Rudenstam CM, Zettergren L (1966) Vascularization of liver tumours and the effect of artery ligature. 4th European Conference on Microcirculation, Cambridge 1966, pp 425–431

Persson B, Jeppsson B, Ekelund L, Nagasue N, Szeleczky M (1982) A new device for temporary occlusion of the hepatic artery. Surg Gynecol Obstet

Segall HN (1923) An Experimental anatomical investigation of the liver. Surg Gynecol Obstet 37: 152–178

von Haberer H (1905) Experimentelle Unterbindung der Leberarterie. Arch Klin Chir 78: 557–587

Wright RD (1937) The blood supply of newly developed epithelial tissue in the liver. J Path Bact 45: 405–414

Intra-Arterial Chemotherapy of the Liver with Transient, Repeated Hypoxia

F. Wopfner

Abteilung für Chirurgie, Universität Erlangen, Maximiliansplatz, 8520 Erlangen, FRG

Introduction

The prognosis for patients with disseminated liver tumors, primary or metastatic, and especially with cancer of portal organs is very poor; the 3-year survival rate approximates 3% for colorectal cancer. Individual prognosis depends mainly on the tumor load of the liver but a generally accepted staging system is not yet available (Bengmark and Jeppson 1982a; Cady 1982; Goligher 1975).

The prognosis for surgically resectable liver metastases is clearly better, showing survival rates of about 40% for 3 years (Adson 1978; Bengmark and Jeppson 1982b; Fortner and Papachristou 1979; Mühe et al. 1979). Systemic chemotherapy with 5-fluorouracil (5-FU) has an overall response rate of 20% (Moertel 1981). No other drug or combination to date has demonstrated any advantage over 5-FU alone (Moertel 1981).

With regional chemotherapy a higher drug concentration within the tumor is reached; the mainly arterial blood supply of overt liver metastases (Ackermann 1982; Lundberg 1977) and some pharmacological data (Ensminger et al. 1978) (Table 1) supply the rationale for

Table 1. Drugs used for regional chemotherapy

	Metabolization by liver during first passage (%)
Regional perfusion	
5-Fluorouracil	30−60
5-Desoxyuridin	30−70
Dichloromethotrexate	up to 90
Methotrexate	up to 10
Adriamycin	app. 30
Actinomycin-D	−
cis-Platin	−
Dacarbazine (DTIC)	−
Etoposide (VP-16-213)	−
Isolated perfusion	
Phenyl-alanin-mustard	
Actinomycin-D	
Methotrexate	
DTIC	

intra-arterial chemotherapy (Ensminger et al. 1978; Fortner and Papachristou 1979; Lundberg 1977; Oberfield et al. 1979; Raming et al. 1977; Ramirez and Ansfield 1982; Siebner and Hagemann 1978). Ligation of the hepatic artery or total liver dearterialization causes tumor necrosis (Bengmark and Jeppson 1982b; Fortner and Papachristou 1979), but transient arterial hypoxia seems to avoid the development of sufficient arterial collaterals (Aronson et al. 1979; Fortner and Papachristou 1979; El-Domeiri 1980) and is just as effective (Fortner and Papachristou 1979; El-Domeiri 1980).

Table 2. Patients with disseminated liver metastases (tumors) treated by intrahepatic chemotherapy as of April 1982 ($n = 33$)

Primary cancer	Patient		Metastases	Catheter	Drug
	Age	Sex			
Colorectal	48	M	S	S-G	5-FU
	48	M	ME	R	5-FU
	40	M	ME	EM	5-FU
	52	M	S	EM	5-FU
	54	M	ME	S-G	5-FU
	55	M	ME	EM	5-FU
	56	M	ME	EM	5-FU
	56	M	ME	EM	5-FU
	59	M	S	EM	5-FU
	61	M	ME	EM	5-FU
	64	M	ME	EM	5-FU
	66	M	ME	EM	5-FU
	71	M	ME	S-G	5-FU
	74	M	S	S-G	5-FU
	25	F	S	EM	5-FU
	43	F	S	EM	5-FU
	43	F	S	EM	5-FU
	48	F	S	R	5-FU
	51	F	ME	EM	5-FU
	51	F	ME	EM	5-FU
	52	F	ME	EM	5-FU
	53	F	ME	EM	5-FU
	56	F	ME	EM	5-FU
	69	F	S	EM	5-FU
Malignoma Breast	51	F	ME	S-G	Prothoate, i.v. and intrahepatic
Gastric	58	M	S	EM	5-FU
Pancreatic	62	F	S	EM	5-FU
Carcinoid	25	F	S	EM	5-FU
	45	F	S	EM	5-FU
	49	M	S	EM	5-FU
	58	M	S	EM	5-FU
Hepatoma	48	M	ME	EM	VP-16-213
	62	F	ME	EM	5-FU

S, synchronous; ME, metachronous; S-G, Swan-Ganz; R, Raimondi; EM, Erlanger model

Our experiences using intrahepatic chemotherapy with transient repeated arterial hypoxia — mainly via a newly developed indwelling double-lumen catheter — are presented here.

Patients and Methods

Between 1978 and 1982 intrahepatic chemotherapy was performed on 33 patients (see Table 2) in whom the liver was 50%−70% involved with disseminated metastases. All patients had local control of the primary and no other distant metastases. Only one patient with hepatoma had cirrhosis of the liver. The technical details on the insertion of catheters have been outlined earlier (Wopfner 1981).

Chemotherapy was begun at some point within the first postoperative week, depending on the clinical status of the patient. Each patient received 250−500 mg 5-FU intrahepatically every other day, according to subjective tolerance, the limit being determined by the appearance of nausea, vomiting, or profuse diarrhea. After dismissal from the hospital, patients were treated exclusively as outpatients by their family doctors, receiving weekly infusions increasing with subjective tolerance. During each treatment a 30-min dearterialization was performed (except in cases of carcinoid syndrome). If less than 1000 mg was tolerated, the patient received 750 or 500 mg, twice or three times as week respectively, according to tolerance, achieving 1000−2000 mg/week, or approximately 20−30 mg/kg body wt.

With careful instruction and close cooperation neither the patients nor the family doctors had major problems with catheter care or handling.

Results

Toxicity of Chemotherapy

By adjustment of dose to individual subjective tolerance the toxicity during intrahepatic chemotherapy was kept within acceptable limits (Table 3), and the patients did very well on the whole. In one case, bone marrow toxicity caused a short pause. In another patient, with a known history of chronic duodenal ulcer a short interruption of therapy was also necessary; the treatment could be continued with protection from cimetidine and antacids without further complications. We observed symptoms of gastritis in two patients and diarrhea in another two. Reversible elevations of serum transaminases were seen nine times; no patient developed chemical hepatitis. Wound healing was not affected.

Duration of Therapy

Table 4 charts the reasons for cessation of therapy in 31 of 33 patients. In 21 cases cessation was due to catheter problems. One patient with carcinoid syndrome died postoperatively of liver necrosis; this followed renal failure after a thrombosis caused by catheter dislocation. The case has been reported previously (Wopfner 1981). Of the nine cases in which progression of disease was a factor, one involved synchronous thrombosis and sepsis. Among the 16 cases in which thrombosis itself was the cause of cessation, there were two in which the thrombosis was due to catheter dislocation. Clinical signs of thrombosis were

Table 3. Incidence of toxicity with intrahepatic chemotherapy for metastases from colorectal primary

Toxicity after subjective tolerance was reached	Grade	Time		No. of patients
		From administration of drug (days)	From beginning of treatment (months)	
Loss of appetite	Light[a]	1–2		4
Nausea	Light	1–2		3
Vomiting	None	–		0
Diarrhea	Light	1–2	2,3	2
Gastritis (without history)		1–2	1,1	2
Duodenal ulcer (with history)			6	1
Leukopenia	< 2,500			0
Thrombopenia	< 80,000		6	1
Elevated transaminases	Light-moderate (reversible)		2	9
Wound healing	Not affected			0
Subjective status during treatment[b]	1–3			24

[a] Grading: light, moderate, severe, life-threatening

[b] *1*, fully active; *2*, good general condition but not active; *3*, disabled but active; *4*, disabled, not active; *5*, bedridden

Table 4. Duration of intrahepatic chemotherapy for 33 patients

Reason for cessation	No. of patients	Duration (months)	Average (months)
Dislocation of			
Swan-Ganz catheter	4	3	3
Watkins catheter (Chronofusor)	1	12	12
Disease progression	9	3–12	7.1
Thrombosis	16	3–24	10
None	2	5, 6	–
Death	1		

Table 5. Therapy administered following thrombosis to 11 patients with metastases from colorectal primary

Treatment	No. of patients	Duration (months)
Second implantation		
Hepatic artery	1	3
Portal vein	3	> 12, 4, 2
Intravenous chemotherapy		
Methotrexate and 5-FU	3	5, > 4, 5
5-FU	3	> 1, > 6, 7
None	1	> 6

pain on administration of the drug or reflux outside of the catheter. No patient developed hepatic failure or chronic hepatic disease later on. In two of 33 cases, therapy could be completed without premature cessation. Table 5 details therapy following thrombosis for those patients with colorectal primary.

Clinical

CT scans following therapy showed complete disapperance of liver metastases in five patients (four colorectal primary, one breast) 2−7 months after the start of treatment. This

Table 6. Follow-up over 4−36 months in 33 patients

Malignancy	Examination method	Total regression	Partial regression or stable disease	Disease progression	
		(Months from the start of treatment)		Liver	Extra-hepatic
Colorectal	CT scan	3−10		−	−
(n = 24)	(n = 8)	4−18 +		−	−
		7−12		−	−
		2−16		×	×
			1−3	−	×
			2−6 +	−	−
			12	×	×
			6 +	−	−
	Ultrasound		3−8	×	×
	(n = 6)		2−6	×	×
			4 +	−	−
			5 +	−	−
			8 +	−	−
			8 +	−	−
	Clinical, laboratory		3−6 (weeks)	×	×
	(n = 10)		7	×	−
			6 +	−	−
			6 +	−	−
			5 +	−	−
			3 +	−	−
			3	×	×
			3	−	×
			3 +	−	−
			4 +	−	−
Breast	CT scan, ultrasound	4−36		−	−
Gastric	Ultrasound		8	−	×
Pancreatic	CT scan		5	×	−
Carcinoid[a]	CT scan		24 +	−	−
			24 +	−	−
Hepatoma	Clinical		6 +	−	−
			4	×	−
			6	×	−

+, continuing; ×, yes; −, no
[a] Decreased 5-HIAA, one postoperative death

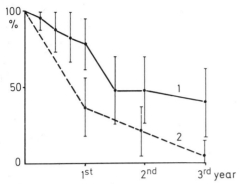

Fig. 1. Survival rates of (*1*) 24 patients as compared with (*2*) 29 controls. Rates are uncorrected, and calculated by the actuarial method with 95% confidence intervals. Group *1* received intrahepatic chemotherapy from May 1, 1978 to Dec. 31, 1981. Group *2* received no postoperative therapy; they were followed up from Jan. 1, 1969 to Dec. 31, 1981. All patients in each group presented disseminated liver metastases from colorectal primary. The primary was treated locally by radical excision and there were no other distant metastases known at the time of operation. Mean survival rate for Group 1 was 79% ± 17% for the first year, 48% ± 22% for the second. For Group 2 it was 37% ± 19% for the first year, and 21% ± 17% for the second

total regression lasted as long as 36 months in one patient. Partial regression was determined in seven patients by means of CT scanning or ultrasound. There were 18 patients with clinically stable disease and two who showed rapid disease progression.

One patient with ascites, jaundice, and pain recovered shortly from his symptoms, but only for a few weeks. Three patients with carcinoids showed a rapid decrease in previously elevated 5-HIAA, back to normal or only slightly elevated levels. In cases of hepatoma only brief responses were seen (see Table 6).

Careful analysis of the survival rates for the 24 patients with colorectal liver metastases (Fig. 1) shows a significant improvement in the first year for the treated patients; the untreated patients are "historical (nonrandomized) controls".

Discussion

The treatment of disseminated liver tumors, primary or metastatic, as yet is only of a palliative nature (Mitteilungen der Deutschen Gesellschaft für Chirurgie 1978). The morbidity caused by the treatment, as outlined in this paper, seems to be acceptable for the patients, allowing good quality of life; the treatment seems to be palliatively effective.

Controlled studies are undoubtedly needed (Bengmark and Jeppson 1982a, b; Cady 1982; Ramirez and Ansfield 1982). Addition of other modalities (Boddie et al. 1979; Ensminger et al. 1978, 1981; Fortner et al. 1975; Grundmann 1979; Order and Leibel 1982; Sherman and Weichselbaum 1982; Taylor et al. 1981; Webber et al. 1978) also seems justified.

Additional treatment might include isolated hypothermal or hyperthermal perfusion, followed by continuous or intermittent intrahepatic, intra-arterial, or intraportal regional perfusion. This might be combined with systemic chemotherapy and/or local irradiation.

Totally implantable pump systems are needed, as well as other types of catheters. The value and necessary duration of arterial hypoxia should be determined, and the effectiveness of both new and established drugs should be studied, alone and in combinations.

Summary

Intra-arterial liver perfusion with transient repeated hypoxia via an indwelling double-lumen polyurethane catheter was undertaken in 25 of 33 patients with diffuse metastases involving 50% − 70% of the liver, and whose primary cancer had previously been treated by local radical resections. Treatment continued over 3 − 12 months until disease progression and over 3 − 24 months until thrombosis. In 24 patients with colorectal carcinoma the 1-year survival rate (using the actuarial method) was 79% ± 17%.
The treatment morbidity was low. It is concluded that this form of treatment improves the quality of life and gives safe and effective palliation to the patients.

References

Ackermann NB (1982) The blood supply of liver metastases. In: Weiss L, Gilbert HA (eds) Liver metastases. Hall, Boston, pp 96−125

Adson MA (1978) Liver tumors-surgical treatment. Digestive cancer, vol IX. Pergamon Press, Oxford

Aronson KF, Hellekant J, Holmberg U, Rothmann H, Teder T (1979) Controlled blocking of hepatic artery flow with enzymatically degradable microspheres combined with oncolytic drugs. Eur Surg Res 11: 99

Bengmark S, Jeppson B (1982a) Staging of liver metastases. In: Weiss L, Gilbert HA (eds) Liver metastases. Hall, Boston, pp 268−274

Bengmark S, Jönsson RE (1982b) Surgical treatment of liver metastases. In: Weiss L, Gilbert HA (eds) Liver metastases. Hall, Boston, pp 294−321

Boddie AW, Booker L, Mullins JD, Buckley CJ, McBride CM (1979) Hepatic hyperthermia by total isolation and regional perfusion in vivo. J Surg Res 26: 447−457

Cady B (1982) Selection of treatment for liver metastases. In: Weiss L, Gilbert HA (eds) Liver metastases. Hall, Boston, pp 275−293

El-Domeiri AA (1980) Treatment of hepatic metastases in cancer of the colon and rectum. A preliminary report. Cancer 45: 2245

Ensminger WD, Rosowsky A, Raso V, Levin DC, Glode M, Come ST, Steele G, Frei E (1978) A clinical-pharmacological evaluation of hepatic arterial infusions of 5-fluoro-2-deoxyuridine and 5-fluorouracil. Cancer Res 38: 3784−3792

Ensminger W, Niederhuber J, Dakhil S, Thrall J, Wheeler R (1981) Totally implanted drug delivery system for hepatic arterial chemotherapy. Cancer Treat Rep 56: 393−400

Fortner JG, Papachristou DN (1979) Surgery of liver tumors. Int Adv Surg Oncol 2: 251

Fortner JG, Penneman R, Krakoff IH (1975) Actinomycin-D perfusion of the isolated lever for cancer. Bull Soc Int Chir 5: 399−403

Goligher JC (1975) Surgery of the anus, rectum and colon. Bailliere Tindal, London

Grundmann R (1979) Der Verschluß der Arteria hepatica. Dtsch Med Wochenschr 104: 848

Lundberg B (1977) Intra-arterial chemotherapy. Cancer, vol V. Plenum Press, New York

Mitteilungen der Deutschen Gesellschaft für Chirurgie, Beilage 3, 1978

Moertel CG (1981) Adjuvant therapy of gastrointestinal carcinoma, an overview. In: Salmon SE, Jones SE (eds) Adjuvant therapy of cancer III. Grune and Stratton, New York

Mühe E, Gall FP, Angermann B (1979) Resektionen von Lebermetastasen. Klinikarzt 8:602

Oberfield RA, McCaffrey JA, Polio J, Clouse ME, Hamilton TH (1979) Prolonged and continous percutaneous intra-arterial hepatic infusion chemotherapy in advanced metastatic liver adeno-carcinoma from colorectal primary cancer. Cancer 44:414

Order SE, Leibel SA (1982) Combined hepatic irradiation and misinidazole for palliation of liver metastases. In: Weiss L, Gilbert HA (eds) Liver metastases. Hall, Boston, pp 360–368

Raming KP, Sparks FC, Eilber FR, Morton DL (1977) management of hepatic metastases. Semin Oncol 4:71

Ramirez G, Ansfield FJ (1982) Chemotherapy of liver metastases. In: Weiss L, Gilbert HA (eds) Liver metastases. Hall, Boston, pp 348–359

Sherman DM, Weichselbaum RR (1982) Hepatic metastasis: the role of radiotherapy. In: Weiss L, Gilbert HA (eds) Liver metastases. Hall, Boston, pp 337–347

Siebner M, Hagemann U (1978) Perfusionstherapie der Arteria hepatica bei Lebermetastasen mit 5-Fluorouracil. Therapiewoche 28:8639

Taylor I, West C, Rowling J (1981) Can colorectal liver metastases be prevented? In: Gerard A (ed) Progress and perspectives in the treatment of gastrointestinal tumors. Pergamon Press, Oxford, p 89

Webber BM, Soderberg CH, Leone LA, Rege VB, Glicksman AS (1978) A combined treatment approach to management of hepatic metastases. Cancer 42:1087

Wopfner F (1981) Therapie inoperabler Lebermetastasen. Dtsch Med Wochenschr 106:1099–1102

Intrahepatic Chemotherapy in Isolated Liver Metastases

R. Hinterberger[1], J. Fischer[1], J. Preiß[1], and H. Weigand[2]

1 Abteilung für Hämatologie, Universität Mainz, Langenbeckstrasse 1, 6500 Mainz, FRG
2 Abteilung für Radiologie, Universität Mainz, Langenbeckstrasse 1, 6500 Mainz, FRG

Most malignant liver tumors in Europe are of metastatic origin. The failure of early detection renders most of these tumors nonresectable at the time of diagnosis.

Although in colorectal cancer especially some liver metastases grow very slowly, and survival of more than 5 years without treatment has been reported, the mean survival rate is less than 1 year. Systemic chemotherapy does not seem to be effective, and one short course of intrahepatic infusion of cytostatic drugs followed by systemic chemotherapy is not superior to systemic therapy alone (Grage et al. 1979).

In various studies, prolonged intra-arterial liver infusion with cytostatics, mostly 5-fluorouracil (5-FU) or floxuridine (FUDR), resulted in a remission rate in the range of 50%. However, a lack of randomized trials makes it a definitive statement on survival with this approach impossible.

Materials and Methods

In 1978 we started regional continuous intrahepatic chemotherapy of isolated liver metastases of carcinomas of various origins. Of the 25 patients treated, 16 were males and nine were females; the mean age was 51 years.

The time between the operation of the primary tumor and the diagnosis of liver metastases was 15 months on average, in a range of 0−84 months.

The duration of regional liver infusion was 5.7 months on the average; the longest infusion time was 23 months. We have used several different approaches for the permanent catheter. The hepatic artery was used for 18 implantations, and the portal vein for 12, of which four were done during laparotomy, and eight via transumbilical insertion according to the recently published method (Weigand et al., this volume). In the most suitable method, the hepatic artery was cannulated, following angiography, with the catheter inserted via the femoral artery. The catheter remained in place and the liver was perfused with 5-FU for a period of 5−10 days.

In 18 cases the hepatic artery was cannulated; two patients received two catheters each because of vascular anomalies. In 12 cases the portal vein was cannulated; three of the four patients in whom this was done surgically had had a previous arterial catheter which spontaneously dislocated.

We chose the transumbilical approach for perfusion through the portal vein for all those patients for whom resection of the liver metastases was impossible because of size.

We have found that infusion of the portal vein system is effective without prior ligation of the hepatic artery in spite of reports to the contrary (Taylor et al. 1979).

In this we agree with the findings that ligation of the hepatic artery leads to only temporary dearterilization because new collateral vessels are formed in 4 days to a few weeks (Grundmann 1979).

An additional reason for choosing the transumbilical, portal vein access for certain groups of patients is that this method is technically easier to handle, and carries a smaller operative risk.

Among our group of 25 patients, the primary tumor was a colorectal carcinoma in 18 cases; there was a mammary carcinoma in one case, one gall-bladder, one stomach, and two pancreatic carcinomas, and two carcinoids of unknown primary localization.

Administration of Therapy

Chemotherapy was administered continously through a portable CORMED-infusionpump ML 6-4. We used either regional therapy alone (until complications arose) or regional therapy combined with systemic therapy in those cases where (a) the extrahepatic metastases appeared during regional therapy, or (b) where the CEA-level rose continuously in spite of the hepatic metastases decreasing in size and without extrahepatic metastases being demonstrable. ˙

Each patient received 5-FU and FUDR given by continuous infusion for 7 days, and vincristine, carmustine (BCNU), and dacarbazine (DTIC) given systemically as shown in Table 1. During the interval or when the side effects of the cytostatic drugs used became too severe, normal physiological saline solution was perfused. As standard procedure 1000−5000 IU heparin was added to the perfused solution for 24 h. It only took a short time to train all our patients, who then managed to deal with their pumps on their own, with the effect that chemotherapy could be continued on an outpatient basis. The family physician looked after the patients during the time between regular visits every 4−6 weeks at the outpatient clinic of our department.

Therapy was postponed when the following side effects occured:

1. Agranulocytosis.
2. Stomatitis and gastrointestinal complications.
3. Gastric or duodenal ulcers.
4. Gastrointestinal bleeding.
5. Intractable diarrhea.

Table 1. Regional and combined (regional and systemic) chemotherapy

Therapy	Drug	Dose $(mg/m^2/day)$	No. of days
Regional	5-FU or FUDR	500 8−12	Daily until complications arose
Regional combined with systemic	Vincristine DTIC BCNU	1 300 100	1 (first day) 2 (first 2 days) 1 (first day)

There were 17 serious complications for 15 patients. Agranulocytosis with sepsis occurred in six patients, two of whom died as a result. Two other patients suffered sepsis from infection due to the inserted catheter. In both cases the complications could treated with antibiotic infusions through the catheter, which remained in position and could be used further for cytostatic treatment. There were two patients with ulcers – one gastric, the other gastric and duodenal.
Eight arterial catheters dislocated into the surrounding liver parenchyma; in three cases the catheter was found to be situated in the biliary tract. There was one occluded catheter and one portal veinthrombosis, both of which conditions were resolved spontaneously.

Results

Responses to therapy and the degree of remission were assessed 6 months after the beginning of therapy using clinical findings, CEA-level, CT-scans, and abdominal sonography.
In nine patients no response to therapy was observed (Fig. 1). No nonresponder lived more than 12 months, the mean survival time being 6.8 months. This is in accordance with the survival times for the control study without therapy performed by Jaffe et al. (1968). Good response was seen in 16 patients; one patient achieved complete remission, proven by laparotomy, and has been symptom free for 22 months. Mean survival time in the group of responders is 25 months. Periods of remission ranged from 1 to 22 months. In most cases tumor relapses occurred at extrahepatic sites such as the lungs or the skin.
This study provides evidence for the assumption that if the tumor is responding well to intrahepatic therapy survival time can be increased. During this time the quality of patient's life is not so badly disturbed by the therapy.

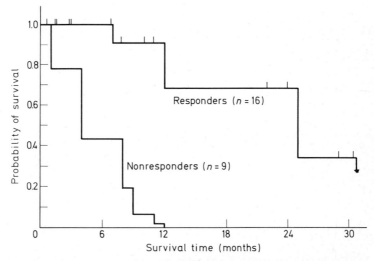

Fig. 1. Survival time and probability of survival for 25 patients (nine nonresponders and 16 responders) who received intrahepatic infusion chemotherapy for isolated liver metastases. The *small vertical lines* represent patients still living and the length of time since the start of individual treatment

References

Grage TB, Shingleton WW, Jubert AV, Elias EG, Aust JB, Moss SE (1979) Results of a prospective
    randomized study of hepatic artery infusion with 5-fluorouracil vs. Intravenous 5-fluorouracil in
    patients with hepatic metastases from colorectal cancer. Front Gastrointest Res 5: 116−119,
    129
Grundmann R (1979) Der Verschluß der A. hepatica. Dtsch Med Wochenschr 104: 848−855
Jaffe BM, Donegan WL, Watson F (1968) An investigation of the factors which influence the survival
    in patients with untreated hepatic metastases. Surg Gynecol Obstet 127: 1
Taylor J, Bennett R, Sherriff S (1979) The blood supply of colorectal liver metastases. Br J Cancer
    39: 749

Improved Quality of Life with an Implantable Pump for Liver Perfusion

P. Kempf, M. Olbermann, and J. Fischer

Abteilung für Chirurgie, Stadtkrankenhaus, 6090 Rüsselsheim, FRG

Introduction

The treatment of liver metastases in colorectal cancer can in no way be regarded as standardized. All therapeutic methods offered to date are attempts to prolong life. Survival time with liver metastases averages 4–6 months after diagnosis is established. Systemic treatment with cytostatic agents has not shown any marked effect. For example, Oberfield et al. (1979) achieved an 8.5-month survival time in his patients by liver perfusion, but the extracorporal pump used offers many disadvantages and possible complications.
Egeli et al. (this volume) describe surgical removal of the tumor and perfusion of the liver as the best method. Simultaneous temporary or total hypoxia of the liver achieved by ligation of the artery (EORTC 1980) or by the method presented by Bengmark and Fredlund (1978) may also result in some success. Wopfner (this volume), too, achieved a prolonged survival time for patients with metastases by inducing intermittent hypoxia with an inserted ballon catheter.

Material and Method

During the past 3 years we performed 16 liver perfusions in patients with liver metastases from colorectal cancer. In 13 cases we chose arterial perfusion via the gastroduodenal artery and the hepatic artery itself. In three cases we used the portal vein and ligated the hepatic arteries according to the EORTC protocol. One patient died after the operation of hepatic necrosis.
The indication for liver perfusion was to destroy either surgically inoperable liver metastases – postoperatively – micrometastases in resectable liver metastases. The rate of infections was high, but identical with the frequency of complications noted by Oberfield et al. (1979) and Egeli et al. (this volume).
Dislocation of the catheter was considered a severe complication, as the aim of the operation was not fulfilled. Since the beginning of 1982 the implantable pump of the Infusaid Company, Boston offers the possibility of avoiding many complications. The Infusaid pump is marketed as model 100 and as model 400; the function of the pump is explained in the figures.
The catheter of the pump (Fig. 1) is a tube made of Teflon; special rings enclosed guarantee exact fixation of the perfusion tube in the vessel and deter dislocation. As the tube is of very

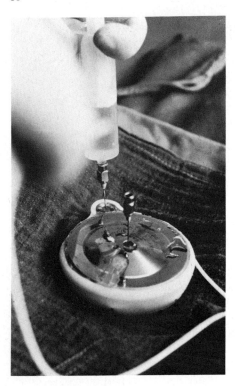

Fig. 1. The Infusaid pump, model 400; one needle is placed in the main compartment and the second in the sideboard

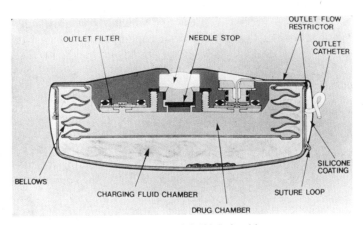

Fig. 2. A cross section of the model-100 Infusaid pump

soft material, it will not break as former catheters did. The pump itself consists of titanium and does not cause foreign-boddy reactions as do pacemakers. The pump is inserted into the abdominal wall above the fascia and below the skin and is refilled percutaneously at 2-week intervals. The pump is set so that up to 900 ml floxuridine can be infused into the liver daily in a constant flow. Working totally mechanically and without any electronic devices, there are few defects, and no service is necessary (Figs. 2 and 3).

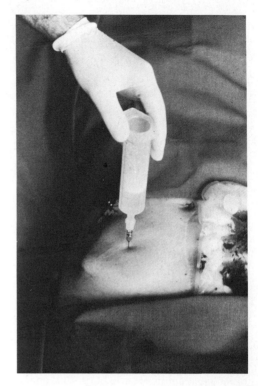

Fig. 3. The abdomen of a patient with rectal cancer and liver metastases during the refilling procedure

Summary

In spite of the current discussion on whether liver perfusion is effective (Grage et al. 1979; Ansfield et al. 1975), the implantable perfusion pump offers the possibility of combining the still questionable therapeutic success with a high quality of life during the time remaining to such patients.

References

Ansfield FJ et al. (1975) Further clinical studies with intrahepatic arterial infusion with 5-Fluorouracil. Cancer 36: 2413−2417

Bengmark S, Fredlund PE (1978) Temporary dearterialization combined with intra-arterial infusion of oncolytic drugs in the treatment of liver tumors. Prog Clin Cancer 7: 207−216

EORTC Gastro-Intestinal Group (1980) Chirurgisches Universitätsklinikum, Zürich. Liver metastases of Colorectal origin, October 1980

Fortner JC et al. (1973) Treatment of primary and secondary liver cancer by hepatic artery ligation and infusion chemotherapy. Ann Surg 178: 162−178

Grage TB et al. (1979) Results of a prospective randomized study of hepatic artery infusion with 5-FU versus intravenous 5-fluorouracil in patients with hepatic metastases from colorectal cancer. Surgery 86: 550−555

Oberfield RA et al. (1979) Prolonged and continuous percutaneous intra-arterial hepatic infusion chemotherapy in advanced metastatic liver adenocarcinoma from colorectal primary. Cancer 44: 414−423

Pettavel J, Morgenthaler F (1978) Protracted arterial chemotherapy of liver tumours: an experience of 107 cases over a 12-year period. Prog Clin Cancer 7: 217−233 (1978)

Catheterization of the Portal Vein by the Transumbilical Approach for Intrahepatic Chemotherapy

H. Weigand[1], M. Stahlschmidt[2], and J. Fischer[3]

1 Abteilung für Radiologie, Universität Mainz, Langenbeckstrasse 1, 6500 Mainz, FRG
2 Abteilung für Chirurgie, Universität Mainz, Langenbeckstrasse 1, 6500 Mainz, FRG
3 Abteilung für Hämatologie, Universität Mainz, Langenbeckstrasse 1, 6500 Mainz, FRG

For patients with colorectal malignomas and surgically nonresectable metastases, regional long-term perfusion with chemotherapeutic drugs may be valuable, according to the current view. Several techniques are used for regional long-term liver perfusion; either the arterial approach via the hepatic artery or a venous approach via the portal vein can be chosen. A long-term catheter can be implanted in the hepatic artery or the portal vein during the resection of the primary tumor or during the "second-look" procedure. In either case a laparotomy has to be done.

A less invasive but equally safe approach to the liver is by recannulation of the central vein of the ligamentum teres hepatis. This anatomical approach to the portal vein was described by Doviner (1954) and Carbalhaes (1959) for the first time. In the literature, the technique is considered to be a safe and simple procedure which has no serious complications.

The left umbilical vein disappears about 2 weeks post partum. It persists as a cord located at the free edge of the ligamentum teres hepatis between the umbilicus and the hilus hepatis. If the liver is of normal size, in almost 90% of cases the ligamentum teres hepatis can be prepared cranial to the paramedian of the umbilicus. This can be done with the patient under local anaesthesia. Most of the ligamentum (about 5−10 cm) is located extraperitoneally in the fat tissue, so that an opening of the peritoneum can be avoided in nearly all cases.

The ligamentum is exposed and prepared free from the fatty tissue, as far as possible in the direction of the hilus hepatis. Directly retroumbilically there is the change from the very thin, fibrous tissue of the central vein to a more solid texture, comparable to that of the ureter or the ductus deferens. It is here that a partial transsection of the central vein must be done. The former lumen of the central vein can then be obliterated stepwise by use of either flexible or inflexible bougies of increasing diameter. Additionally, a special lubricant should be used. At the passage into the left ramus principalis of the portal system inside the left liver lobe the catheter meets with sphincter-like resistance, which can be overcome with increased force. The catheter reaches the portal system via the ramus ventroflexus. The structure of this passage can be examined with either a flexible or an inflexible endoscope.

If the intraportal position of the first catheter is documented by the first injection of contrast medium, a normal French-7 angiographic catheter is pushed forward into the ramus principalis sinister, using the guide wire. Turning to the right, the tip of the catheter should be positioned so far into the portal system that the guide wire is forced to run into the main branch of the portal vein retrograde.

Recent Results in Cancer Research, Vol. 86
© Springer-Verlag Berlin · Heidelberg 1983

By means of the guide wire, the long-term catheter (CAVE-Fix-MT) is inserted the portal vein in a definite position in exchange for the first catheter. The distal end of the catheter leads of the incision percutaneously. Its intravenous end should not cause any pressure on the veinous wall. Care should be taken to avoid destruction of a thin drainage vessel of the pancreatic head by the catheter tip. On closing the incision stepwise, the transumbilical exploratory (TUS) catheter should be ligated within the central vein and should be fixed on the skin in a loop by two sutures. To increase the efficiency of portal vein perfusion the hepatic artery can also be embolized, because on the one hand, the portal vein allowes sufficient liver function, and on the other hand, most of the metastases are supplied with blood chiefly from the hepatic artery. Within only a few weeks of occlusion of the hepatic artery alone a new supply of blood to the liver has been established via rearterialization.

Since 1981, 11 patients have been treated by means of transumbilical exploration for long-term perfusion of liver metastases. As of 10 months after the start of therapy no complications had occurred. It is too soon to evaluate the effectiveness of this treatment in general, but several patients have experienced an impressive decrease in metastases without any significant side effects.

Compared with other cannulation procedures, TUS has the advantage of being an anatomical approach. Only local anesthesia is required, and the catheter can be changed as often as necessary on an outpatient basis.

In our opinion, TUS should be the technique of choice for regional, long-term perfusion of the liver, using cytostatic drugs via the portal venous system. It is preferable to other approaches − intraoperative, as well as postoperative − in that it provides easy ambulant care of the perfusion apparatus.

References

Doviner DG (1954) Topographical study of the possibilities for angiography of the liver via the nonobliterated part of the umbilical vein. (in Russian) Tes dokl Nautsch Ges St v Rost med Inst

Gonzales Carbalhaes O (1959) Una nueva via de acceso al sistema porta con grandes posibilidades diagnósticas, terapeúticas de investigación. Rev Sanid Mil (Mex) 42:42

Discussion

As catheters are placed via the portal venous route, portal venous thromboses are seen quite often, but they are usually asymptomatic and disappear soon after the infusion is stopped.

The longest interval between the start of an intra-arterial infusion and measurable regression is about 3 months. Generally if there is no response by 6 weeks it is unlikely that regression will occur.

After partial hepatectomy for liver metastases, chances are that a few nodules remain in the rest of the liver tissue. For this reason, infusion of the rest of the liver seems valuable.

Isolated Liver Perfusion in Dogs

F. Ghussen, K. Nagel, and W. Isselhard

Chirurgische Universitätsklinik E16, Institut für experimentelle Medizin,
Joseph-Stelzmann-Strasse 9, 5000 Köln 41, FRG

The surgical treatment of liver tumors has been complemented by regional infusion therapy with cytostatics in many centres over the past few years (Ansfield et al. 1971; Misra et al. 1977; Ramming et al. 1976; Taylor 1978). The liver is thus supplied with high doses of cytostatics via the arterial or portal system. However, after passing through the liver these drugs enter the systemic circulation and cause the familiar side effects. Moreover, the results of controlled studies which have become available show that survival times could not be substantially prolonged.

We therefore developed a new surgical procedure for isolated liver perfusion in which the advantages of the direct and high-dose cytostatic regimen can be utilized, the disadvantage of the systemic effect avoided, and the action of the cytostatic agent enhanced by recirculation. In addition, there is the possibility of regional hyperthermia. Here we present the procedure, and show that the catheter system developed by us provides an adequate venous reflux from the lower half of the body and from the portal area, and that a 1-h liver perfusion can be performed under normothermic conditions without irreversibly damaging healthy liver tissue.

Method

Catheter System and Perfusion Aggregate

In Fig. 1 the catheter system is schematically presented. The perfusion aggregate consists of a roller pump, a heat exchanger and an oxygenator with a maximum fill volume of 1.5 l. The perfusion system is filled with 2,000 U heparin, 300 ml of the animal's blood and 300 ml Ringer solution.

Surgical Technique

The studies were conducted with 10 Alsatians of both sexes with a mean body weight of 26.9 ± 1.7 kg. After premedication, initiation of anaesthesia with pentobarbital (10–15 mg/kg body wt.) and endotracheal intubation, we respirated the animals, using an Engström respirator, with a mixture of nitrous oxide and oxygen at a ratio of 3 : 1. Analgesia was continued by administration of fentanyl. The arterial systemic pressure was

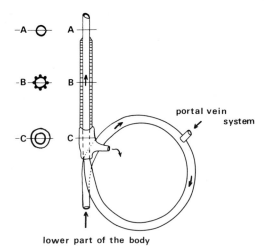

Fig. 1. The catheter system

measured via a polyethylene catheter inserted in the A. brachialis using an electromagnetic Statham bridge. We inserted a second polyethylene catheter through a side branch of the V. brachialis up to the height of the right atrium, and another in a similar manner into the V. brachialis on the opposite side. After heparinising the animals by administering 0.1 mg heparin potassium per kg body wt., we opened the abdomen by a median incision. All ligament connections to the liver were detached (Ll. triangulare dextrum and sinistrum, L. coronarium hepatis, L. teres hepatis, L. falciforme hepatis, L. hepatoduodenale, and the Omentum minus), and collateral vessels, in particular the Vasa phrenica, were ligated and severed.

Via a 2.5-cm-long incision we inserted the double-lumen part of the catheter cranially in the suprarenal section of the inferior Vena cava, and the single-lumen part caudally, then released the blood flow from the lower half of the body centripetally via the interior lumen of the catheter. To divert the portal flow into the inner caval shunt we opened the portal vein lengthwise for a distance of 2.5 cm and placed a catheter 6 mm in diameter in a distal position.

Via the same incision of the portal vein we placed another catheter in the direction of the hilus. After clamping the hepatic artery and the bile duct and applying a suprahepatic tourniquet to the inferior Vena cava we initiated the isolated, 1-h normothermic perfusion of the liver with the aid of the perfusion aggregate, via silicon tube connections to the portal vein catheter pointing towards the hilus and via the outer lumen of the caval catheter back to the aggregate (Fig. 2).

At the end of the perfusion we removed the tourniquets from the suprahepatic section of the Vena cava, the hepatic artery and the bile duct, decannulated and closed first the portal vein (running suture) then the inferior Vena vava, and after closing the abdomen, observed the animals postoperatively for 24 h.

Parameters Measured

The following parameters were measured: Flow rates in the infrahepatic Vena cava and the portal vein, perfusion flow and perfusion pressure, intra-arterial systemic pressure, blood gases in the arterial and venous branches of the perfusion circuit, rectal and liver

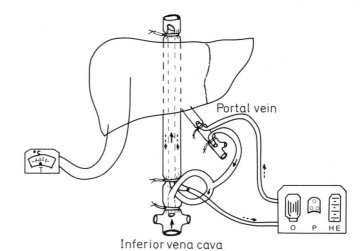

Portal vein

Fig. 2. The experimental
setup. *O*, oxygenator;
P, roller pump; *HE*, heat
exchanger

Inferior vena cava

O   P   HE

temperatures, the content of adenosine triphosphate (ATP), glycogen and glucose in the
tissue.

Four other dogs served as controls for the metabolic studies. They were anaesthetised,
their livers were prepared and their vessels clamped as described above; however, no
catheters were inserted and perfusion was not done. With a modified dye dilution method
we examined the isolation of the liver from the systemic circulation (Ghussen et al.
1982).

Results

The flow through the interior shunt remained at a median value of 1.113 ± 0.147 l/min, the
flow from the portal system being 0.635 ± 0.097 l/min, and from the lower half of the body
0.583 ± 0.092 l/min. The values measured during perfusion did not differ significantly from
the physiological flow rates prior to perfusion.

The perfusion flow through the liver was 0.549 ± 0.062 l/min (0.55 ± 0.03 ml/min per
g tissue) at a perfusion pressure of 10.00 ± 2.4 cm H_2O.

After the Vena cava was clamped, the systemic arterial pressure dropped from 120 mm Hg
to 90 mm Hg, after the portal vein was clamped, to 60 mm Hg, but it recovered each time
the catheter was inserted and the blood flow released. During perfusion arterial pressure
remained constant at about 100 mm Hg. After decannulation and closure of the vessels,
baseline values were achieved (Fig. 3).

Liver temperature immediately after the abdomen had been opened was $38.08 \pm 0.16°$ C.
This temperature could be maintained at a constant level during perfusion. The tissue
contents of ATP, glycogen and glucose in the liver of the control animals and of the
perfused animals are shown in Fig. 4. The ATP content, which in the control animals
amounted to 2.73 µmol/g wet weight (WW), dropped to 1.92 µmol/g WW after a 1-h
perfusion period (not significant), but rose again to 2.40 µmol/g WW 24 h after perfusion
was stopped. The glycogen content in tissue showed a similar behaviour at almost
consistent values (Fig. 4).

With the dilution method we determined leakage between the perfusion circuit and the
systemic circulation on the order of 6%−7% of the total perfusion circuit volume.

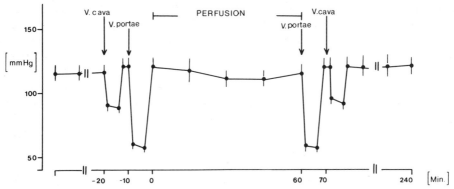

Fig. 3. Systemic arterial pressure during regional perfusion of the liver

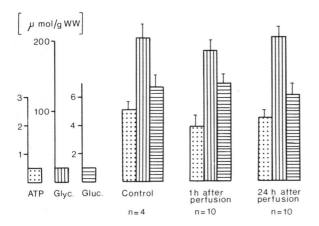

Fig. 4. Tissue levels of adenosine triphosphate (*ATP*), glycogen (*Glyc*), and glucose (*Gluc*) in the liver after regional perfusion. *WW*, wet weight

Discussion

Reports on regionally isolated liver perfusion have hitherto been rare (Ausman 1961; Chung et al. 1962; Healey et al. 1961; Mulcare et al. 1973). In published papers only study models without detailed information on results are described. Only Boddie et al. (1979) have presented a technically simple and practical model.

Because the hepatic veins discharge immediately into the inferior Vena cava, diverting the venous blood of the liver is as a rule only feasible by clamping off the hepatic section of the V. cava, which makes an extra-anatomic bypass necessary for the return of the caval blood.

However, with the catheter system we developed we were able to return an adequate volume of blood from the lower half of the body and the portal flow area without an additional porto-caval anastomosis or an extra-anatomic diversion.

The flow rates did not differ from the physiological values. After clamping the inferior Vena cava and the portal vein, we observed a fall in the arterial systemic pressure to 90 mm Hg or 60 mm Hg under otherwise physiological conditions. Because of the absence of collateral circulatory systems in the dog, an interruption of the portal flow is particularly effective haemodynamically (Child et al. 1950; Jonstone 1957). We also observed these falls in pressure during the clamping phase. Since the venous reflux to the heart was assured through the internal shunt, the arterial systemic mean pressure returned to normal after the blood flow was released.

The main problem in using a double-lumen caval catheter is to provide a sufficient volume of venous reflux from the liver. Only then are adequate perfusion rates assured. The flow rates in the perfusion circuit we measured correspond to the values under physiological conditions (Brauer 1963; Drapanas et al. 1966; Martins et al. 1956). The perfusion pressure values necessary for this were also within the physiological pressure range of the portal vein under our perfusion conditions. Boddie et al. (1979) perfused the liver with substantially higher pressure (150 mm Hg) and markedly lower flow rates (150−275 ml/min). In our opinion, these poor perfusion conditions are the cause of liver damage and the 25% mortality these authors reported.

The intra-operatively determined blood gases in the perfusate as well as the content of metabolites in the tissue confirm that the liver was adequately perfused under our trial conditions. In no case did we observe an "outflow block phenomenon", a sign of hypoxic liver-cell damage in the dog (Andrews et al. 1955; Chapman et al. 1960; Eiseman et al. 1961; Kestens and McDermott 1961).

By "skeletising" and clamping the supplying and discharging vessels and the bile duct it was possible to isolate the liver almost completely from the systemic circulation. The amount of leakage corresponds to that reported by other authors (Ausman 1961; Boddie et al. 1979; Mulcare et al. 1973).

The present results encourage us to clarify further questions on the perfusion of the liver under normothermic and hyperthermic conditions, using cytostatics in trials with longer observation times.

References

Andrews WHH, Hecker R, Macgrath GB, Ritchie HO (1955) The action of adrenaline, 1-noradrenaline, acetylcholine and other substances of the perfused canine liver. J Physiol 128:413−418

Ansfield FJ, Ramirez G, Skibba JL, Bryan GT, Davis HL, Wirtanen W (1971) Intrahepatic arterial infusion with 5-fluorouracil. Cancer 28:1147−1151

Ausman RK (1961) Development of a technique for isolated perfusion of the liver. NY State J Med 61:3993−3997

Boddie AW, Booker L, Mullins JD, Buckley CJ, McBride CM (1979) Hepatic hyperthermia by total isolation and regional perfusion in vivo. J Surg Res 26:447−457

Brauer RW (1963) Liver circulation and function. Physiol Rev 43:115−121

Chapman ND, Goldsworthy PD, Nyphus L, Volweiler W, Harkins H (1960) Studies in isolated organ physiology: B.S.B. clearance in bovine liver. Surgery 48:111−118

Child CG, Milness RF, Holswade GR, Gore Al (1950) Sudden and complete occlusion of the portal vein in the *Macaca mulatta* monkey. Ann Surg 132:474−479

Chung WB, Moore JR, Merseran W (1962) A technique of isolated perfusion of the liver. Surgery 51:508−511

Drapanas T, Zemel R, Vang JO (1966) Hemodynamics of isolated perfused pig liver. Ann Surg 164:522−537

Eiseman B, Knipe P, McCall H, Orloff M (1961) Isolated liver perfusion for reducing blood ammonia. Arch Surg 83:356−363

Ghussen F, Nagel K, Sturz I, Isselhard W (1982) A modified dye dilution method to estimate regional isolated perfusion of the extremity. Res Exp Med (Berl) 180:179−187

Healey JF, Smith JL, Clark RL, Stehlin JS, White EC (1961) Hepatic tissue tolerance to Thio-TEPA administered by isolation perfusion technique. J Surg Res 1:111−116

Hickman R, Saunders SJ, Terblanche J (1971) Liver function in the pig. Total hepatic and portal flow values in vivo. S Afr Med J 48: 1197–1200

Johnstone FRC (1957) Acute ligation of the portal vein. Surgery 41: 958–969

Kestens PJ, McDermott WF (1961) Perfusion and replacement of the canine liver. Surgery 50: 196–201

Martins AJ, Goldsworthy DD, Jones TW, Nyphus LM, Devito RN, Volweiler W, Harkins HN (1956) Studies of hepatic physiology in the isolated perfused calf liver. Surg Forum 7: 489–493

Misra NC, Jaiswal MSD, Singh RV (1977) Intrahepatic arterial infusion of combination of mitomycin-C and 5-fluorouracil in treatment of primary and metastatic liver carcinoma. Cancer 39: 1425–1429

Mulcare RJ, Solis A, Fortner JG (1973) Isolation and perfusion of the liver for cancer chemotherapy. J Surg Res 15: 87–95

Ramming KP, Sparks FC, Eibler FR (1976) Hepatic artery ligation and 5-fluorouracil infusion for metastatic colon carcinoma and primary hepatoma. Am J Surg 132: 236–242

Taylor J (1978) Cytotoxic perfusion for colorectal liver metastases. Br J Surg 65: 109–114

First Experimental and Clinical Results of Isolated Liver Perfusion with Cytotoxics in Metastases from Colorectal Primary

K. Aigner, H. Walther, J. Tonn, A. Wenzl, R. Hechtel, G. Merker, and K. Schwemmle

Allgemeinchirurgische Klinik des Zentrums für Chirurgie, Justus-Liebig-Universität, Klinikstrasse 29, 6300 Giessen, FRG

Up to now the most effective treatment of disseminated liver metastases of colorectal primary has been intra-arterial infusion chemotherapy. The concept of delivering large doses of cytostatics to malignant tumors via vascular isolation was introduced in the 1950s. In an isolated perfusion system, the tumor-bearing liver may be supplied with a high concentration of cytostatics during the perfusion period, while systemic side effects of the drug can be avoided by complete isolation of the perfused area.

Ausman (1961) and Healy (1961) first described techniques for isolated perfusion of the liver using an extracorporeal circuit. Ausman tried this method on 12 dogs and five patients, using nitrogen mustard. However, clinical data and therapeutic effects of the perfusion were not presented.

Method

In an attempt to develop a standardized technique for isolated perfusion of the liver, we operated on a total of 34 dogs, using various drugs such as dacarbazine, methotrexate, and 5-fluorouracil. By means of an extracorporeal pump oxygenator circuit the venous blood was oxygenated and returned to the liver via the hepatic artery and the portal vein through two separate arterial lines (Fig. 1). The portal blood was filtered in a portocaval shunt in order to lower ammonia levels.

Although metastases from colorectal cancer spread to the liver via the portal vein, they tend to acquire an exclusively arterial blood supply. Breedis and Young (1953) showed that the neoplasm is nourished almost completely by arterial blood. Thus, in isolated perfusion, both the hepatic artery and the portal vein are perfused separately with arterialized blood. The venous hepatic outflow through a special catheter which is inserted from below the renal veins is collected by gravity in the oxygenator.

The double-channel catheter consists of a vena caval shunt tube to maintain cardiac venous return and a second tube for isolated hepatic venous return (Fig. 2). The portocaval shunt tube inserts in the vena cava tube. Two additional openings collect the venous return from the kidneys, as the vena cava is cannulated from below the renal veins.

After the cannulation procedure the tubing set is connected to the heart-lung machine (Fig. 3). The hepatic artery is cannulated via the gastroduodenal artery and perfused at a maximum flow rate of 300 ml/min, the portal vein with 250 ml/min for 1 h at a temperature of 38.1° C.

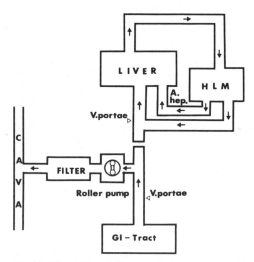

Fig. 1. The isolated liver perfusion system with a portocaval shunt. HLM, heart-lung machine

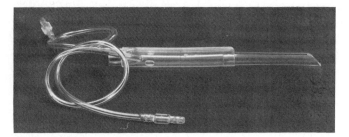

Fig. 2. Double-channel catheter for cannulation of the vena cava

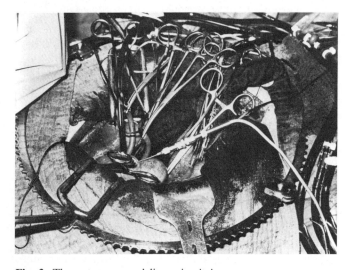

Fig. 3. The extracorporeal liver circuit in man

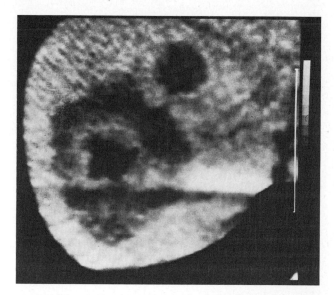

Fig. 4. The so-called target phenomenon of a liver metastasis in computed tomography 2 weeks after isolated liver perfusion

In November, 1981 we performed two isolated liver perfusions in patients suffering from multiple liver metastases from colorectal cancer. The doses administered to the two patients were 300 and 450 mg 5-fluorouracil respectively. The primary tumors had been resected 5 weeks in one and 11 months in the other prior to the perfusion treatment.

Results

Both patients recovered from the operation without complications. Postoperative sonographic measurements showed areas of colliquation in the tumors. In the CAT scan the so-called target phenomenon was observed, showing central necrosis of metastases (Fig. 4).

These findings were confirmed in second-look operations in both patients, 2 and 4 months respectively after the first operation. In both cases several metastases had disappeared and in the second case, especially, the remaining tumors showed extended necrotic areas. One patient unfortunately suffers from local tumor recurrence in the anastomosis of the rectum.

By means of pulse cytophotometry we have demonstrated that there is no tumor growth at the present time. An impressive lowering of the 2-C peak has been noted. Tumor growth was obviously stopped in the premitotic phase.

Discussion

The presence of hepatic metastases of colorectal primary has been an indication for treatment by hepatic artery infusion, which is superior to systemic chemotherapy (Oberfield et al. 1979; Pettavel and Morgenthaler 1976). Beginning in 1957, several attempts have been made to completely isolate and perfuse the liver in situ (Ausman 1961; Aust and Ausman 1960; Healy et al. 1961; Ryan et al. 1958). The cases we have presented here show that complete isolation of the liver can be obtained without complications, provided the correct technique is used (Aigner et al. to be published, Aigner et al. 1982). This may be a useful addition to the treatment of neoplasms of the liver, as high concentrations of cytotoxins can be administered to the tumor-bearing tissue. Our two patients who underwent isolated liver perfusion were classified Lausanne stages II and III (Pettavel and Morgenthaler 1976) with a spontaneous survival time of 1.4–4.7 months. Considering the 6 months' follow-up period and all clinical findings, we conclude that isolated liver perfusion does prolong survival rates without systemic side effects to the patient.

Summary

In two patients suffering from numerous liver metastases in both lobes from colorectal primary isolated liverperfusion with 5-fluorouracil was performed. By means of a special cannulation system the hepatic artery and the portal vein were arterialized. The patients recovered rapidly after the operation. Sonographic measurements, CAT scans, pulse cytophotometry, and second-look operations with histological examinations of metastatic tissue verified extensive tumor regression. No complications occured within 6 months after the perfusion treatment.

References

Aigner K, Tonn JC, Krahl M, Walther H, Wizemann V, Breithaupt H, Merker G, Schwemmle K (to be published) Die portocavale Hämofiltration bei der isolierten Leberperfusion. Langenbecks Arch Chir

Aigner K, Walther H, Tonn J-C, Krahl M, Wenzl A, Merker G, Schwemmle K (1982) Die isolierte Leberperfusion mit 5-Fluorouracil (5-FU) beim Menschen. Chirurg 53: 571

Ausman RK (1961) Development of a technique for isolated perfusion of the liver. NY State J Med 61: 3993

Aust JB, Ausman RK (1960) The technique of liver perfusion. Cancer Chemother Rep 10: 23

Breedis C, Young G (1953) The blood supply of neoplasms in the liver. Am J Pathol 30: 969

Healy JE, Smith JL, Clar RL, Stehlin JS, White EC (1961) Hepatic tissue tolerance to thio-TEPA administered by the isolation-perfusion technique. J Surg Res 1: 111

Oberfield RA, McCaffrey JA, Polio J, Clouse ME, Hamilton T (1979) Prolonged and continuous percutaneous intra-arterial hepatic infusion chemotherapy in advanced metastatic liver adeno-carcinoma from colorectal primary. Cancer 44: 414

Pettavel J, Morgenthaler FR (1976) Dix ans d'experience de chimiothérapi artérielle des tumeurs primaires et secondaires du foie. Ann Gastroenterol Hepatol 12: 349

Ryan RF, Krementz ET, Creech O, Winblad N, Chamblee W, Check H (1958) Selected perfusion of isolated viscera with chemotherapeutic agents. Surg Forum 8: 158

Ultrastructural Changes in the Dog Liver Cell After Isolated Liver Perfusion with Various Cytotoxins*

G. Merker[1], H.-J. Helling[1], M. Krahl[1], and K. Aigner[2]**

1 Abteilung für Physiologie, Klinik für Chirurgie, Justus-Liebig-Universität,
  Aulweg 129, 6300 Giessen, FRG
2 Allgemeinchirurgische Klinik im Zentrum für Chirurgie, Justus-Liebig-Universität,
  Klinikstrasse 29, 6300 Giessen, FRG

Before isolated liver perfusion could be done in patients suffering from tumors, detailed information on the reaction of the intact liver tissue to different cytotoxins had to be obtained in experimental animals, using the perfusion method elsewhere elaborated (Aigner et al. to be published).

The special conditions of local blood circulation in the liver are of advantage for a direct cellular action of drugs administered by portal perfusion. The sinusoids form an uninterrupted three-dimensional network among the liver cells. The lumen of the sinusoids is enclosed by endothelial cells or Kupffer cells and these are surrounded by the perisinusoidal space of Disse. The endothelial cells are therefore not in contact with a basement membrane. The structure of the sinusoidal border in the liver provides evidence that substances transported in the sinusoidal fluid − physiological constituents as well as drugs − directly contact the liver parenchymal cells. Entrance into the liver cells is assumed to involve the microvilli, as well as the formation of pinocytotic vesicles.

Materials and Methods

Structural injuries induced by cytotoxins were examined in the parenchymal liver cells of 19 mongrel dogs (1−4 years old, body weight 25−40 kg) with the electron microscope following isolated liver perfusion for 30−40 min with 5-fluorouracil (5-FU; $n = 5$, 100−1,000 mg/kg liver weight), dacarbazine DTIC; $n = 6$, 50−150 mg/kg liver weight), methotrexate (MTX; $n = 5$, 100−1,000 mg/kg liver weight) or cis-platinum (cis-PT; $n = 3$, 3−20 mg/kg liver weight). For the controls ($n = 5$), perfusion was performed for 20−80 min without cytotoxic agents added to the perfusion fluid.

For the electron-microscopic examination small pieces of liver tissue were excised (a) before the onset of perfusion, both pre- and postoperatively, (b) directly after perfusion, and (c) following perfusion with 5-FU and DTIC only, after a survival time of 4 weeks.

*   A portion of this work was performed by H.-J. Helling (5-FU, MTX, dacarbazine) and by M. Krahl (cis-PT) in partial fulfilment of the degree of Dr. med., Justus Liebig-University, Giessen
** The authors are greatly indebted to Dr. Syed Ali, Department of Anatomy and Cytobiology, Justus Liebig-University, Giessen, for valuable technical advice and for stimulating discussions. The efficient technical contributions of Mrs. I. Stei are also gratefully acknowledged

Tissue samples were fixed by immersion in 5% phosphate-buffered glutaraldehyde; postfixation was in 1% osmium tetroxide. The material was dehydrated in alcohol, then in propylenoxide and embedded in Durcupan (Fluka). Ultrathin sections were stained with uranyl acetate and lead citrate. The electron-microscopic examinations were performed at the Department of Anatomy and Cytobiology, University of Giessen, using a Phillips 201 electron microscope.

Results

No significant structural changes occurred in the controls except for a reduction of the cellular glycogen content after perfusion times longer than 30 min. In the normal liver cell glycogen usually occurs in the form of α-particles or "rosettes". Mitochondrial granules are scattered in the electron-dense mitochondrial matrix between the cristae (Fig. 1). Only occasionally are mitochondria observed in close proximity to the areas of granular endoplasmic reticulum. Cellular reactions can be observed immediately after perfusion

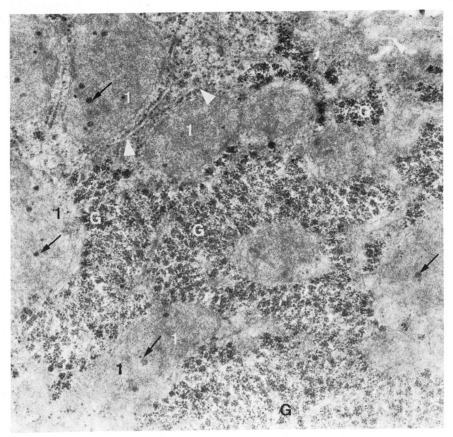

Fig. 1. Liver cell of a dog (control) after perfusion without cytotoxins (20 min). Glycogen occurs in the form of α-particles (*G*). Mitochondrial granules (*arrows*) are scattered through the mitochondrial matrix. The granular endoplasmic reticulum (*arrowheads*) is not especially prominent. *1*, mitochondria; Durcupan, × 19,500

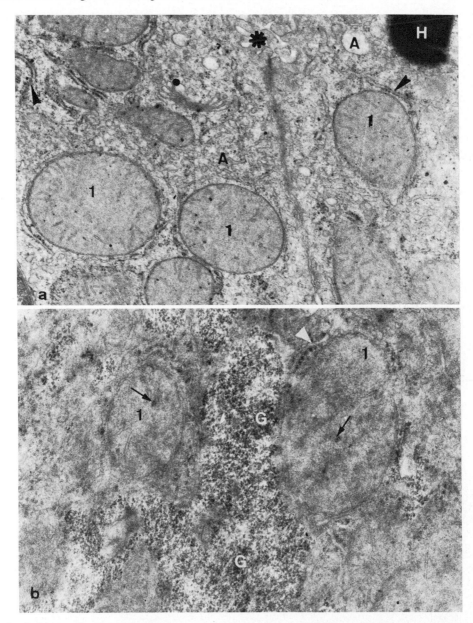

Fig. 2a, b. Liver cells of a dog. **a** Acute reaction after perfusion with 500 mg 5-FU/kg liver weight; note the cellular vacuolization in (a) due to hypertrophy of the agranular reticulum (*A*). From the slightly swollen mitochondria (*1*) mitochondrial granules have disappeared. **b** Recovery of the cellular structures 4 weeks after the perfusion; the vacuolization is regressive, and glycogen stores (*G*) are refilled, mostly containing β-particles. Mitochondrial granules have reappeared (*arrows*). *Arrowheads*, rough endoplasmic reticulum; *dot*, Golgi complex; *asterisk*, bile canaliculus; *H*, hemosiderin inclusion; Durcupan, **a** and **b** × 60,600

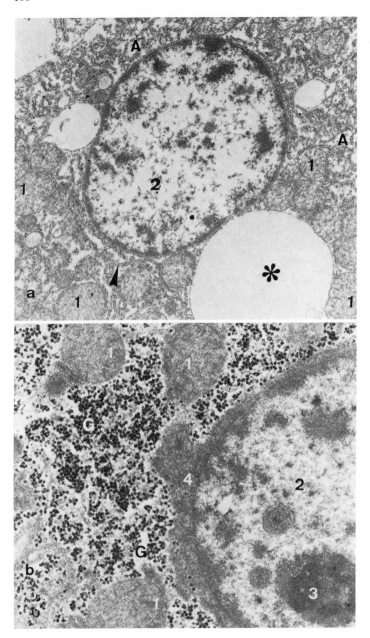

Fig. 3a, b. Liver cells of dogs showing acute effects of perfusion with 400 mg. MTX/kg liver weight (**a**) and of perfusion with 10 mg *cis*-PT/kg liver weight (**b**). General cellular vacuolization (*A*) characterizes the acute reaction to MTX. Huge vacuoles occur frequently in the cellular matrix (*asterix*). Mitochondrial structures are severely damaged (*1*). *cis*-Pt induces acute accumulation of glycogen (*G*), mitochondrial swelling, and condensation of electron-dense material in the mitochondrial matrix (*1*) and also in the circumnuclear area (*4*). *2*, nucleus; *3*, nucleolus; Durcupan, **a** × 8,800, **b** × 13,200

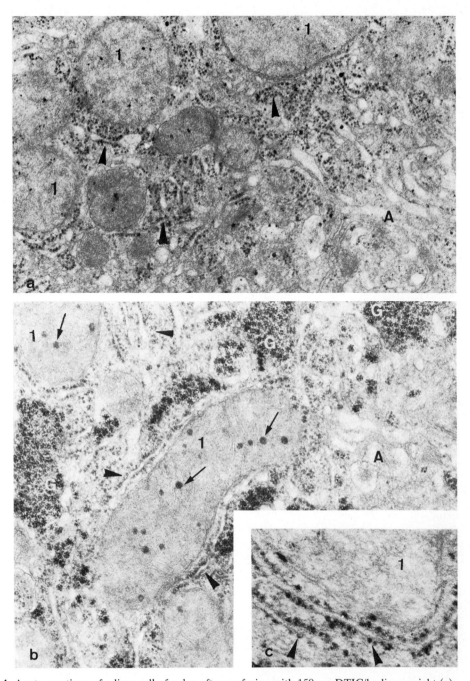

Fig. 4. Acute reactions of a liver cell of a dog after perfusion with 150 mg DTIC/kg liver weight (**a**), and recovery of cellular structures 4 weeks after perfusion (**b, c**). Acute loss of glycogen can be seen in **a,** accompanied by disintegration of the rough endoplasmic reticulum. Remainders of the granular endoplasmic reticulum bear prominent ribosomes (*arrowheads*). The swollen mitochondria (*1*) contain no granules. After a survival time of 4 weeks (**b**) rapid regeneration of the glycogen stores containing α-particles and of the components of the granular endoplasmic reticulum (**b, c,** *arrowheads*) is observed. Cisternal profiles of the granular endoplasmic reticulum in close relationship to mitochondria (**b, c,** *1*) occur frequently. Mitochondrial granules (*arrows*) are remarkably prominent in (**b**). *A,* agranular endoplasmic reticulum; Durcupan, **a** × 19,500, **b** × 60,600, **c** × 88,000

with cytotoxic agents, especially in liver cells bordering the sinusoids. Sublethal injuries increase with rising concentrations of the cytotoxins, the cellular reactions induced by the antimetabolic compounds 5-FU and MTX being quite similar. Administration of 500 mg 5-FU/kg liver weight is survived without complications, while 250 mg MTX/kg liver weight is just tolerated.

The acute cellular injuries resulting from liver perfusion with 500 mg 5-FU/kg liver weight consist in depletion of glycogen, disintegration of the rough endoplasmic reticulum, the remainders of which are scattered throughout the cytoplasm, and general vacuolization due to swelling of the agranular endoplasmic reticulum. Although their internal structures appear intact, mitochondria are moderately swollen (Fig. 2a).

Four weeks after perfusion with 500 mg 5-FU all liver cells examined reveal distinct signs of recovery, with the structures of the granular endoplasmic reticulum mostly restored. Glycogen stores reappear and contain mostly individual β-particles, rosette-like structures being rare. In the cellular matrix a moderate vacuolization is still observed. In the Kupffer cells as well as in the parenchymal liver cells hemosiderin inclusions occur frequently (Fig. 2b).

Although its general effect is similar to that of 5-FU, treatment with MTX induces acute mitochondrial deformation, generalized vacuolization, and a greater degree of lipid accumulation (Fig. 3a).

With respect to the cytotoxic agents cis-PT and DTIC, cis-PT induces acute mitochondrial swelling, progressive disintegration of the granular endoplasmic reticulum, and a circumnuclear condensation of electron-dense material. Instead of the general depletion of the glycogen stores and cellular vacuolization observed after administration of the two antimetabolic compounds examined, cis-PT treatment results in an obvious, acute accumulation of cellular glycogen (Fig. 3b). The examination of the action of this drug is not yet completed. The acute effects of perfusion with 150 mg DTIC/kg liver weight, a concentration which is survived, consist in a general loss of glycogen, mitochondrial swelling, accumulation of lipid droplets, and partial to total disintegration of the granular endoplasmic reticulum. Remainders of apparently intact cisternal profiles of the granular endoplasmic reticulum bearing prominent ribosomes frequently wrap around mitochondria (Fig. 4a).

Four weeks after liver perfusion with 150 mg DTIC, Kupffer cells containing hemosiderin inclusions occur frequently in markedly increased numbers. Occasionally, focal centri-lobular necrosis is observed. Most parenchymal cells, however, show signs of rapid recovery. The glycogen deposits are restored, consisting mostly of α-particles. Nuclear structures and components of the granular endoplasmic reticulum are particularly prominent, with the cisternal system containing electron-dense material and free ribosomes (Fig. 4b, c).

Discussion

Former examinations of drug action in the liver cell (Rees 1964; for review see Hargreaves 1968) have shown primary effects to concern the endoplasmic reticulum. As the site of amino-acid incorporation into protein the granular endoplasmic reticulum is of obvious importance. The disorganization of the granular endoplasmic reticulum accompanied by hypertrophy of the smooth membranes observed after liver perfusion with different cytotoxins appears to be a generalized pathophysiological response of the liver cell to toxic agents (Figs. 2—4; Mikata and Luse 1964). Extensive mitochondrial damage (Fig. 3a) seems to be secondary to other intracellular changes in liver cell injury.

In the parenchymal liver cell the agranular endoplasmic reticulum seems to be concerned with detoxification mechanisms (Fawcett 1966), a substantial increase in drug-metabolizing enzymes being correlated with an increase in smooth-surfaced membranes.

Prominent ribosomes and structures of the rough endoplasmic reticulum observed in close proximity to mitochondria 4 weeks after liver perfusion with DTIC probably indicate increased protein synthesis, a finding which presents an intriguing problem. According to clinical experience in perfusion of extremities using DTIC for therapy of melanomas and sarcomas, early tumor regression was followed by rapid tumor recurrence. The possible signs of cellular hyperactivity observed 4 weeks after liver perfusion with DTIC require attention and further elucidation.

Comparing the effects of the cytotoxic agents examined, 5-FU exhibited the best balanced action on the parenchymal liver cell. Therefore, 5-FU was the cytotoxin of choice for the first isolated liver perfusions in patients.

Summary

Following isolated liver perfusion with different cytotoxins — 5-fluorouracil (5-FU), methotrexate (MTX), dacarbazine (DTIC) *cis*-platinum (*cis*-PT) — liver tissue of dogs was examined with the electron microscope (a) directly after the perfusion and (b) after a survival time of 4 weeks (5-FU and DTIC). Acute disintegration of the granular endoplasmic reticulum and depletion of the glycogen stores occurred after perfusion with 5-FU, MTX, and DTIC, while *cis*-PT induced disintegration of the granular endoplasmic reticulum accompanied by an accumulation of glycogen. Four weeks after perfusion with DTIC signs of remarkably increased cellular activity were observed, while 4 weeks after perfusion with 5-FU the parenchymal liver cells revealed a well-balanced and moderate recovery of the cellular structures.

References

Aigner K, Tonn JC, Krahl M, Walther H, Wizemann V, Breithaupt H, Merker G, Schwemmle K (to be published) Die portocavale Hämofiltration bei der isolierten Leberperfusion. Langenbecks Arch Chir

Fawcett DW (1966) An atlas of fine structure. The cell. Saunders, Philadelphia

Hargreaves T (1968) The liver and bile metabolism. North-Holland, Amsterdam

Mikata A, Luse SA (1964) Ultrastructural changes in the rat liver produced by N-2-fluorenyldia-cetamide. Am J Path 44: 455—480

Rees KR (1964) Mechanism of action of certain exogenous toxic agents in liver cells. In: de Rueck AVS, Knight J (eds) Cellular injury. Churchill, London, pp 53—66

Anesthesia for Isolated Liver Perfusion in Man

J. Biscoping, F. Mikus, and G. Hempelmann

Abteilung für Anästhesiologie, Justus-Liebig-Universität, Klinikstrasse 29, 6300 Giessen, FRG

Anesthesia for isolated liver perfusion in man must take into account that the surgeon intends to exclude the liver for a certain time from systemic circulation, thus compromising filtration and deactivation of potentially toxic products. Venous return will be blocked temporarily, and after reinstallation of normal circulation remaining doses of highly cytostatic drugs will enter the systemic circulation, thus influencing cardiac performance in a negative inotropic way.

To a certain extent the hemodynamic situation (venous return is inhibited) in this surgical procedure is similar to the anhepatic phase during liver transplantation (Schaps et al. 1978). To date, our anesthesiological know-how is based on experimental (Ausman and Aust 1960; Healy 1960) and clinical experiences in liver transplantation, and on the experimental results of our group in isolated liver perfusion (Aigner et al. 1980, 1983; Kluge et al. 1981a, b; Reinacher et al. 1981). Thus far, this procedure has been performed in only three patients.

Preoperative Procedures

In our opinion, anesthesia in isolated liver perfusion should be performed according to anesthesiological procedures in liver transplantation or in those operations for severe liver insufficiency.

Preoperative screening and premedication is performed as for any other patient presenting for major surgical intervention; special emphasis, however, should be put upon liver function tests and clotting parameters. For premedication, any analgesic and sedative in addition to atropine is sufficient; intravenous induction of a hypnotic such as etomidate, and a high dose of fentanyl anesthesia in connection with benzodiazepines, such as diazepam (5–10 mg) or flunitrazepam (1–2 mg), and the muscle relaxant pancuronium bromide is preferred. Controlled ventilation with oxygen and nitrous oxide (1:1) and application of a positive endexpiratory pressure of 5–10 cm H_2O should be mandatory, intermittently checked by blood gas analysis.

The anesthesiological apparatus should include four large i.v. lines, a central venous catheter, a pulmonary artery catheter (if possible a thermodilution catheter), an arterial cannula for the radial artery, a gastric tube, a urinary catheter, rectal and esophageal temperature sensors, an ECG, a warming device for the patient (e.g., a water mattress), and blood units.

Recent Results in Cancer Research, Vol. 86
© Springer-Verlag Berlin · Heidelberg 1983

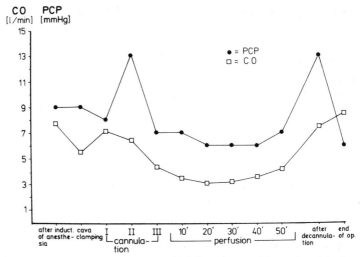

Fig. 1. Cardiac output (*CO*) and pulmonary capillary pressure (*PCP*) as measured for patient 1 during isolated liver perfusion procedure. *I*, insertion of caudal tourniguet; *II*, cannulation of portal vein; *II*, cannulation of hepatic artery

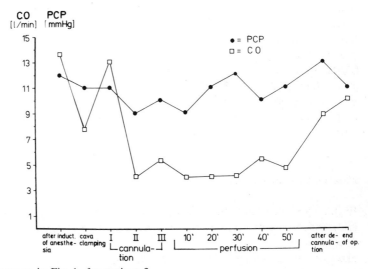

Fig. 2. Same measurements as in Fig. 1, for patient 2

The heart rate, and ECG (V_5), systemic arterial pressure, right atrial pressure, and pulmonary arterial pressure are monitored continuously, whereas cardiac output and pulmonary capillary pressure (see Figs. 1 and 2), as well as the following laboratory data, are monitored intermittently: blood gas parameters, serum electrolytes, blood sugar, hematocrit and hemoglobin, metabolism, respiration, body temperature, and urine output.

Hemodynamic Problems

Because of the surgical procedure, the lower caval vein has to be blocked for a rather short period — approximately 5 min — while a special perfusion catheter is installed. Induced

Table 1. Fluid replacement

	Patient 1	Patient 2
Crystalloids	2,000 ml	2,250 ml
Colloids	600 ml	1,650 ml
Packed red cells	4,000 ml	4,000 ml
Fresh-frozen plasma	500 ml	500 ml
Total	6,100 ml	8,400 ml
	≙ 124 ml/kg body wt.	≙ 92 ml/kg body wt.

hypervolemia should precede this measure in order to guarantee sufficient venous return via collateral veins. Especially during this period, volume and/or catecholamine therapy can be guided most effectively by left ventricular filling pressure, indicated by the pulmonary capillary wedge pressure. Right ventricular filling pressure (central venous pressure) is a poor guide for the adjustment of therapeutic measures during this period; systolic pressure, heart rate, cardiac output, and pulmonary capillary wedge pressure are the most appropriate tools in this situation.

After installation of the separate liver perfusion catheter, reported already in detail by Dr. Aigner (this volume), venous return is still compromised to a significant extent, resulting in a constant decrease in cardiac output, especially when surplus-volume substitution is not sufficient, In all three of our patients, low-dose catecholamine therapy was necessary during this period to improve both hemodynamics and urinary output, which almost ceased in all patients during the second part of the selective liver perfusion. After decannulation, however, urination resumed in all three patients.

Disregarding isovolumetric fluid replacement within the separate liver perfusion circuit, volume replacement and fluid therapy (Table 1) in all patients far exceeded blood loss and urinary output. Totals of 7.1, 8.4, and 8.7 liters respectively were necessary in our three patients, half of the volume being blood, the other half consisting of electrolyte solutions, plasma expanders, and albumin solutions.

Metabolic Changes

There was a tendency to metabolic acidosis in all patients (Fig. 3); although in our normoventilated patients moderate acidosis around pH values of 7.3 is usual because of a better stability of the cytostatic substances (Chang et al. 1979; Ghussen et al. 1981), 400−500 mEq sodium bicarbonate was necessary for these three. This implies that there is a need to control blood gas parameters and acid-base parameters in arterial blood samples and mixed venous blood samples, as well as in the liver perfusion circuit, intermittently, especially during the period of isolated liver perfusion.

Some authours have reported a decrease in blood sugar during the anhepatic phase of liver transplantation; this is not in accordance with our own results in orthotopic liver transplantation (Schaps et al. 1978). In isolated liver perfusion, too, there was no decrease in blood sugar (Fig. 3), therefore there was no need for glucose infusions. On the contrary, increases slightly above 300 mg% were treated by increments of insulin.

The metabolic derangement may be influenced to a significant extent by body temperature (Fig. 4). In all patients there was a severe drop in temperature to 33° C, although infusions

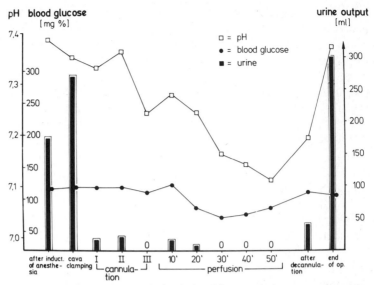

Fig. 3. Arterial pH, blood glucose, and urine output during isolated liver perfusion, as measured for patient 2. *I, II,* and *III,* as for Fig. 1

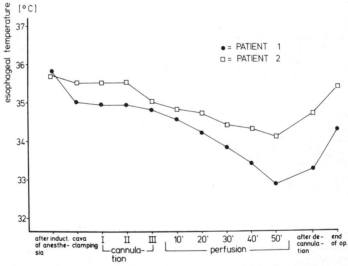

Fig. 4. Esophageal temperature, measured for patients 1 and 2, during isolated liver perfusion procedure. *I, II,* and *III,* as for Fig. 1

and blood units were warmed up prior to administration and water mattresses were used to keep the patient's body temperature near normal. Before being delivered to the intensive care ward, all patients were warmed by additional water mattresses and other heating devices immediately after the end of the surgical procedure. No high-risk patient should be transported from the operating room to any intensive care ward as long as he or she is hypothermic.

In our opinion, the most dangerous period seems to be when the liver is reconnected to the patient's systemic circulation. At this moment 1−1.5 l of blood volume may be necessary to adequately refill the liver. On the other hand, despite the fact that the cytostatics are washed out of the liver circulation, a small amount of these negative inotropic drugs do enter the systemic circulation and influence the hemodynamics. In addition, the temperature loss within the isolated liver circuit and thus the liver itself seems to be more severe; therefore, after reconnection of the liver to the systemic circulation an acute temperature loss might influence hemodynamics as well. Catecholamines and rapid volume therapy are important at this point!

Blood Coagulation

Although the patients have to be heparinized before cannulation (200 U/kg body wt., repeated 1 h later at 50% of the initial dose) for this sophisticated surgical precedure, and mass transfusions must be performed, clotting parameters were not significantly changed after protamine hydrochloride had been given in a ratio of 1 : 1. Warm blood or fresh blood units were not necessary for our patients; one unit of fresh-frozen plasma, however, was infused after every third blood unit.

All patients were ventilated postoperatively for several hours until most of the anesthetics and muscle relaxants had been metabolized and/or excreted. Antagonization of opioids and muscle relaxants does not seem to be appropriate as therapy for such patients, because rebound phenomena in case of liver insufficiency could be dangerous. On the other hand, induced hypervolemia during the surgical procedure and membrane derangement because of the cytostatics may cause an interstitial edema. Fluid input is therefore restricted during the immediate postoperative period and extubation is performed according to generally accepted respiratory parameters.

Anesthesiological management in patients undergoing selective liver perfusion is comparable to problems in orthotopic liver transplantation − the anhepatic period, however, is much shorter. From the hemodynamic point of view, more severe changes might be due to the cytostatic drugs, which do influence myocardial inotropy. Changes in metabolic and coagulatory parameters are of lesser importance, especially during the postoperative period, because liver function is influenced only to a small extent. According to our experience, intensive care treatment for 1 or 2 days after the operation is of benefit to the patient.

References

Aigner K, Hild P, Henneking K, Paul E, Hundeiker M, Breithaupt H, Merker G, Jungbluth A (1980) DTIC − studies in isolated perfusion of the leg and the liver in dogs. Speech at the EORTC Melanoma Symposium, April 24−25, 1980, Lausanne

Aigner K, Hild P, Hundeiker M (1983) Neue Entwicklungen in der isolierten Extremitätenperfusion. Z Hautkr (in press)

Ausman RK, Aust JB (1960) Isolated perfusion of the liver with NH_2. Surg Forum 10: 77

Chang SY, Evans TL, Alberts DS (1979) The stability of melphalan in the presence of chloride ion. J Pharm Pharmacol 31: 853

Ghussen F, Nagel F, Groth W (1981) Regionale hypertherme Zytostatikaperfusion bei malignen Melanomen der Extremitäten. Dtsch Med Wochenschr 106: 1612

Healy JE (1960) The technique of liver perfusion. Cancer Chemother Rep 10:24

Kluge E, Reinacher S, Aigner K, Rieder W, Hempelmann G (1981a) Hemodynamic changes during hyperthermic perfusion (upper/lower extremity) in patients with melanomaa. Speech at the EORTC Melanoma Symposium, April 24–25, 1981, Hamburg

Kluge E, Reinacher S, Rieder W, Aigner K, Hild P, Hempelmann G (1981b) Verhalten von Hämodynamik und Stoffwechselgrößen bei der hyperthermen Zytostatikaperfusion der unteren Extremität unter Neuroleptanalgesie (NLA) und Kombinationsnarkose (NLA+PDA). Vortrag ZAK, Sept. 15–18, 1981, Berlin

Reinacher S, Kluge E, Aigner K, Hild P, Hempelmann G (1981) Metabolic changes during hyperthermic perfusion (upper/ lower extremity) in patients with melanoma. Speech at the EORTC Melanoma Symposium April 24–25, 1981, Hamburg

Schaps D, Hempelmann G, Pichlmayr R (1978) Zur orthotopen Lebertransplantation aus anaesthesiologischer Sicht. Anaesthesist 27:405

Kinetics of Methotrexate, Dacarbazine and 5-Fluorouracil During Isolated Liver Perfusion

H. Breithaupt[1], K. Aigner[2], and R. Hechtel[2]

1 Medizinische Klinik, Justus-Liebig-Universität, Klinikstrasse 36, 6300 Giessen, FRG
2 Allgemeinchirurgische Klinik des Zentrums für Chirurgie, Justus-Liebig-Universität, Klinikstrasse 29, 6300 Giessen, FRG

Methotrexate (MTX) is an antineoplastic agent which competitively inhibits dihydrofolate reductase, thus inducing a deficiency of tetrahydrofolate (folinic acid, Leucovorin), an important coenzyme in the biosynthesis of amino acids and the purine and pyrimidine units of DNA. Following intravenous administration, MTX disappears rapidly from plasma with a half-life ($t_{1/2}$) of about 2 h, mainly by renal elimination. After high doses of MTX (> 1 g/m^2) a variable portion of MTX undergoes metabolic transformation to 7-hydroxy-MTX, a potentially nephrotoxic compound. MTX, 7-hydroxy-MTX and 2,4-diamino-N^{10}-methylpteroic acid (APA), an enteric metabolite of MTX, can be precisely determined in biological fluids within 8 min by means of a high-pressure liquid chromatographic (HPLC) method.

During continuous 6-h infusions of high-dose MTX, peak plasma levels of MTX were obtained at 10^{-3} M. The metabolite 7-hydroxy-MTX was detectable in plasma 30−60 min after infusions were started, and reached a maximum of 5×10^{-4} M 3 h after infusions were stopped.

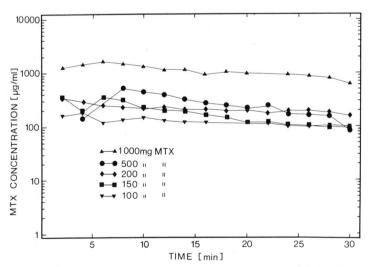

Fig. 1. Concentration of MTX in the perfusate during isolated dog liver perfusion, following bolus administration of 100−1,000 mg MTX into the extracorporeal circuit

Isolated dog liver perfusion experiments were performed, with 100–1,000 mg MTX injected into the extracorporeal circulation. Under these conditions MTX concentrations in the perfusate peaked at 160–1,600 µg/ml (3.5×10^{-4}–3.5×10^{-3} M; Fig. 1). The metabolite 7-hydroxy-MTX was not detectable in the perfusate as well as MTX and 7-hydroxy-MTX in plasma samples obtained from systemic circulation. The limit of sensitivity of the HPLC assay used was about 20 ng/ml (4×10^{-8} M).

Methotrexate disappearance from the perfusate was monoexponential with $t_{1/2}$ values ranging from 10 to 39 min (Table 1). The volume of distribution was about 600 ml, and the clearance values were at 18 ml/min.

When, however, a bolus of the cytotoxic agent dacarbazine (DTIC) was injected into the extracorporeal circuit, rapid formation of its metabolic derivative 5-aminoimidazole-4-carboxamide (AIC) was observed. DTIC, a useful cytostatic agent in the treatment of malignant melanoma, soft tissue sarcoma, and Hodgkin's disease, undergoes microsomal N-demethylation in the liver, giving rise to AIC and a methyl carbonium ion, an agent presumably alkylating DNA.

Table 1. Kinetic data from isolated dog liver perfusion with MTX

Dose of MTX (mg)	C_{max} (µg/ml)	V_D (ml)	$T_{1/2}$ (min)	Clearance (ml/min)
100	162	608	39	11
150	311	576	13	19
200	342	666	34	14
500	832	546	10	36
1,000	1,642	601	25	11
Mean		599	24	18
S.E.		44	13	10

Fig. 2. HPLC determination of DTIC and AIC in plasma. Amounts chromatographed were 5 µg DTIC, AIC, and 2-azahypoxanthine (AHX) per milliliter plasma. Stationary phase: Spherisor ODS, 5 µm as reverse-phase material packed in stainless-steel columns 7 cm long and with 0.4 cm internal diameter (ID) for DTIC, 30 cm long with 0.4 cm ID each for AIC and AHX. Mobile phase: tetrabutyl-ammonium phosphate 0.005 M (PIC A, Waters) for DTIC, and 1-heptane sulfonic acid 0.005 M (PIC B7, Waters) for both AIC and AHX. Sample volume, 20 µl; flow rate, 2 ml/min; back pressure, 800 psi for DTIC and < 500 psi for AIC; room temperature; detection at 326 nm for DTIC and 270 nm for AIC; 0.02 AUFS

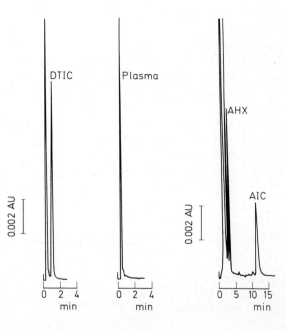

The pharmacokinetics of DTIC and AIC have been studied using a rapid, sensitive HPLC method developed in our laboratory (Fig. 2).

Following intravenous bolus injection of DTIC into the systemic circulation, disappearance from plasma was biphasic for DTIC with a terminal $t_{1/2}$ of 30—52 min, whereas plasma decay of AIC was monoexponential, with a $t_{1/2}$ of 43—116 min.

During isolated liver perfusion with DTIC (50—250 mg) maximal plasma levels of DTIC ranged from 40 to 300 μg/ml, decreasing monoexponentially with $t_{1/2}$ values of 30—150 min, similar to $t_{1/2}$ values observed following systemic administration (Fig. 3). AIC was demonstrable in the perfusate immediately after liver perfusion with DTIC had been started. The AIC levels increased continuously, reaching 30 μg/ml at the end of the perfusion experiments. Altogether, about 30% of DTIC that had left extracorporeal circulation reappeared as AIC. The photodegradation product 2-azahypoxanthine was not detected in the samples analyzed.

The overall kinetic data from isolated liver perfusion experiments with DTIC in six dogs are depicted in Table 2. The clearance values for DTIC (18.4 ± 10.2 ml/min; x̄ ± SD) compare favorably with clearance values reported for systemic application. The rate of formation of AIC was 18.5 ± 6.6 min, and its entrance into the extracorporeal circuit was 56.6 ± 27.5 ml/min.

The kinetics of 5-fluorouracil (5-FU) during isolated liver perfusion was analyzed in four dogs and two patients. The pyrimidine analogue 5-FU is by itself inactive and requires metabolic activation to the nucleotide 5-fluoro-2'-dioxyuridine-5'-monophosphate (5-FdUMP), which inhibits DNA synthesis by a blockade of thymidylate synthetase activity. Intravenous bolus injection of 5-FU in man produces 5-FU plasma concentrations of 10—100 μg/ml, which decrease rapidly with a $t_{1/2}$ of 10—20 min. Following bolus administration of 100—700 mg 5-FU in isolated dog liver experiments, maximal concentrations of 5-FU in the perfusate were at 60—400 μg/ml (Fig. 4). Disappearance from the extracorporeal circuit was monophasic with $t_{1/2}$ values of 12—164 min. The

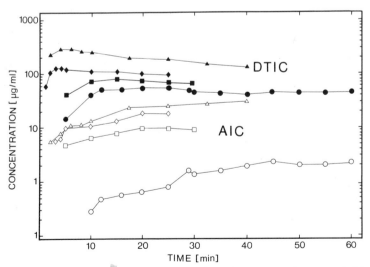

Fig. 3. Concentration of DTIC (*closed symbols*) and AIC (*open symbols*) during isolated dog liver perfusion following bolus administration of 50 (●, ○), 100 (■, □), 150 (♦, ◇), and 250 (▲, △) mg DTIC into the extracorporeal circuit

metabolite 5-FdUMP was not detected in the perfusate at concentrations above 0.2 µg/ml.

Similar plasma levels and disappearance rates were observed in two patients who received 300 and 400 mg 5-FU respectively during isolated liver perfusion for treatment of liver metastases (Fig. 5). In plasma samples collected from the systemic circulation 5-FU and 5-FdUMP were not detectable at concentrations above 0.2 µg/ml.

The kinetic data of 5-FU demonstrate values similar to those reported for systemic bolus injections of 5-FU (Table 3).

Table 2. Kinetic data from isolated dog liver perfusion with DTIC

Dose of DTIC (mg)	DTIC			AIC		
	C_{max} (µg/ml)	$T_{1/2}$ (min)	Clearance (ml/min)	C_{max} (µg/ml)	Rate of formation (min)	Entrance (ml/min)
50	38.3	29.8	30.3	5.2	11.4	79.4
100	55.1	147	8.5	5.2	18.1	69.1
100	53.2	43.1	30.5	7.4	15.2	86.9
150	132	44.3	17.2	18.4	13.4	56.7
150	151	102	6.8	9.7	25.5	27.2
250	295	32.2	17.2	31.0	27.5	20.2
Mean		66.4	18.4		18.5	56.6
S.E.		47.5	10.2		6.6	27.5

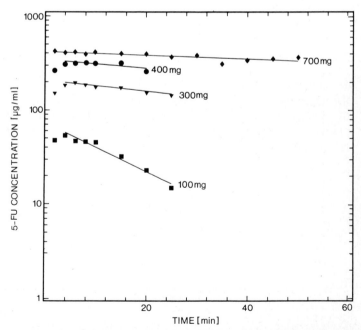

Fig. 4. Concentration of 5-FU during isolated dog liver perfusion following bolus administration of 100–700 mg 5-FU into the extracorporeal circuit

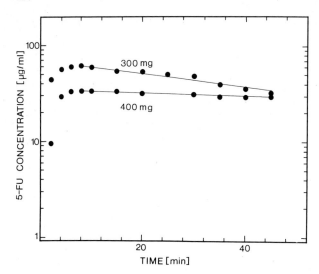

Fig. 5. Concentration of 5-FU during isolated liver perfusion in two patients for treatment of colorectal liver metastases. A bolus of 300 or 400 mg 5-FU respectively was administered into the extracorporeal circuit

Table 3. Kinetic data from isolated liver perfusion with 5-FU

	Dose of 5-FU (mg)	C_{max} (µg/min)	V_D (ml)	$T_{1/2}$ (min)	Clearance (µg/min)
Dog	100	59	1,370	12	82
	300	197	1,460	52	19
	400	313	1,210	74	11
	700	423	1,670	164	7
Man	300	61	4,170	42	69
	400	34	11,670	258	31

In summary, the kinetics of MTX, DTIC, and 5-FU in isolated liver perfusion revealed plasma levels 10–100 times higher than those in conventional therapy. The drugs disappeared from the perfusate monoexponentially, usually with $t_{1/2}$ values of 20–60 min and with clearances ranging from 10 to 30 ml/min. The formation of a metabolite was demonstrated for DTIC only.

Discussion

Neither infusion chemotherapy nor any other chemotherapy is as effective in previously irradiated tumors, because the blood flow does not reach them as well.

In pelvic tumors, epidural opiate as well as intra-arterial nitrogen mustard can be used for pain treatment.

Inner ligation of the artery and additional intra-arterial cytostatic treatment was discussed as being an adjuvant step in cancer treatment.

The pain-relieving effect of nitrogen mustard is presumed to be due to nerve damage rather than to tumor damage.

Implantable infusion pumps work on a system of expansion of gases compressed in a chamber. The disadvantage is that they are very expensive.

Surgically placed catheters which can be inserted in an immobile skin area allow the patient more flexibility in terms of being out of the hospital for long-term infusion. More complications were found from percutaneously placed intra-arterial catheters.

Clinical Experience in the Use of Intra-Arterial Infusion Chemotherapy in the Treatment of Cancers in the Head and Neck, the Extremities, the Breast and the Stomach

F. O. Stephens

Department of Surgery, Sydney Hospital, University of Sidney, Sydney, N.S.W., 2000, Australia

With head and neck tumours local recurrence of disease is the common cause of treatment failure. Anti-cancer drugs have been used to treat these tumour recurrences, but in general results have been poor, whether the drugs were given systemically of by intra-arterial regional infusion. This may be due to the presence of tumour in poorly vascularised scar tissue resulting from previous attempts at surgical excision or from previous radiotherapy (Stephens 1974).

The most common use of anti-cancer drugs has been in the treatment of patients with widely disseminated malignancies, and more recently as adjuvant chemotherapy following resection of local primary malignancies, especially of the breast or the stomach, or of other less common tumours such as osteogenic sarcoma. However, there are an increasing number of reports on the possibility of using chemotherapy as primary of "basal" treatment to reduce the size, extent or viability of advanced or aggressive, but localised, malignancies to allow for more effective eradication by subsequent radiotherapy and/or surgical excision (Stephens 1974; von Essen et al. 1968; Jussawalla and Shetty 1978; Nervi et al. 1970).

Squamous Cell Carcinoma

Advanced, of Lower Lip, Previously Untreated

World wide statistics suggest that tumour eradication by radiotherapy and/or surgery may be expected in about two-thirds of patients with advanced, but localised, previously untreated squamous cell carcinoma (SCC) of the lower lip greater than 2 cm in diameter and penetrating muscle (stage III and stage IV) (Hornback and Shidnia 1978; Jesse et al. 1976). Our experience has confirmed this. Since January 1974, however, six such patients with the most advanced lesions were treated first with "basal" chemotherapy (in four cases given intra-arterially and in two cases intravenously) prior to radiotherapy. The treatment regimen has been reported elsewhere (Stephens et al. 1981a). The basal chemotherapy reduced the lesions significantly in all cases, and subsequent radiotherapy with or without surgery has been able to eradicate the residual tumour in all patients to date (Fig. 1). The minimum follow-up period of these apparent "cures" is 3 years.

Recent Results in Cancer Research, Vol. 86
© Springer-Verlag Berlin · Heidelberg 1983

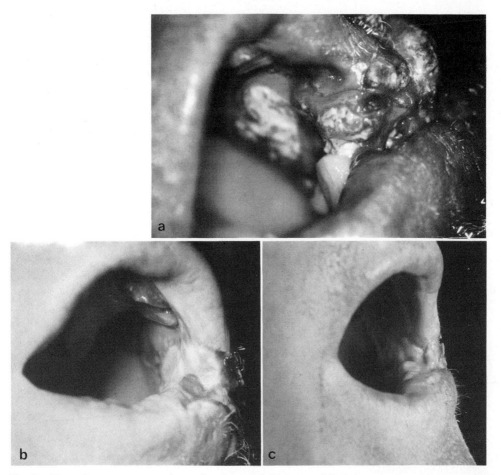

Fig. 1. a Extensive squamous carcinoma involving full thickness of the left angle of mouth and buccal mucosa, as well as skin, and extending into both upper and lower lips. **b** After intra-arterial infusion chemotherapy, the lesion is considerably smaller. **c** After follow-up radiotherapy, the lesion shows complete regression with some puckered scarring only. Multiple biopsies taken 3 months after treatment were negative and there has been no further evidence of tumour

Advanced of Lower Lip, Recurrent Tumours

For similarly advanced cancers of the lower lip which are recurrent after previous attempts at tumour eradication by radiotherapy and/or surgery, the success rate has been pathetically low at most clinics. Only three of 14 2-year "cures" were reported from the Mayo Clinic, and only three in14 from Roswell Park (Brown et al. 1976; Hendricks et al. 1977). Indiana teaching hospitals reported no cures in eight similar patients (Hornback and Shidnia 1978). Although basal chemotherapy given by intra-arterial infusion is less effective after previous treatment by radiotherapy or surgery, in our clinic we have nonetheless used basal chemotherapy as initial treatment for seven such patients presenting with recurrent tumours; in four of these cases regression was sufficient to allow apparent total tumour eradication by subsequent surgical resection or radiotherapy with a minimum follow-up period of 2 years (Stephens et al. 1981a).

Of Anterior Two-thirds of Tongue and Floor of Mouth

Over the same period of time 43 patients with similarly advanced cancers of the tongue and the floor of the mouth have also been treated in our clinic. Of these, 15 patients who presented since 1971 with the worst lesions were initially treated with basal chemotherapy given intra-arterially as the first modality of treatment, followed by radiotherapy and/or surgical resection, and the remaining 28 patients were treated with radiotherapy and/or surgery alone. The plan of therapy has been reported elsewhere (Stephens et al. 1981b). Of the 28 patients treated with either radiotherapy alone or radiotherapy with operation, six were alive and apparently free of disease after 2 or more years. Of the 15 patients treated initially with intra-arterial infusion chemotherapy prior to radiotherapy and/or surgery, eight were alive and apparently free of disease after the same amount of time. Though the number of patients in this series is small, the difference is significant ($p = 0.05$).

Of Posterior Tongue and Oropharynx

The outlook for patients with cancer of the oropharynx, including the tonsillar fossa and posterior third of the tongue, is even worse than for those with cancer of the anterior tongue of floor of the mouth. A similar plan of treatment by initial basal chemotherapy given by intra-arterial infusion was followed, with follow-up radiotherapy and with or without surgical excision, and the results compared with our results in similar patients treated with radiotherapy and/or surgery alone. For those patients with carcinoma limited to the tonsillar fossa, results were satisfactory with radiotherapy alone and there was no apparent difference in those patients given prior infusion chemotherapy. For the small number of patients in our series who presented with carcinoma of the oropharynx and fixed nodes in the neck, we have not been able to effect a cure regardless of whether initial basal chemotherapy was used. However, 19 patients presented with carcinoma extending beyond the tonsillar fossa, with or without palpable, but mobile, nodes in the neck. Of these, 11 were treated with radiotherapy, with or without surgery, alone, and in only one patient has there been an apparent "cure" after 2 years. Eight of the 19 patients were treated with initial basal chemotherapy followed by radiotherapy, with or without surgery, and four of them were apparently "cured" after a 2 year follow-up period.

Advanced Malignant Tumours of Extremities

A number of advanced and aggressive malignant tumours in the limbs have been similarly treated with a preliminary course of infusion chemotherapy, to reduce the extent or viability of the tumours prior to surgical excision. The treatment schedule and results have been recorded elsewhere (Stephens et al. 1980a). The series included not only patients with advanced squamous carcinoma but also two with soft tissue sarcoma and one with mycosis fungoides, most advanced in the right liver limb, causing extreme pain and debility. In all six patients who had originally been advised to undergo amputation, response to infusion chemotherapy reduced the tumours to such an extent that amputation was avoided completely in five cases and reduced from above the knee to below the knee in one. Five of these six people remain alive and well; one who presented with a large liposarcoma of the thigh died with pulmonary metastases but without evidence of local tumour recurrence.

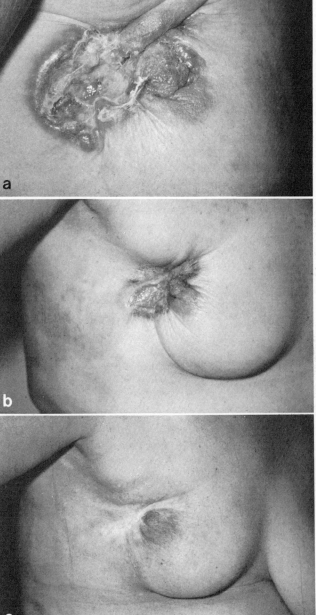

Fig. 2. a Ulceration of skin of breast adjacent to nipple. On presentation, the breast contained a large carcinoma, occupying most of the breast tissue and fixed to the chest wall. There was brawny induration of the axilla, which contained fixed nodes. There was oedema in the arm. Biopsy showed poorly differentiated breast carcinoma. **b** After infusion chemotherapy, the masses in breast and axilla became smaller, as did the area of ulceration. **c** After follow-up radiotherapy, the masses further resolved and were mobile, and the ulcer healed. However, a small, hard mobile mass remained in both breast and axilla. Mastectomy with axillary clearance was carried out. The residual lumps consisted predominantly of fibrous tissue, but also contained foci of malignant cells. The patient was given 1 year of adjuvant systemic chemotherapy, and remains well and apparently tumour free 4 years later

Advanced Stage III Breast Cancer

Fifteen patients with advanced breast cancer involving virtually the whole of the breast with either attachment to or fungation through overlying skin were first treated by infusion chemotherapy administered over a period of about 4 weeks, followed by a rest period of 3 weeks and then radiotherapy. Infusion chemotherapy was given by cannulation of the subclavian artery through a branch of the axillary or brachial artery, but in cases where infusion of the medial aspect of the breast was not achieved, cannulation of the internal mammary artery was also carried out, usually via the superior epigastric artery in the upper abdomen. Patients were reassesed 8 weeks after completion of radiotherapy, and if the tumour had not completely disappeared from the breast and the axilla, a mastectomy with axillary clearance was also performed (Fig. 2). Subsequently each patient was given a course of adjuvant chemotherapy for 1 year, consisting of cyclophosphamide, methotrexate and 5-fluorouracil (Bonadonna et al. 1976). Other details of treatment have been reported elsewhere (Stephens et al. 1980b).

In 13 of these 15 patients, local control of tumour was achieved and 11 of the 15 were alive, without evidence of tumour, from 1 to 6 years after presentation.

Gastric Cancer

Since May 1976, 27 patients with gastric cancer have been treated initially with "basal" chemotherapy in preparation of subsequent gastric resection where feasible. In 25 of the patients the chemotherapy was given by intra-arterial infusion by cannulation of the coeliac axis via a percutaneous transfemoral approach. In the other two patients the lower oesophagus was involved, and the same programme of chemotherapy was given systemically.

Ten of the 27 patients were considered to be doubtfully resectable when they first presented because of involvement of the entire stomach (including linitis plastica), involvement of the pancreas or the presence of a fixed abdominal mass. The tumours of the other 17 patients were considered to be resectable by subtotal gastrectomy, total gastrectomy or gastrectomy with partial oesophagectomy.

For the 17 patients with potentially resectable cancers, basal chemotherapy was given over a period of 4–5 weeks prior to surgery, as outlined elsewhere (Stephens et al. 1979). In all patients pain and nausea, when present could be relieved during the first 2 weeks of basal chemotherapy, but after a further 2 weeks of chemotherapy, anorexia and nausea usually recurred. After 4–5 weeks most patients were nauseated to a degree where chemotherapy had to be suspended. After 2 weeks at home the patients were once again examined by gastroscopy. In about half of the patients investigations, including gastroscopy, revealed significant evidence of tumour regression; there was apparent total disappearance of tumour in two.

In two of the ten patients who initially presented with lesions considered not resectable the tumours were reduced to an extent where laparotomy could be performed and gastrectomy was achieved. However, none of these patients achieved long-term survival; all died within 3 years.

For the 17 patients who initially presented with tumours judged resectable, gastrectomy was carried out 3–4 weeks after completion of the chemotherapy programme. There were two postoperative deaths — one from pulmonary embolus and one from pancreatitis. Of the 15 patients who survived the operative procedure, 11 are alive and well and have been apparently free of disease for between 1 and 6 years postoperatively.

Discussion

The use of chemotherapy — given either systemically or by intra-arterial infusion — to attempt to eradicate tumours which are recurrent in scar tissue following previous surgery or radiotherapy has been disappointing. The poor results achieved, in fact, caused most surgeons who were first interested in the technique of infusion chemotherapy to lose interest in this modality of treatment.

There is a growing body of experience which suggests that the most appropriate use of infusion chemotherapy is as "basal" treatment to reduce the viability and extent of advanced lesions. The objective is to reduce the tumours to proportions which are more controllable by subsequent radiotherapy and/or surgical excision.

Although in our series the number of patients with any one type of localised lesion previoulsy untreated is small, our experience with basal chemotherapy as the first modality of treatment has encouraged us to believe that the approach is worthy of further studies. This is especially so for treatment of advanced cancers in the head and neck region, the breast, and the extremities or for gastric cancer. These are situations in which the results of standard treatment are unsatisfactory because of the high incidence of recurrent disease, or because the only prospect of cure is by amputation of a limb or by some other mutilating surgical procedure.

References

Bonadonna G, Brusamolino E, Valagussa P, Rossi A, Brugnatelli L, Brambilla C, De Lena M, Tancini G, Bajetta E, Musumeci B, Veronesi U (1976) Combination chemotherapy as an adjuvant treatment in operable breast cancer. N Engl J Med 294: 405–410

Brown RG, Poole MD, Calamel PM, Bakamijian VY (1976) Advanced and recurrent squamous carcinoma of the lower lip. Am J Surg 132: 492–497

Hendricks JL, Mendelson BC, Woods JE (1977) Invasive carcinoma of the lower lip. Surg Clin North Am 57: 837–844

Hornback NB, Shidnia H (1978) Carcinoma of the lower lip: treatment results at Indiana University Hospitals. Cancer 41: 352–357

Jesse RH, Fletcher GH, Lindberg RD, Daly TE, Matalon V, Luna MA (1976) In: Clarke RL, Howe CD (eds) Cancer patient care. Year Book Medical Publ., Chicago, p 120

Jussawalla DJ, Shetty PA (1978) Experiences with intra-arterial chemotherapy for head and neck cancer. J Surg Oncol 10: 33–37

Nervi C, Arcangeli G, Casale C, Cortese M, Guadagni A, Le Pera V (1970) A reappraisal of intra-arterial chemotherapy. Results obtained in 145 patients with head and neck cancer treated during 1963–1966 with intra-arterial chemotherapy followed by radical radiotherapy. Cancer 26: 577–582

Stephens FO (1974) Combined chemotherapy, radiotherapy, and surgery in the treatment of advanced but localised solid malignant tumours. Aust NZ J Surg 44: 343–353

Stephens FO, Harker GJS, Dickinson RTJ, Roberts BA (1979) Preoperative basal chemotherapy in the management of cancer of the stomach: A preliminary report. Aust NZ J Surg 49: 331–335

Stephens FO, Crea P, Harker GJS, Lonegran DM (1980a) Intraarterial infusion chemotherapy in salvage of limbs involved with advanced neoplasms. Aust NZ J Surg 50: 387–392

Stephens FO, Crea P, Harker GJS, Roberts BA, Hambly CK (1980b) Intra-arterial chemotherapy as basal treatment in advanced and fungating primary breast cancer. Lancet 2: 435–438

Stephens FO, Harker GJS, Hambly CK (1981a) Treatment of advanced cancer of the lower lip – the use of intraarterial or intravenous chemotherapy as basal treatment. Cancer 48: 1309–1314

Stephens FO, Kalnins IK, Harker GJS, Crea P, Smith ER (1981b) Intra-arterial infusion chemotherapy in the treatment of advanced squamous carcinoma of the tongue and floor of the mouth. Surg Gynecol Obstet 152: 816–818

von Essen CF, Joseph LBM, Simon GT, Singh AD, Singh SP (1968) Sequential chemotherapy and radiation therapy of buccal mucosa carcinoma in South India. Methods and preliminary results. Am J Roentgenol 102: 530–540

Intra-Arterial Infusion Therapy for Pulmonary Tumours

O. Kokron and F. Olbert

Ludwig-Boltzmann-Institut für experimentelle Traumatologie,
Donaueschinger Strasse 13, 1200 Wien, Austria

Introduction

The infusion of cytostatic substances into the tumour via the tumour-feeding artery permits a selective increase in the concentration of drug in the tumour. Based on the unsatisfactory therapeutic results so far achieved in cases of advanced pulmonary tumours – in particular with non-small-cell bronchogenic carcinomas and in the admittedly rare cases of primary pulmonary sarcoma – we decided to use this method with selected patients in order to intensify cytostatic action.

The following are regarded as indications for this method:

1. The tumour has to be located in an area supplied by an artery; it must be demonstrable and measurable by angiography.
2. The clinical picture must not be dominated by metastases or secondary diseases.
3. Other more promising methods of therapy must not be interfered with.
4. Scintigraphic perfusion pattern of the other lung has to be normal.
5. Conditions must be suitable from the internist's point of view.

Arteriosclerosis is essentially regarded as a contraindication.

Since 1977, 49 patients with pulmonary tumours have fulfilled these criteria, and they will be dealt with in our paper.

Vascular Route of Access

The arterial approach to primary and secondary pulmonary tumours can be either via the pulmonary artery or via a nutrient vessel (bronchial artery, intercostal arteries, internal thoracic artery and, in rare cases, other arteries).

Theoretically, a nutrient vessel would be the ideal route of access to a primary tumour. Placing of the catheter is relatively difficult , however, since the specific route of access varies with the anatomic variations frequently encountered. Due to the difficulties in fixing the catheter in vessels with a small lumen the duration of infusion is limited to 4−6 h under clinical routine conditions. Because of rapidly developing stenosis of the vessel, repeated infusions will not always be possible.

Placing a catheter in the pulmonary artery, on the other hand, does not pose any technical problems and can almost always be repeated. The affected pulmonary segment may be expected to be reached in the vast majority of cases. Since the catheter can be adequately fixed, infusions may last for several days. The insertion of the catheter via the right atrium is considered a disadvantage, since it may give rise to cardiac side effects. The main argument advanced against this route, however, is the assumption that cytostatic drugs introduced via the pulmonary circulation will be absorbed by the tumour to only a limited extent, but results of recent animal experiments using adriamycin in dogs argue against this assumption.

Choice of Drugs

Even in cases the customary systemic route is used, the optimal choice and dosage of cytostatic drugs is still under discussion. In the case of intra-arterial therapy additional aspects have to be taken into consideration. The method will be of advantage only if the drug can act upon the tumour during the first passage, i.e., very rapidly. By the second passage of the drug concentrations will be equivalent to those obtained after intravenous infusion. In planning the arterial approach it would therefore be useful to know how fast the cytostatic drug penetrates the cell, whether and in what way the penetration rate depends on the concentration, and how long the drug remains inactive. In the absence of such specific information we have to rely for our orientation on such general data as tissue fixation, possible endothelial lesions, and half-life. Our treatment plans are therefore based largely on empirical findings and observations.

Our approach was as follows: To permit an unambiquous assessment of therapeutic effects, arterial infusion was performed wherever possible only on patients who had not been previously treated with cytostatic drugs. For the same reason, single-drug therapy was preferred. The drugs were chosen on the basis of their known systemic potency, but dosages were reduced by approximately $\frac{1}{2}$ or $\frac{1}{4}$. If the therapy failed i.e., the tumour progressed) systemic chemotherapy was subsequently resorted to unless other therapeutic regimes were indicated.

Problems to be Resolved

The questions we asked ourselves concerning intra-arterial infusion treatment, and which we shall attempt to answer on the basis of our findings, were the following:

1. Is the intervention practicable under routine hospital conditions?
2. Is the technique such that a patient may be reasonably subjected to it? What side effects and risks might be incurred?
3. What are the differences as to effects and side effects between infusions via the pulmonary route and those via the nutrient circulation?
4. Is there any evidence for an increased potency of intra-arterial doses as compared with identical doses administered intravenously?

Materials and Methods

Initial intra-arterial infusion treatment has so far been indicated for 49 of our patients. In two cases, however, catheterisation of the bronchial artery proved to be impossible, in one

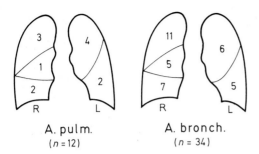

Fig. 1. The location of the pulmonary tumors in the 47 patients of our study. In 11 cases access was via the pulmonary artery; in 34, via the bronchial artery; in one via the internal thoracic artery; and in one via the intercostal artery

for technical reasons and in the other because of a collapse of the patient forcing us to discontinue the procedure. The remaining group of 47 patients comprised 37 men and ten women, aged 24—71 (median: 56). The diagnoses included 45 cases of carcinoma (16 small-cell and two large-cell carcinomas, 12 squamous cell carcinomas, 12 adenocarcinomas, two alveolar cell carcinomas and one cylindromatous carcinoma) and two cases of primary pulmonary sarcoma (one leiomyosarcoma and one fibrosarcoma). Figure 1 shows the locations of tumours. As to the stage, 34 cases were classified as "limited" (i.e., limited to one side of the chest including the ipsilateral supraclavicular fossa) and 13 as "extensive" (i.e., extending beyond the hemithorax). While three patients showed poorer ratings and significantly impaired performance, 44 were well nourished and in good general condition with only slightly reduced performance. The periods of hospitalisation prior to the first intra-arterial infusion ranged from 9 to 1613 days (median: 44). Three of the 47 patients had previously been subjected to chemotherapy.

In 11 cases the catheter was introduced via the pulmonary artery, in 34 cases via the bronchial artery (unilateral bronchial artery in 12 cases, pulmonary trunk in seven cases, and Truncus intercostobronchialis in 15 cases), in one case via an intercostal artery, and in one case via the internal thoracic artery.

Infusions via the pulmonary artery were performed 1—5 times (in each case for 3 days), total treatment time ranging from 2 to 289 days (median: 31.5).

Infusions via a branch of the bronchial artery were performed 1—3 times, lasting for 3—6 h, total treatment times ranging from 1 to 76 days (median: 1 day).

While catheterisation of the pulmonary artery succeeded in all cases, problems were encountered in eight of the 37 cases selected for bronchial artery catheterisation: in three cases the first catheterisation failed (in one of these cases subsequent insertion via the pulmonary artery was successfully performed); one infusion had to be discontinued because of severe side effects; in three patients a second, and in one patient a third intervention was no longer possible.

Table 1 lists the substances used for infusion for each of the routes of access. In the majority of cases single-drug therapy was performed; exceptions were two pulmonary sarcomas, one Pancoast tumor (intercostal artery), and three advanced bronchocarcinomas, where initial polychemotherapy was believed to be required. Further exceptions were four patients (two with adenocarcinoma and two with squamous cell carcinoma) in whom we used a preparation of proteolytic enzymes (Wobemugos, Mucos-Emulsionsgesellschaft, Grünwald b. München. FRG) for infusion via the pulmonary artery.

Table 1. Forms of treatment for 47 patients

Access route	Drug	Dose (mg)	No. of patients
Bronchial artery	cis-Platinum	50– 100	8
	DTIC	500–1,000	7
	Adriamycin	50– 100	4
	Bleomycin	15	4
	VP–16–213	200	2
	VM–26	200	2
	Actinomycin-D	0.5	1
	5-Fluorouracil	1,000	1
	ADR with	50	
	VM-26	100	1
	VP-16 with	100	
	DDP and	50	
	IFA	3,000	1
	VP-16 with	200	
	VCR and	1	
	IFA	2,000	1
	VP-16 with	200	
	VCR and	1	
	ADR	80	1
	VCR with	1	
	ADR and	50	
	DTIC	500	1
Pulmonary artery	Wobemugos	1,000	4
	VM-26	150– 200	2
	cis-Platinum	90– 100	2
	Adriamycin	80	1
	Ifosfamide	3 × 1,000	1
	Bleomycin	3 × 15	1
Internal thoracic arthery	VCR with	1	
	ADR and	80	
	DTIC	500	1
Intercostal artery	VM-26 with	50	
	5-FU and	500	
	DTIC	200	1

DTIC, dacarbazine; VP-16-213, etoposide; VM-26, teniposide; 5-FU, 5-fluorouracil; DDP, cis-platinum

Results

After intra-arterial therapy and prior to intravenous chemotherapy, if any, the following changes in the tumours were observed upon radiology: one complete remission (confirmed by postmortem), five partial remissions (size reduced by more than 50%), eight minor

Table 2. Characteristics of cases in which treatment was followed by partial remission

Type of carcinoma	TNM classification	Stage	Vascularisation of tumour	Access route	Drug	Dose (mg)	No. of infusions	Duration of therapy (days)
Small cell	221	Extensive	Poor	Tr. communis	VM	150	3	42[a]
Large cell	221	Extensive	Very poor	Tr. intercosto-bronchialis	DDP	100	1	1
Adenocarcinoma	210	Limited	High	A. bronchialis sinus	DTIC	600	3	76
Alveolar cell	211	Extensive	Poor	Tr. intercosto-bronchidis	DDP	50	1	1
Squamous cell	220	Limited	Poor	Tr. intercosto-bronchialis	DDP	100	2	23

VM, teniposide; *DDP*, cis-platinum; *DTIC*, dacarbazine

[a] Only the first infusion was via the bronchial artery; the second and third were via the pulmonary artery

remissions (size reduced by less than 50%), no measurable change in 18 cases, and progression of the tumour in nine cases; six cases were not possible to evaluate.

Complete remission of the tumour was achieved after a single application of 50 mg adriamycin and 100 mg VM-26 (teniposide) into the right. Tr. intercostobronchialis in one case of central cylindromatous carcinoma of the right basal lobe with metastases in the mediastinal lymph nodes. The characteristics of the cases showing partial remission are listed in Table 2.

Side effects varied according to vascular route, as well as to type and dosage of cytostatic drug. In general, however, they were more pronounced than after intravenous infusion of the same drug. No side effects were observed in only three cases; there were minor ones in 23 patients, marked side effects in 12, and massive side effects in eight. In one patient a fistula developed between an aortic wall necrosis and an oesophageal necrosis on the 50th day after infusion, with a fatal haemorrhage into the gastrointestinal tract. This

Table 3. Side effects observed in 47 patients who received intra-arterial infusion chemotherapy

Side effect	No. of patients
Chest pain	21
Nausea	20
Raised temperature	10
Dry cough	5
Weakness	5
Outbreak of sweat	3
Sensation of giddiness	3
Haemoptysis	3
Pleurodynia	2
Arterial occlusion	1
Chill	1
Regional histological lesion	3
Agitation, anxiety	1
Coruscation	1
Thrombo-embolism	1

Table 4. Side effects according to drug administered

Drug	No. of patients	0	+	+ +	+ + +	Lethal
Adriamycin	5	−	4	1	−	−
VP-16-213	2	−	2	−	−	−
VM-26	4	−	−	3	1	−
Bleomycin	5	−	4	−	1	−
DTIC	7	1	1	2	3	−
cis-Platinum	10	−	5	3	2	−
Actinomycin-D	1	−	1	−	−	−
5-Fluorouracil	1	1	−	−	−	−
Ifosfamide	1	−	1	−	−	−
ADR + VM-26	1	−	−	−	−	1
3-drug combin.	6	1	4	−	1	−

Table 5. Survival times of patients according to tumor-feeding artery (days)

A. pulmonaris (n = 11)	A. bronchialis (n = 34)		A. thorac. int. (n = 1)	A. intercost (n = 1)
10	11	174	353	363
23	27	176		
–	33	196		
47	50	198		
135	51 <	224		
198	55	245		
203	71	289		
209	74	297		
299	75	302		
307	84	344		
496	88	350 <		
842 <	122	355		
	133	355 <		
	141	364 <		
	146	365		
	150	365 <		
	169 <	391		

<, still alive

complication occurred in the patient who showed complete remission, which was confirmed by both radiology and postmortem. See Table 3 for details about side effects and Table 4 for side effects as a function of the form of therapy. Survival times from the first infusion ranged from 11 to 391 days (median: 197 days) for small-cell carcinomas; the two patients with large-cell carcinomas survived for 27 and 299 days respectively, patients with squamous cell carcinoma for between 33 and more than 842 days (median: 139.5), those with adenocarcinoma for 71–565 days (median: 232.5), patients with alveolar cell carcinoma for 10 and 245 days respectively, the patient with cylindromatous carcinoma for 50 days and the sarcoma patients for 84 and 353 days respectively. Table 5 relates survival times to the type of arterial access and Table 6 to the form of therapy.

Discussion

While our group of patients is relatively large, the conclusions to be drawn require detailed descriptions of the individual cases involved. Along with other factors of prognosis the results have to be broken down according to type of tumour cell, route of access and form of therapy. Since systemic chemotherapy was subsequently used in the majority of cases, we can only evaluate the acute and subacute effects and side effects in connection with intra-arterial treatment. The survival times of the patients six of whom are still alive) form only a marginal factor in our consideration.

It may be noted that the median survival time of patients with small-cell bronchocarcinomas is slightly longer than that of our total group, while it is shorter for those with adenocarcinomas and squamous cell carcinomas. Remissions by more than 50% of the original tumour size were found only after infusion via a branch of the bronchial artery and only after cytostatic therapy.

Table 6. Survival times according to therapy (days)

WOBE (n = 4)	ADR (n = 5)	VP (n = 2)	VM (n = 4)	BLM (n = 5)	DTIC (n = 7)	DDP (n = 10)	ACD (n = 1)	5FU (n = 1)	IFA (n = 1)	ADR (n = 1)	3-Drug (n = 6)
98	11	88	10	47	51 <	27	33	364 <	23	50	74
307	141	344	135	55	133	71					84
412	174		150	75	302	146					297
496	224		198	122	350 <	169 <					353
	842 <			196	355 <	176					363
					365	203					391
					365 <	245					
						289					
						299					
						355					

WOBE, Wobemugos; *ADR*, adriamycin; *VP*, VP-16-213 (etoposide); *VM*, VM-26 (teniposide); *BLM*, bleomycin; *DTIC*, dacarbazine; *DDP*, cis-platin; *ACD*, actinomycin-D; *5FU*, 5-fluorouracil; *IFA*, ifosfamide

Strikingly, these tumours were − with one exception − poorly vascularised, and all cell types were represented.

Following the infusion of proteolytic enzymes two minimal remissions were noted and in two further cases no change was observed. While survival times are relatively long with this type of treatment a conclusive evaluation is difficult for a number of reasons.

The questions raised initially may be answered as follows:

1. Intra-arterial infusion therapy can be performed under routine hospital conditions.
2. Side effects and risks are higher than with equivalent intravenous chemotherapy. The justification of such treatment in spite of side effects and risks depends on the advantages and the effectiveness of the method − questions that cannot as yet be answered.
3. Both the effects and the side effects of the treatment are more pronounced in cases of infusion via a nutrient vessel than via the pulmonary artery.
4. While our results suggest that intra-arterial infusion is more effective on tumours than an equivalent intravenous infusion, the evidence so far available is not conclusive.

Summary

On a total of 47 patients with pulmonary tumours (45 carcinomas and two pulmonary sarcomas) intra-arterial infusion therapy was performed via the bronchial artery (34 cases), the pulmonary artery (11 cases), the internal thoracic artery (1 case) and the intercostal artery (1 case). Cytostatic drugs were given to 43 patients (mainly in the form of single-drug therapy) and four patients received a preparation of proteolytic enzymes. In the majority of cases (34 of 47 patients) intra-arterial therapy was followed by intravenous cytostatic treatment. We can evaluate the effect of the intra-arterial therapy on the basis of the number and extent of tumour remissions, as well as of acute or subacute side effects. Effects over longer period and the survival times of patients can only be evaluated to a limited extent. We observed one complete tumour remission, five partial remissions (size of tumour reduced by more than 50%) and eight minor remissions (reduction by less than 50%); in 18 cases there was no measurable change in the tumour and in nine cases progression was observed (six cases cannot be evaluated.) Complete or partial remissions were observed only after treatment via the bronchial artery and after cytostatic therapy. These tumours were rather poorly vascularised and remissions occurred irrespective of cell type. There are certain indications that intra-arterial chemotherapy may be superior to equivalent intravenous chemotherapy, but the evidence so far available is not conclusive.

Scintigraphic Documentation of Lymph Drainage of Cutaneous Tumours

H. Müller, S. F. Grebe, E. L. Sattler, and G.-L. Fängewisch*

Abteilung für Nuklearmedizin, Universitätskliniken, Friedrichstrasse 25, 6300 Giessen, FRG

Since its development several years ago, lymphoscintigraphy has not been widely used. Originally the method employed a radiogold colloid; however, the more recent use of radiotechnetium colloids has facilitated the development of a new diagnostic technique which visualises the subcutaneous drainage of lymph from any skin region. Using scintigrams, it is possible to illustrate the different, often a priori not easily predicted crossed directions of lymphatic drainage. Variations in the lymphatic system may be demonstrated in each individual patient.

The lymph nodes are clearly visible, providing the surgeon with preoperative information about the sites of the nodes which are potentially involved in the drainage of lymph from the tumour cells.

With the initiative and close cooperation of our colleagues in the dermatology department, we have modified the technique of lymphoscintigraphy and adapted it for the investigation of skin tumours. Other universities have also been working on similar projects.

Method

We prepare small aliquots of radiotechnetium colloid, which are mixed with hyaluronidase; 3−5 mCi of technetium Tc 99m sulfur colloid (Lymphoscint, Nuclear GmbH, Grenzach-Wyhlen) with 150 U hyaluronidase (Kinetin, Schering AG, Berlin) is administered in a total volume of 1.0−3.0 ml, depending on the number of individual injection sites.

Initially, we surrounded the main tumour with 4−8 subcutaneous depots of radioactivity within a radius of 4−5 cm. More recently we have chosen the location and the number of radioactive depots individually for each subject. Our studies have shown that it is normally possible to reduce the time required for a scintigram sequence from a maximum of 24 h down to 4−6 h. We also scan the contralateral side of the body in every case, to investigate any crossover in lymph drainage.

Results

During the past 18 months, we have been able to carry out lymphoscintigrams on more than 20 patients with melanomas, most of the tumours being in the trunk of the body. Figures 1−6 demonstrate some lymphscans obtained with a gamma camera.

* Many thanks to our technician, Mrs. C. Schuster, for her dedication and for the accurate production of the scintigrams

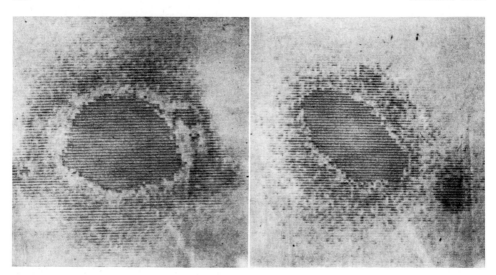

Fig. 1 (*Left*). Photograph of scintigram (and original) of patient Sch., 67-year-old male, with melanoma at the median line of the nape of the neck, later excised. The view is from the dorsal side of the patient, and shows drainage to the cervical lymph node

Fig. 2 (*Right*). Photograph of scintigram (and original) of patient Kr., 23-year-old male, with melanoma of the right scapula region, above the spine. Drainage is shown to the equilateral right axilla, and to the equilateral supraclavicular lymph node

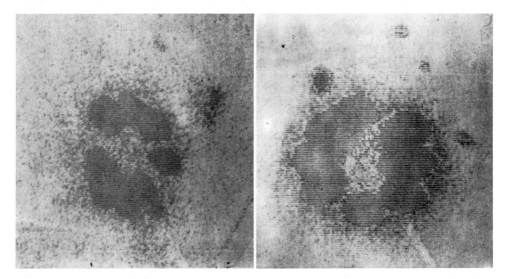

Fig. 3 (*Left*). Photograph of scintigram (and original) of patient He., 61-year-old female, with melanoma of the right scapula region, below the spine. The view is from the patient's dorsal side, and shows drainage to the equilateral right axilla, as well as to the contralateral left axilla (crossover drainage)

Fig. 4 (*Right*). Photograph of scintigram (and original) of patient He., 31-year-old female, with left paravertebral cranial melanoma. View is from patient's dorsal side and shows drainage to the equilateral left axilla, to the contralateral right axilla (crossover), to the equilateral supraclavicular lymph node, and to the contralateral right supraclavicular and cervical lymph node (crossover)

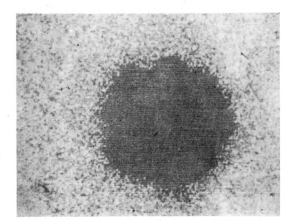

Fig. 5. Photograph of scintigram (and original) of patient Ho., 41-year-old female, with right paravertebral lumbar melanoma. View from the patient's dorsal side shows drainage to the equilateral right axilla and crossover drainage to the contralateral left axilla

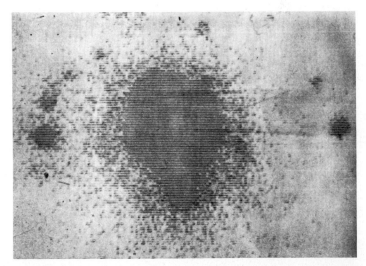

Fig. 6. Photograph of scintigraph (and original) of patient Ha., 42-year-old female, with right parasternal melanoma. View is from the patient's ventral side. Drainage is to the equilateral right axilla, to the contralateral left axilla (crossover), to the equilateral right supraclavicular lymph node, and to the contralateral left supraclavicular lymph node (crossover)

Summary

A method of lymphoscintigraphy is described which provides additional diagnostic information, of particular value prior to surgery for the removal of cutaneous tumours. The technique demonstrates the individual physiology of the lymphatic drainage system from a particular region of the skin. However, it is not the aim of the method to diagnose possible lymph node metastases

References

Altmeyer P, Node F, Merkel H (1980) Lymphogene Metastasierungsbereitschaft des malignen Melanoms. Dtsch Med Wochenschr 105: 1769

Ege GE, Warbick A (1979) Lymphoscintigraphy: A comparison of 99m-Tc antimony sulphide colloid and 99m-Tc stannous phytate. Br J Radiol 52: 124

Free HJ, Robinson DS, Sample WF, Graham LS, Homes CE, Morton DL (1978) The determination of lymph shed by colloidal gold scanning in patients with malignant melanoma. Surgery 84: 626

Kaplan WD, Davis MA, Rose CM (1979) A comparison of two technetium-99m-labeled radiopharmaceuticals for lymphoscintigraphy. J Nucl Med 20: 933

Meyer CM, Lecklittner ML, Balch CE, Bessey PQ, Tauxe WN (1979) Technetium 99m-colloid cutaneous lymphoscintigraphy in the management of truncal melanoma. Radiology 131: 205

Munz DL, Altmeyer P, Holzmann H, Encke A, Hör H (1982) Der Stellenwert der Lympho-scintigraphie in der Behandlung maligner Melanome der Haut. Dtsch Med Wochenschr 107: 86

Sherman AI, Ter Pogossain M (1953) Lymphonode concentrative colloidal gold following interstitial injection. Cancer 6: 1238

Strand SE, Jönsson PE, Berquist L, Dawiskiba S, Hafström LO, Persson B (1981) Preoperative 99m-Tc-antimony sulphide colloid scintigraphy for identification of the lymph drainage in patients with malignant melanoma. In: Cox PH (ed) Progress in radiopharmacology, vol 2, p 293

Weidner F, Tonak J (1981) Das maligne Melanom der Haut. Perimed, Erlangen, S 186

Winkel zum K, Priwitzer U, Jancke N, Schnyder UW (1972) Lymphoszintigraphie beim malignen Melanom. Hautarzt 23: 394

Winkel zum K (1972) Lymphologie mit Radionukliden. Hoffmann, Berlin

Kinetics of ^{57}Co-Bleomycin in Sheep
After Intra-Arterial Injection in the Head and Neck Region

J. Bier[1], E. Loer[1], and J. Franke[2]

1 Abteilung für Kiefernchirurgie und plastische Chirurgie, Klinikum Steglitz,
  Freie Universität Berlin, Hindenburgdamm 30, 1000 Berlin 45, FRG
2 Institut für Nuklearmedizin, Klinikum Steglitz, Freie Universität Berlin,
  Hindenburgdamm 30, 1000 Berlin 45, FRG

Introduction

For the therapy of squamous cell carcinomas of the head and neck area several cytostatics have been used to date, which were administered either systemically or by intravenous injection or infusion. In order to improve the therapeutic range of these drugs, several possibilities of regionalizing the treatment of these tumors were tested. For this purpose, intra-arterial chemotherapy was introduced for bleomycin, among other drugs, by Huntington et al. (1973), Bertino et al. (1973), Bitter (1973), and Höltje et al. (1974). The hypothetical goal of this regional type of therapy is to bind more of the active substance in the tumor region than is normal after systemic administration, thereby increasing the cytostatic effect on the tumor while decreasing the systemic-toxic side effects.

Insufficient experimental confirmation of intra-arterial chemotherapy and the lack of convincing clinical data have induced us to further clarify this complex by kinetic examinations of the head and neck region. In the present study, tests were performed to determine whether variations in the mode of administration (local, intra-arterial, systemic) of ^{57}Co-bleomycin have an influence on the elimination kinetics, blood plasma activity, and organ distribution of the labeled cytostatic. The aim was first to obtain data about the general load for the organism, which would allow conclusions regarding the systemic toxicity of intra-arterially applied cytostatics in comparison with other modes of injection.

Second, the experimental procedure was based on the idea of detecting possible changes in cytostatic activity at the required site of action by variations of drug administration. To this end, ^{57}Co-bleomycin activities over a hypothetical tumor area in the buccal plane in a live animal were continuously recorded during the entire experimental period. After the animal had been killed, ^{57}Co-bleomycin activities were determined in the hypothetical tumor area and the adjacent draining lymph nodes of the first and second orders. The disadvantages of the experimental system was that no transplantable tumors were available for the animals.

Material and Methods

Female merino sheep weighing between 40 and 50 kg were obtained from the Winkelmann Animal Breeding Institute, Paderborn, Germany.

Recent Results in Cancer Research, Vol. 86
© Springer-Verlag Berlin · Heidelberg 1983

Lyophilized bleomycin sulfate (Mack, Illertissen, Germany) was radioactively labeled with $^{57}Co^{2+}$ according to the method reported earlier (Bier et al. 1979).

The activity measurements of urine, blood plasma, and tissue samples were performed after weight determinations in the drill hole of an NaI crystal (Baird Atomic, The Hague, Netherlands) under defined geometric conditions. Externally, ^{57}Co-bleomycin activities were determined over the hypothetical tumor region in the buccal plane, again with an NaI crystal. All measurements were corrected according to the background counting and the half-life of $^{57}Co^{2+}$ related to the injection time.

The experiments were performed with five groups of five animals each (Fig. 1). The right buccal plane of the oral cavity was taken as the hypothetical tumor site. The submandibular and parotid lymph nodes are considered draining lymph nodes of the first order for the hypothetical tumor region, while the lateral retropharyngeal lymph node is regarded as a draining lymph node of the second order. This tumor region is supplied by arterial vessels in the following sequence: external carotid artery, superficial temporal artery, transverse facial artery.

Aqueous ^{57}Co-bleomycin was administered as a bolus injection in five ways:

1. Submucosally (s.m.) into the right buccal plane (hypothetical tumor site; Fig. 2).
2. Intra-arterially (i.a.) into the right transverse facial artery (Fig. 3).
3. Intra-arterially into the right superficial temporal artery (Fig. 4).
4. Intra-arterially into the right external carotid artery (Fig. 5).
5. Intravenously (i.v.) into the right saphenous vein.

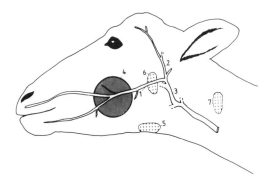

Fig. 1. Hypothetical tumor region (*4*) in the planum buccale of a sheep's head with arterial blood-vessel supply (*1–3*) and draining lymph nodes of the first (*5,6*) and second (*7*) orders. *1*, transverse facial artery; *2*, superficial temporal artery; *3*, external carotid artery; *4*, hypothetical tumor site; *5*, submandibular lymph node; *6*, parotid lymph node; *7*, lateral retropharyngeal lymph node

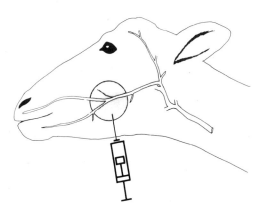

Fig. 2. Submucous ^{57}Co-bleomycin administration into the buccal plane (hypothetical tumor region)

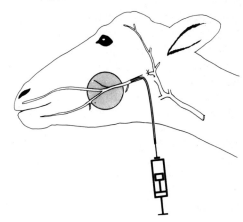

Fig. 3. Intra-arterial ^{57}Co-bleomycin administration into the transverse facial artery

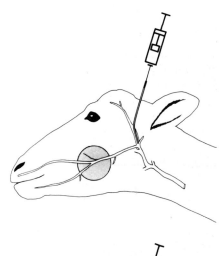

Fig. 4. Intra-arterial ^{57}Co-bleomycin administration into the superficial temporal artery

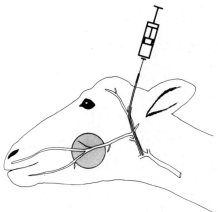

Fig. 5. Intra-arterial ^{57}Co-bleomycin administration into the external carotid artery

The correct position of the catheter was tested by injection of 2.5% patent blue (Byk Gulden, Constance, Germany). The animals received 0.3 mg ^{57}Co-bleomycin/kg body wt. The injection volume amounted to 2 ml/animal, corresponding to an activity of 100 µCi.

The results were checked for significant ($p < 0.05$) differences using the Wilcoxon test. In addition, the median values ($\bar{x}$), the 20th (x_{20}) and the 80th (x_{80}) percentiles were determined.

Results

⁵⁷Co-Bleomycin Elimination

The elimination of ⁵⁷Co-bleomycin was determined by activity measurement of the urine catheter from the experimental animals. The results are shown in Fig. 6. Six hours after ⁵⁷Co-bleomycin application, no significant differences could be detected between the various test groups. Elimination was $\bar{x} = 77\%$ for group I (buccal plane), $\bar{x} = 81\%$ for group II (transverse facial artery), $\bar{x} = 82\%$ for group III (superficial temporal artery), $\bar{x} = 76\%$ for group IV (common carotid artery), and $\bar{x} = 78\%$ for group V (saphenous vein).

⁵⁷Co-Bleomycin Blood Plasma Level

The plasma levels of ⁵⁷Co-bleomycin were determined at 17 different times between 1 and 360 min. Figure 7 shows the concentration time curves of ⁵⁷Co-bleomycin in the inferior vena cava.

Up to the 30th min after the start of the experiment, significantly ($2\alpha < 0.05$) lower ⁵⁷Co-bleomycin blood plasma activities could be detected for s.m. injection of ⁵⁷Co-bleomycin (group I) compared with i.a. (groups II–IV) and i.v. (group V) administration. From the 60th min until the end of the experiment, the activity differences between the individual test groups were no longer significant. During the entire test period of 360 min the ⁵⁷Co-bleomycin blood plasma activities of the i.a. variations tested (groups II–IV) did not differ from the values obtained after i.v. administration (group V).

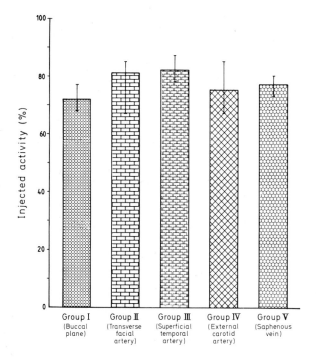

Fig. 6. Elimination of ⁵⁷Co-bleomycin in urine

[57]Co-Bleomycin Organ Distribution

The decrease in [57]Co-bleomycin activities in the hypothetical tumor area for the individual groups is presented in Fig. 8. Compared with all other groups (II−V), group I (buccal plane) showed significantly ($2\alpha < 0.01$) higher [57]Co-bleomycin activities in the hypothetical

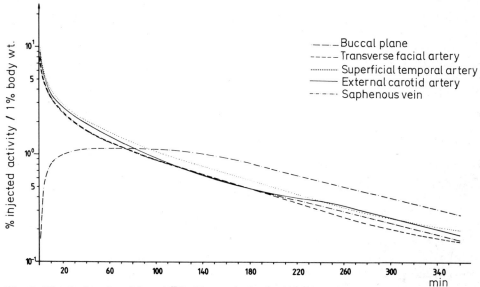

Fig. 7. Blood plasma activity of [57]Co-bleomycin in the inferior vena cava

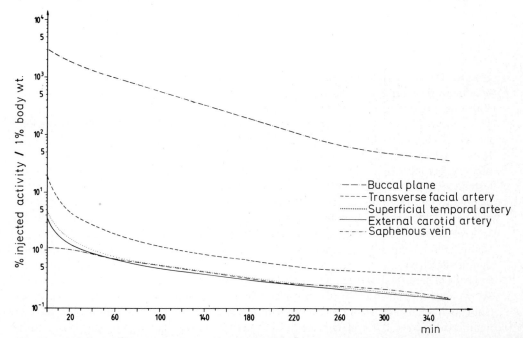

Fig. 8. Activities of [57]Co-bleomycin in the hypothetical tumor area (buccal plane)

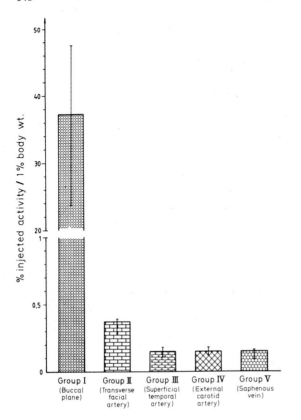

y-axis: % injected activity / 1% body wt.

Group I (Buccal plane), Group II (Transverse facial artery), Group III (Superficial temporal artery), Group IV (External carotid artery), Group V (Saphenous vein)

Fig. 9. Activities of ^{57}Co-bleomycin in the hypothetical tumor area 6 h after administration

tumor region over the entire test period of 360 min. Activities measured in the buccal plane for group II (transverse facial artery) were also higher ($2\alpha < 0.01$) during the entire experiment than for groups III (superficial temporal artery), IV (external carotid artery), and V (saphenous vein). No significant ($2\alpha < 0.05$) differences were detected between groups III and IV. Compared with group V, the absolute values determined in the hypothetical tumor area were significantly ($2\alpha < 0.05$) increased for group III up to the 30th min and for group IV for the 1st min.

The tissue distribution ^{57}Co-bleomycin in the head and neck region 6 h after the various modes of administration is presented in Figs. 9 and 10.

In the hypothetical tumor area (buccal plane), ^{57}Co-bleomycin activity was significantly ($2\alpha < 0.01$) increased after s.m. (group I) administration in comparison with all other tested variations (i.a., groups II–IV; i.v., group V). The injection of radioactively labeled bleomycin into the transverse facial artery (group II) resulted in significantly ($2\alpha < 0.01$) higher activities in the hypothetical tumor area than did i.a. administration into the superficial temporal artery (group III) and the external carotid artery (group IV), or i.v. administration into the saphenous vein (group V). On the other hand, no statistically significant activity differences for ^{57}Co-bleomycin were detectable between groups III (superficial temporal artery), IV (external carotid artery), and V (saphenous vein).

Six h after administration of ^{57}Co-bleomycin, the lymph nodes of the first order (submandibular and parotid lymph nodes) draining the hypothetical tumor area showed significantly ($2\alpha < 0.01$) higher activities in group I (s.m.) than in all other test groups. Comparison of groups II–V (transverse facial artery, superficial temporal artery, external

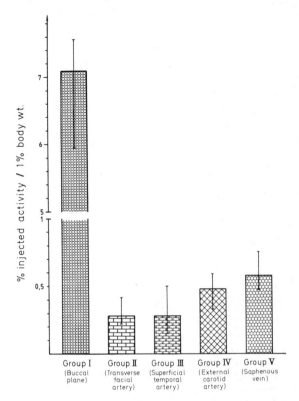

Fig. 10. Activities of [57]Co-bleomycin in the draining submandibular lymph node 6 h after administration

artery, saphenous vein) revealed no significant differences for the draining lymph nodes of the first order.

In all test groups, the lymph node of the second order (lateral retropharyngeal) draining the hypothetical tumor area evidenced no significant activity difference for [57]Co-bleomycin on either the hypothetical tumor side or the contralateral control side.

Discussion

The use of i.a. chemotherapy in the treatment of head and neck carcinomas goes back to reports by Klopp et al. (1950), who coincidentally observed an intensified therapeutic effect in comparison with systemic administration after i.a. injection of a cytostatic in a patient with Hodgkin's disease. In the same year Bierman et al. (1950) reported higher remission rates after i.a. cytostatic administration in the treatment of skin tumors. Independently of one another, both groups of authors attributed the effects they had observed to higher active cytostatic concentrations in the tumor area after i.a. application.

Up to now it has not been possible, either experimentally or clinically, to produce clear evidence for an advantage of the principle of regionalized chemotherapy of head and neck tumors in the form of i.a. treatment over the systemic i.v. administration method. The pros and cons of both are still being discussed.

It was the purpose of the present study to test whether, compared with systemic or local ^{57}Co-bleomycin administration, various modes of i.a. administration lead to lower systemic drug load and to higher drug activities in a hypothetical tumor area and in the lymph nodes draining it.

^{57}Co-Bleomycin Elimination

For the elimination of ^{57}Co-bleomycin in relation to the mode of administration, no significant differences could be detected between the s.m. group (I), the i.a. groups (II−IV) and the i.v. group (V). During the 6-h test period, the animals in the individual test groups had eliminated between 72% and 82% of ^{57}Co-bleomycin activity via the kidneys. Thus, evidence was provided for the fact that renal elimination of ^{57}Co-bleomycin does not depend on the mode of administration.

From these findings it can be concluded that the total body load for animals with a labeled cytostatic − at least for a 6-h period − is identical regardless of different modes of administration. This means that the intra-arterial test variants do not result in an administration mode-dependent change in the total load for the organism with ^{57}Co-bleomycin. This statement is also confirmed by previous examinations (Bier et al. 1979). Therefore, the hypothesis is that variations in the distribution have to occur if the total body activity is identical. Thus, the blood plasma values of ^{57}Co-bleomycin were determined as a measurement of the general systemic load.

^{57}Co-Bleomycin Blood Plasma Level

For animals injected i.a. (groups II−IV) and i.v. (group V) with ^{57}Co-bleomycin, no significant activity differences could be detected between the individual groups in any of the total of 17 measurements of vena cava blood between 1 and 360 min. Even at the first measurement − 1 min after the ^{57}Co-bleomycin injection − the blood plasma activities of i.a.- and i.v.-treated animals were identical. These findings indicate that no major blood plasma activity-changing ^{57}Co-bleomycin binding in the perfused hypothetical tumor site (buccal plane) occurred with any of the tested i.a. administration variations. Another possible conclusion is that the identical blood plasma levels lead to an equally identical general organ load. This means that by the tested i.a. variations no reduction in systemic toxicity is obtained as compared with i.v. systemic administration.

Findings comparable to our results were reported by Didolkar et al. (1978) for both animal experiments and clinical investigations.

Our results are also confirmed by tests performed as early as 1966 by Scheunemann. For rabbits, which were treated either i.v. or i.a. with triaziquone − a cytostatic with a strongly myelotoxic effect − no differences could be detected in the extent of bone marrow aplasia or for peripheral leukocytopenia between the two groups.

^{57}Co-Bleomycin Organ Distribution

The highest values in the buccal plane were determined for animals treated s.m. (group I) with ^{57}Co-bleomycin. They remained significantly higher than the values for all other groups (II−V) throughout the entire test period. Activities were determined as higher by the factor 1026 than in the i.v.-treated animals (group V). The differences compared with the i.v. group were considerably smaller after supraselective injection of ^{57}Co-bleomycin into the transverse facial artery (group II). Even though the activities were still increased by the factor 15 at the beginning of the test, they decreased to the factor 2.6 to 2.0 within 60 min. Measured over the entire test period, the activities in the hypothetical tumor area were only three times higher for group II (transverse facial artery) than those for group V (saphenous vein).

This result makes it clear on the one hand that the cytostatic concentration in the hypothetical tumor area after local administration of labeled bleomycin is the highest by far, and on the other hand that supraselective i.a. injection of ^{57}Co-bleomycin leads to a relatively small activity concentration at the required site of action in comparison to i.v. administration. However, the use of this isolated i.a. perfusion method without concomitant blood flow is not of direct clinical relevance.

The clinically relevant administration modes of i.a. chemotherapy are represented by groups III and IV. As already conjectured in the discussion of the relative activities, it is only at the beginning of the experiment that these groups show an increase in absolute values as compared with i.v. administration of ^{57}Co-bleomycin. For group III (superficial temporal artery), a significant difference in comparison with group V (saphenous vein) was only detectable for the time from 1 to 360 min. The differences were even smaller between group IV (external carotid artery) and group V (saphenous vein); 15 min after initiation of the experiment, significant differences were no longer detectable.

In a recent theoretical study by Chen and Gross (1980), attention was called to the decisive influence of drug elimination or inactivation in i.a. chemotherapy. On the basis of kinetic mathematical models, they formed the opinion that i.a. chemotherapy is useful — if at all — only with drugs that are very rapidly eliminated. In addition, they also pointed out the important influence of blood flow in the infused artery. The greater the flow, the smaller the increased concentration of the drug will be after i.a. perfusion in comparison with i.v. administration. This calculation was confirmed by our investigation. With ascending selectivity of the catheter position — external carotid artery, superficial temporal artery, transverse facial artery — higher activities were determined in the hypothetical tumor area shortly after injection of ^{57}Co-bleomycin.

Isolated consideration of the activities in the head and neck region 6 h after administration of ^{57}Co-bleomycin casts further doubt on the value of i.a. chemotherapy. No differences were revealed by a comparison of the activities in the hypothetical tumor area after i.v. administration (group V) and i.a. injection into the superficial temporal artery (group III) or external carotid artery (group IV). Increases in ^{57}Co-bleomycin concentration by the factors 2.6 and 255 respectively only resulted after supraselective catheterization of the transverse facial artery (group II) and direct injection into the hypothetical tumor region (group I).

Findings on i.a. chemotherapy in animal experiments have only seldom been described up to now (Sindram et al. 1974; Didolkar et al. 1978; Karakousis et al. 1979). However, the available data provide indications that support our findings and point towards a trend against i.a. chemotherapy in the treatment of head and neck carcinomas.

Particular importance was attached to the draining lymph nodes of the first and second orders of the hypothetical tumor region. They represent the tissue structures primarily endangered by metastases of squamous cell carcinoma in the head and neck region. No activity differences could be detected in the draining lymph nodes of the first and second orders for all tested modes of i.a. administration of ^{57}Co-bleomycin (groups II–IV) as compared with i.v. administration (group V). It was only for the s.m.-injected animals (group I) that the activities measured were 15–24 times higher for the submandibular lymph node and 8–14 times higher for the parotid lymph node, as compared with the i.v.-

(group V) and i.a.-treated (groups II−IV) animals. Thus, evidence was provided that, compared with i.v. treatment with ^{57}Co-bleomycin, regional i.a. chemotherapy does not lead to any drug enrichment in the lymph nodes draining the hypothetical tumor area which would possibly improve the therapeutic effect. Only local administration seems to offer the possibility of more effectively treating the regional lymph nodes. We have repeatedly pursued this line of argumentation (Bier et al. 1979; 1980, 1981).

The clinical value of i.a. chemotherapy is the subject of controversy. Because prospective randomized comparative studies are lacking, it has not as yet been possible to establish a clear preference for a particular method of intravascular cytostatic administration. However, a study presented by Shanta and Krishnamurthi (1977) makes possible indirect assessment of i.a. therapy with bleomycin. In an initial clinical study, one group of patients was treated i.a. with bleomycin and subsequent radiotherapy, while in a second study the i.a. chemotherapy was replaced by i.v. treatment. No difference was detectable by comparison of the two studies; 78.5% of the i.a.-treated patients reacted to the therapy, while a positive effect was achieved for 77.3% of the i.v.-treated group.

With reference to our own and other data, a rational basis for the clinical application of i.a. chemotherapy is presently not available. This is all the more true since, compared with systemic treatment, i.a. therapy involves excessively high complication rates resulting from faulty handling of the catheter, hemorrhages, and embolisms, leading to increased morbidity of the treated patients (Jesse et al. 1964; Watkins and Sullivan 1964; Tindel 1967; Bertino et al. 1973, 1975).

In contrast to i.a. chemotherapy, intratumoral administration of high cytostatic concentrations in the tumor and in the area of the draining lymph nodes is favored by the present distribution experiments for treatment of head and neck carcinomas.

Summary

Intra-arterial (i.a.) chemotherapy for the treatment of head and neck tumors is performed on the basis of clinical reports. The hypothetical aim of i.a. chemotherapy is to achieve higher drug concentrations in the tumor than are acheived by systemic intravenous (i.v.) administration. Therefore, it is postulated that i.a. chemotherapy leads to an increased therapeutic effect at the tumor site and to a decrease in systemic drug toxicity. The lack of adequate animal experiments and the absence of prospective randomized clinical trials comparing i.a. with i.v. chemotherapy led to the present kinetic study, concerned with various modes of administration of bleomycin with the aim of achieving high cytotoxic concentrations at the required site. Radioactive bleomycin (^{57}Co-bleomycin) was injected locally (buccal plane, group I), intra-arterially (transverse facial artery, group II; superficial temporal artery, group III; external carotid artery, group IV), and intravenously (saphenous vein, group V) in five sheep per group. Between 1 and 360 min after injection of radioactive bleomycin the urine and the systemic blood activities were determined, and the activities in the hypothetical tumor area (buccal plane) were measured continuously. The animals were killed 360 min after injection and the activities in the hypothetical tumor area, in the lymph nodes draining this area (submandibular, parotic, lateral pharyngeal) and in different tissues and organs were determined. For all groups, 70%−80% of the injected bleomycin was eliminated by the kidneys, without any significant differences among the five groups tested. The systemic blood activities measured at 5-min intervals exhibited no differences for the groups injected i.a. (II−IV) and i.v. (V). Only animals which received local injections (group I) showed lower activities for 60 min after injection as compared with the other four groups. The activities of radioactively labeled bleomycin in the hypothetical tumor area during the entire experiment (360 min) were again similar for the groups injected i.a. (II—IV) and those injected i.v. (V). However, only animals injected locally (group I) showed significantly increased activities. After the death of the animals there was again no significant difference between i.a. and i.v. administration. Only local injection led to significantly increased tissue activities. Similar results also obtained for the lymph nodes draining the hypothetical tumor area. Summarizing the results in the sheep model for radioactive bleomycin, the following statement is possible: Compared with i.v. treatment, i.a. chemotherapy is not able to increase the drug activities significantly in the hypothetical tumor area and in the lymph nodes draining this area, and a decrease in systemic drug toxicity could not be detected after i.a. administration.

References

Bertino JR, Mosher MB, DeConti RC (1973) Chemotherapy of cancer of the head and neck. Cancer 31: 1141—1149

Bertino JR, Boston B, Capizzi RL (1975) The role of chemotherapy in the management of cancer of the head and neck. Cancer 36: 752—758

Bier J, Benders P, Bitter K (1979) Ausscheidung und Organverteilung von ^{57}Co-Bleomycin. Dtsch Z Mund Kiefer Gesichts Chir 3: 151—157

Bier J, Bier H, Lathan B, Siegel T, Ohanian S (1980) Tierexperimentelle Untersuchungen zur intratumoralen Chemotherapie mit Bleomycin. Arch Otorhinolaryngol 229: 13—27

Bier J, Bier H, Lathan B, Michel O, Siegel T, Schlesinger S (1981) Intratumorale Chemotherapie mit Bleomycin-Emulsion. Dtsch Z Mund Kiefer Gesichts Chir 5: 335—340

Bierman HR, Shimkin MB, Byron RL, Miller ER (1950) Effects of intraarterial administration of nitrogen mustard. 5th International Cancer Congress, Paris, 1950

Bitter K (1973) Relations between histology, TNM category and results of treatment with methotrexate-bleomycin combination in squamous cell carcinomas of the oral cavity. J Maxillofac Surg 1: 113—115

Chen HS, Gross JF (1980) Intra-arterial infusion of anticancer drugs: theoretic aspects of drug delivery and review of responses. Cancer Treat Rep 1: 31—35

Didolkar MS, Kanter PM, Baffi RR, Schwartz HS, Lopez R, Baez N (1978) Comparison of regional versus systemic chemotherapy with adriamycin. Ann Surg 3: 332—336

Höltje WJ, Lentrodt J, Landbeck G (1974) Störungen der Blutstillung durch Bleomycin nach arterieller Perfusion von Plattenepithelkarzinomen der Mundhöhle. 2nd Congress of the European Association for Maxillofacial Surgery, Zürich, 1974

Huntington MC, Dupriest RW, Fletcher WS (1973) Intraarterial bleomycin therapy in inoperable squamous cell carcinomas. Cancer 31: 153—157

Jesse R, Villarreal R, Latayf V, Rufino C, Hickey R (1964) Intraarterial infusion for head and neck cancer. Arch Surg 88: 618—627

Karakousis CP, Kanter PM, Lopez R, Moore R, Hoyloke ED (1979) Modes of regional chemotherapy. J Surg Res 26: 134—141

Klopp CT, Alford TC, Bateman J, Berry GN, Wipship P (1950) Fractionated intraarterial cancer chemotherapy with methyldiamine hydrochloride; preliminary report. Ann Surg 132: 811—832

Scheunemann H (1966) Experimentelle und klinische Untersuchungen zur intraarteriellen Chemotherapie inoperabler maligner Tumoren im Kiefer- und Gesichtsbereich. Hanser, München

Shanta V, Krishnamurthi S (1977) Combined therapy of oral cancer, bleomycin and radiation: a clinical trial. Clin Radiol 28: 427—429

Sindram PJ, Snow GB, van Putter LM (1974) Intra-arterial infusion with methotrexate in the rat. Br J Cancer 30: 349—354

Tindel S (1967) Intra-arterial chemotherapy for recurrent neoplasms. JAMA 200: 913—917

Watkins E Jr, Sullivan RD (1964) Cancer chemotherapy by prolonged arterial infusion. Surg Gynecol Obstet 118: 1—19

Combined Treatment of Maxillofacial Carcinoma by Intra-Arterial Proliferation Block and Irradiation

J. F. Kreidler[1] and J.-R. Petzel[2]

1 Abteilung VII B Mund- und Kiefer- und Gesichtschirurgie, Bundeswehrkrankenhaus Ulm,
  Postfach 1220, 7900 Ulm, FRG
2 Abteilung für Zahn-, Mund- und Kiefernchirurgie,
  Rheinisch-Westfälische Technische Hochschule Aachen, 5100 Aachen, FRG

Introduction

An extensive retrospective study by the German-Austrian-Swiss Research Group (DÖSAK) on maxillofacial tumors (Fries et al. 1979) revealed the 5-year survival rate for oral carcinoma of all TNM categories to be less than 50%. For T_3N_x tumors survival time was 9−17 months. These unsatisfactory results indicate the necessity for new therapeutic techniques.

Tumors of the maxillofacial region are characterized by three clinical features: superficial location, ease of description and documentation, and good possibility of obtaining biopsy specimen. Blood is supplied to them by the branches of the external carotid artery; this makes the regional administration of cytostatic drugs feasible. Knowledge of the tumors' biological behavior is good; local growth and regional metastases are common features, while distant metastases occur rarely, even with gross tumors.

Tumor chemotherapy has advanced remarkably in the last 10 years. New developments with cytostatic agents, as well as experimental knowledge of the cytokinetic effect of these agents in tumor cells, have provided better clinical results.

The principles of the cytokinetic activity of adriamycin (ADR) and bleomycin (BLM) and quantification of this activity by flow cytometry (FCM) of DNA have been investigated by Schumann and Göhde (1974), Göhde et al. (1975), Barlogie and Drewinko (1978), and Göhde et al. (1979). With the use of ADR and BLM they found a specific blockade in the G_2 phase. According to Sinclair (1968), cells in this phase of the mitotic cycle are hypersensitive to irradiation. Based on this groundwork, our therapeutic regimen consists of a long-lasting blockade of cell proliferation in the G_2 phase by local intra-arterial infusion of the tumor region with ADR and BLM, followed by coordinated irradiation therapy.

Materials and Methods

Platients were chosen for the study here described according to the following criteria:

1. Histologically diagnosed epidermoid carcinoma of the oral cavity or oropharynx, corresponding to the category $T_3N_xM_0$ (UICC 1976).

2. Available access to the primary tumor site through the external carotid artery to allow selective infusion of the chemotherapeutics.
3. Informed consent and cooperation for the planned therapy.
4. Adequate general fitness of the patient.

Normal lung, liver, kidney, and bone marrow function was essential. Pretherapeutic lung function and radiographic examination, and the following laboratory investigations were made: complete blood count, erythrocyte sedimentation rate, blood sugar, electrolytes, creatine, urea, transaminases, phosphate, and coagulation values. Before beginning the therapy the tumor was TNM classified and fully documented.

Therapy Protocol

Under local anesthesia the external carotid artery was catheterized (in a retrograde direction) through the superficial temporal artery. A child's feeding tube with a lateral opening and a resealable cap on the free end was used. A biopsy sample was excised for histological and FCM examination. Today we use a new catheter with antithrombotic coating, specially manufactured by Braun/Melsungen for our purpose.

The extent of the tissue selectively infused was determined by injection of disulfine blue. We strive for super-selective infusion of the primary tumor region. Under continuous infusion of disulfine blue the catheter is inserted until the tumor region is completely stained. For tumors in the area supplied by the maxillary artery this provides selective drug infusion. For tumors in regions supplied by the caudal branches of the external carotid artery, a secondary procedure is necessary to ensure that all of the injected drug is reaching the tumor. This is achieved by ligating the external carotid artery cranially from the branches supplying tumor, and all other branches not supplying the tumor. In this way the total blood flow of the external carotid artery is directed through the tumor region (Kreidler 1976).

The patency and location of the catheter were controlled weekly by disulfine blue injection, and in some cases by angiography.

The tumor was infused via the catheter a maximum of five times a week with ADR and, in some cases, BLM, with the goal of permanent proliferation blockade in the G_2 phase. The infusion was done overnight, running continuously from 8 p.m. until 8 a.m. The dose of ADR was 6–12 mg, that of BLM 7.5–15 mg, per 12-h infusion, depending on the tumor size and the number of carotid branches infused (Fig. 1).

The effectiveness of the block was monitored during the first and second weeks by means of FCM on puncture biopsy samples (Kreidler 1976; Kreidler and Ammon 1979).

When proliferation block was successful (Fig. 2) the tumor was irradiated, using a telecobalt source and a 300-rad single dose. The irradiation therapy was performed on the morning following an infusion and the total irradiation dose was limited to between 3,000 and 4,000 rad.

Following the irradiation therapy we performed a final examination, with the patient usually under general anesthesia, with photodocumentation and biopsy samples for histopathologic evaluation.

If full clinical remission was determined and there was an absence of vital tumor cells in the biopsy samples, the catheter was removed.

The frequency and dose of the cytostatic infusions were varied according to the monitored FCM results. This allowed an initially small dose of cytostatic drug to be increased, when

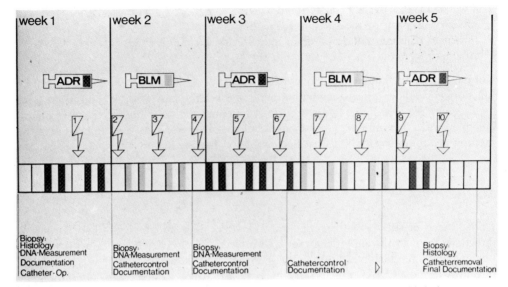

Fig. 1. General treatment regimen. *Shaded portions* of blocks indicate periods of infusion; *arrows,* points at which radiotherapy is administered

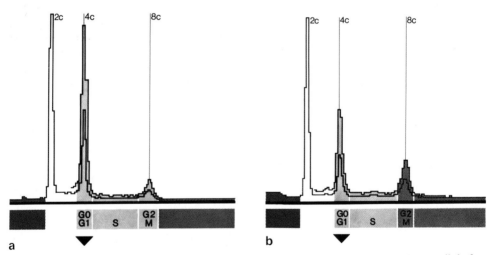

Fig. 2. a Histogram showing DNA distribution of epidermoid carcinoma of the tonsil before treatment. *3C,* diploid nuclei, inflammatory cells; *4C,* tetraploid nuclei, tumor stemline; G_0, G_1, 68.9%; *S,* 18.0%; G_2, *M,* 13.1%. **b** Histogram of same tumor area showing DNA distribution after continuous, super-selective intra-arterial ADR infusion. *8C,* G_2 block; G_0, G_1, 47.8%; *S,* 22.1%; G_2, *M* 30.1%

necessary, to provide effective G_2 block. The resultant partial block of the proliferation cycle during a radiosensitive phase ensures increased effectiveness of subsequent radiation therapy.

Concurrent preventive therapy consisted of:

1. Digitalis therapy with onset of treatment.

2. Low-doses of heparin (15,000−20,000 U/day) and 500 mg acetylsalicylate (Colfarit) twice a day to prevent thromboembolism.
3. A broad-spectrum antibiotic administered prophylactically 3 weeks after the beginning of treatment.
4. Adequate nourishment and fluid balance, ensured by use of a stomach-feeding tube or intravenous catheter.
5. Blood samples taken for laboratory monitoring three times a week.
6. Weekly chest X-rays to examine for lung fibrosis.

Patients generally received physiotherapy, starting with the third week of treatment.

Results

Eleven of the 14 patients treated with the described regimen are alive and free of tumor symptoms. Three patients died because of tumor recurrence or metastases (Table 1, Fig. 3). The median survival time was 30 months.

Primary Tumor

All primary tumors showed complete remission (CR) after cytostatic-radiological treatment. Nine patients remain in remission to date (Figs. 4 and 6). Two patients (nos. 2 and 5) developed residual tumor growth 6−8 weeks following primary tumor treatment (Fig. 5). In both cases the tumor originated in mandibular bone. Surgical removal of the T_1 tumors has been performed without removing the entire scarred area of the former primary tumor. In the meantime, patient no. 2 has died of recurrence and metastases

Table 1. Data on patients treated for carcinoma of the oral cavity

Patient no.	Tumor localisation	TNM	Chemotherapeutic dose (mg)		Radio-therapy (Gy)	Survival time (months)
			ADR	BLM		
1	Floor of the mouth	$T_3N_1M_0$	120	30	30	56
2	Floor of the mouth	$T_3N_1M_0$	246	−	30	37
3	Tonsil	$T_3N_1M_0$	178	105	30	17
4	Tonsil	$T_3N_2M_0$	148	−	30	16
5	Floor of the mouth	$T_3N_1M_0$	168	−	30	45
6	Tongue	$T_3N_0M_0$	108	52.5	30	40
7	Gingiva mandible	$T_3N_1M_0$	120	50	30	36
8	Soft palate	$T_3N_0M_0$	108	150	42	35
9	Lower lip	$T_3N_1M_0$	204	120	25	29
10	Mucosa cheek	$T_3N_1M_0$	164	−	33	26
11	Hard palate	$T_3N_0M_0$	72	165	30	22
12	Floor of the month	$T_2N_1M_0$	27	180	30	21
13	Lower lip	$T_2N_1M_0$	72	90	20	20
14	Floor of the mouth	$T_2N_0M_0$	72	120	30	17

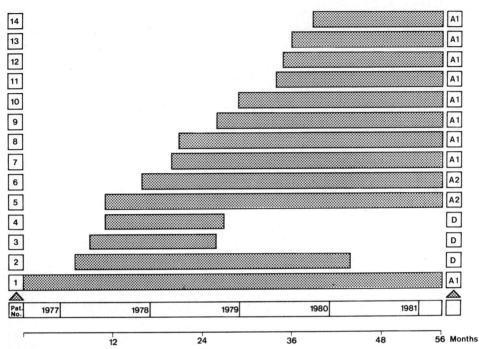

Fig. 3. Survival times for 14 patients in the study. *A,* alive; *D,* dead; *1,* no recurrence of tumor; *2,* free of tumor symptoms after treated recurrence or metastases. Compare with Table 1

(survival time, 37 months). Patient no. 5 has been free of tumor symptoms for 45 months.

Metastases

Six patients with N_1 or N_2 nodes needed radical neck dissection. Patients nos. 2, 3, and 4 at first showed full remission of the regional metastases following cytostatic-radiological treatment. Neck nodes developed 6–12 months later and radical neck dissection had to be performed. Because of this experience we performed primary neck dissection combined with selective catheterization of the external carotid artery in the next such cases. This surgical intervention was followed by simultaneous intra-arterial chemotherapy and radiation (Fig. 6).

Fast reactions in the infused and irradiated area developed beginning in the second week of treatment. Mucositis, superficial necrosis of the mucosa, (Fig. 6d) pain, and hair loss were common. Local alteration of the mucosa healed within 2 weeks after the end of primary therapy.

In two cases we saw reversible hemiparesis as a severe complication. This was probably due to embolization of the internal carotid artery when the catheter position was near the carotid bulbus. In another case (patient no. 3) homolateral partial loss of the visual field occurred several months after the end of primary therapy. In the surgical specimen, total obstruction of the common carotid artery by thrombosis was verified. As a rule, patients lost 5–8 kg although they received high-caloric nutrition. The total duration of inpatient treatment was 5–6 weeks.

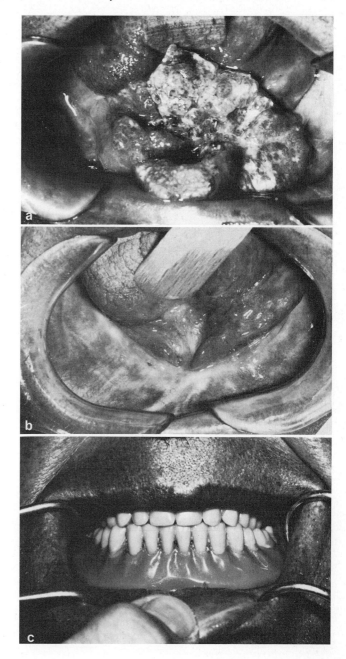

Fig. 4a–c. Patient no. 1 of Table 1. **a** Untreated carcinoma of the floor of the mouth, infiltrating lower lip. **b** Scarred area of primary tumor, 1 year after cytostatic-radiological treatment. **c** Dental prosthetic rehabilitation

Discussion

Nitze (1969) was the first to inaugurate the concept of synchronized radiotherapy of head and neck tumors and report his clinical results (Nitze et al. 1972). Through histologic and autoradiographic examinations he was able to show some probability of synchronization of tumor cells after long-term infusion of 5-fluorouracil.

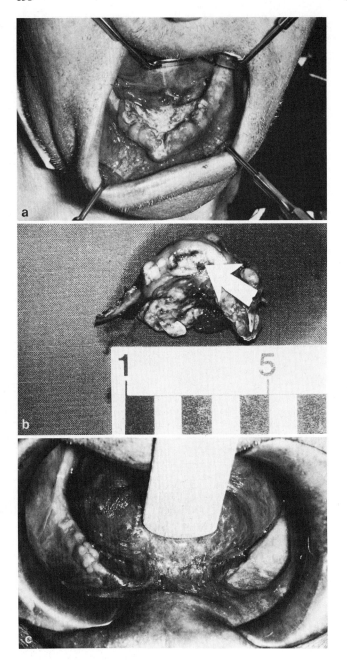

Fig. 5a–c. Patient no. 5 of Table 1. **a** Untreated carcinoma of the floor of the mouth, involving the mandible. **b** Surgical specimen of the recurrent T_1 tumor (*arrow*) originating in the mandibular bone. **c** Healed primary tumor site

The principle of synchronizing therapy is a cytokinetic manipulation of tumor growth in order to get as many or possibly all tumor cells to cycle synchronously through the phases of cell division. As a first step it is necessary to achieve a reversible blockade of the tumor cells during a predetermined cycle phase. Real synchronization means that this block is freed and that tumor cells continue to proliferate simultaneously. In a second step during a later cycle phase, i.e., irradiation in the G_2 phase, specifically effective agents are able to destroy

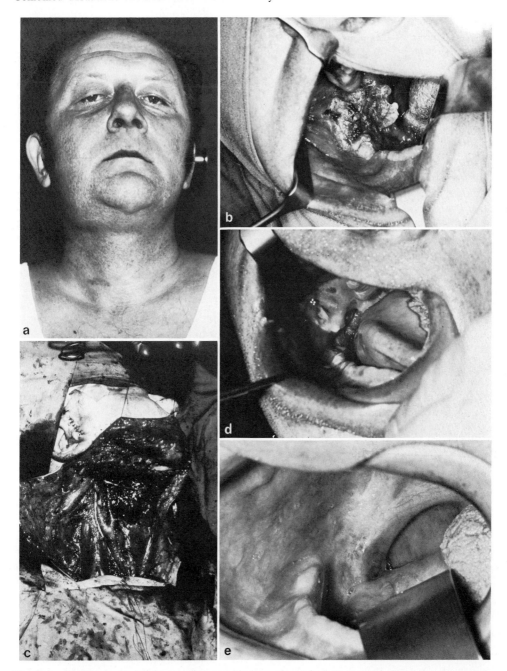

Fig. 6a—e. Patient no. 7 of Table 1. **a** Submandibular node, *right.* **b** Untreated retromolar carcinoma. **c** Disulfine blue injection through the inserted catheter during neck dissection. **d** Mucositis of right side of tongue during therapy; disulfine blue injection. **e** Healed primary tumor site

a high percentage of tumor cells with successful synchronization in the described regimen. The advantage of this concept evidently lies in a higher therapeutic effect achieved by administration of lower doses of cytostatics and irradiation than would otherwise be necessary.

This is in contrast to the principle of medical oncology, which holds that the maximum tolerable dose of chemotherapy should achieve the maximum possible antitumor effect.

Unlike systemic diseases such as malignant lymphoma and leukemia, tumors of the head and neck region are limited locally. Generalized spread occurs only in advanced stages (Fries et al. 1979); therefore, regional chemotherapy and radiotherapy are justified.

Intra-arterial infusion of cytostatic drugs cause tumor cells to accumulate in the radiosensitive G_2 phase, not indirectly by synchronization, but directly by a pharmacological blockade. For this purpose we have chosen the cytostatic antibiotics ADR and BLM, whose interaction in the S phase is well defined, and which lead to a G_2 block in experimental cell systems and human tumors (Schumann and Göhde 1974; Esser et al. 1977; Barlogie and Drevinko 1978; Göhde et al. 1979).

With regard to toxicity, these two agents are a good combination. While ADR produces damage to the blood stem cells and the heart muscle, BLM has its toxic effects on lung and skin.

To control cytokinetic effects of intra-arterial infusion, automatic DNA measurement by FCM is a proven technique. The evidence of G_2 block in random samples after infusion has led us to the reduction of cytostatic doses as shown in Table 1. With these reduced doses we have never seen severe general toxicity. The toxic effects concentrate on the infusion area and have proved to be a good indication of the therapeutic effect.

The median survival time of 30 months in this pilot study of 14 patients encourages us to continue with this combined treatment.

Summary

We investigated the possible potentiation of a regimen of combined cytostatic and radiation therapy for epidermoid carcinoma of the maxillofacial region.

The described combined approach by intra-arterial infusion of ADR and BLM and cytokinetically controlled irradiation was able to produce CR in all treated primary tumors of the head and neck. Regional metastases are not definitely controlled and require surgical intervention.

References

Barlogie B, Drevinko B (1978) Cell cycle stage-dependent induction of G_2-phase arrest by different antitumor agents. Eur J Cancer 14: 741

Esser E, Haut J, Schumann J, Wannenmacher M, Wingenfeld U (1977) Experimentelle Untersuchungen zur Proliferationskinetik und Strahlenbehandlung nach Vincristin und Adriamycin. Strahlentherapie 153: 682

Fries R et al. (German-Austria-Swiss research team on maxillofacial tumors) (1979) Carcinoma of the oral cavity: On the prognostic significance of the primary tumour site. J Maxillofac Surg 7: 15

Göhde W, Schumann J, Büchner T, Barlogie B (1975) Influence of irradiation and cytostatic drugs on proliferation patterns of tumor cells. In: Haanen, Hillen, Wessels (eds) Proc. 1st Int. Symp. Pulse-Cytophotometry. European Press, Ghent

Göhde W, Meistrich M, Meyn R, Schumann J, Johnston D, Barlogie B (1979) Cell-cycle phase-dependence of drug-induced cycle progression delay. J Histochem Cytochem 27: 470

Kreidler JF (1976) DNA-Gehalt und Proliferationskinetik der Carcinome des Kiefer- und Gesichtsbereichs. Impulscytophotometrische Untersuchungen im Hinblick auf die intraarterielle cytostatische Behandlung. Westdeutscher Verlag, Opladen

Kreidler JF, Ammon J (1979) Kombinierte intraarterielle Proliferationshemmung und Bestrahlung. Ein kuratives, zellkinetisches Therapiekonzept für Karzinome des Kiefer- und Gesichtsbereichs. In: Wannenmacher, Gauwerky, Streffer (eds) Kombin. Strahlen- und Chemotherapie. Urban & Schwarzenberg, München, S. 141

Nitze HR (1969) Die Synchronisation menschlichen Gewebes in vivo. Habilitationsschrift, University of Frankfurt a. M.

Nitze HR, Ganzer N, Vosteen K-H (1972) Die Strahlenbehandlung maligner Tumoren nach Synchronisation des Zellteilungsrhythmus. Strahlentherapie 143: 329

Schumann J, Göhde W (1974) Die zellkinetische Wirkung von Bleomycin auf das Ehrlich-Karzinom der Maus in vivo. Strahlentherapie 147: 298

Sinclair WK (1968) Cyclic X-ray responses in mammalian cells in vitro. Radiat Res 33: 620

UICC (1976) TNM-Klassifizierung der malignen Tumoren und allg. Regeln zur Anwendung des TNM-Systems, 2nd edn. Springer, Berlin Heidelberg New York

Intracarotid Artery Infusion of DTIC for Invasive Maxillofacial Melanoma

F. J. Lejeune, A. M. Jortay, and P. Dor

Institut Jules Bordet, Centre des Tumeurs de l'Université Libre de Bruxelles, Service de Chirurgie, Rue Héger-Bordet 1, 1000 Bruxelles, Belgium

Introduction

Malignant melanomas arising in the mucous membranes of the maxillofacial region are often highly invasive, causing bone destruction. Surgery and/or radiotherapy were found to be unsatisfactory treatment for this condition (Castermans et al. 1974; Lejeune et al. 1972) which has a very poor prognosis.

After our experience using intracarotid chemotherapy in the treatment of epidermoid carcinoma of the oral cavity (Jortay 1975), we were tempted to apply this method to malignant melanoma, using dacarbazine (DTIC, dimethyl triazeno imidazole carboxamide). This drug is considered an effective agent against malignant melanoma, with a 20%–25% objective remission rate, and is used after systemic administration in advanced melanoma (Lejeune and De Wasch 1978). However, few papers have been published on intra-arterial infusion of DTIC, and these few have dealt with melanomas of the extremities. Results reported by Savlov et al. (1971) and by Luce (1972) on short series indicated tumor regressions in 30%–50% of treated cases. DTIC was well tolerated by the infused arteries, and bone marrow toxicity was low.

The aim of our study was to evaluate how well tolerated and efficient higher doses of DTIC would be when infused into the external carotid artery system. This is a reappraisal of a study on which we have already made a preliminary report (Jortay et al. 1977).

Patients, Materials, and Methods

DTIC as a lyophilized powder was a gift from Miles Laboratories, Belgium. It was diluted in 5% dextrose in water for a daily dose of 400 mg in 900 ml of solution. The 24-h dose was divided into three fresh solutions, and stored protected from light on the infusion set for a 8-h period at 4° C.

The infusion set was connected to the catheter inserted into the temporal artery by a valve device that prevented the outflow of blood. Solutions containing DTIC were run through an Ivac pump. Correct position of the catheter was checked at 3-day intervals by means of an Evans Patent Blue dye infusion. Patients were checked by complete hematologic studies three times a week during therapy.

Five patients entered the study; all had an inoperable invasive malignant melanoma of the maxillofacial region before infusion. Their characteristics are shown in Table 1.

Recent Results in Cancer Research, Vol. 86
© Springer-Verlag Berlin · Heidelberg 1983

Table 1. Intracarotid artery infusion of DTIC for extensive head and neck melanoma

Case	Sex	Age	Site	DTIC total dose/time	Toxicity	Effect on tumor
1	M	65	Cheek	1. 3.5 g/15 days, 25-day interval	1. None	1. > 50% regression
				2. 3.5 g/15 days	2. None	2. Stabilization then progression
2	F	72	Maxillary sinus	1. 6.3 g/22 days, 8-month interval	1. None	1. > 50% regression
				2. 7 g/23 days	2. None	2. None
3	M	60	Hard palate and upper gingiva (lentigo maligna melanoma)	Bilateral infusion 4.2 g/13 days	None	None
4	F	55	Choroid recurring Orbit ethmoid Antrum cheek	8.5 g/25 days	Leukopenia and thrombopenia	Progression
5	M	48	Ethmoid, sphenoid and orbital extension	8 g/20 days	Leukopenia	Progression

Results

The patients received a total of seven intracarotid artery infusions of DTIC. Table 1 reports the data on dosage, toxicity, and effect on the tumor. All patients received metoclopramide (Primperan) orally. None complained of nausea or vomiting. The two cases of bone marrow toxicity consisted in reversible leukopenia and/or thrombopenia. Two patients received two DTIC infusions each; both responded to the first course but failed to respond to the second when a relapse occurred. Within 6 weeks after the last DTIC carotid infusion, three of the five patients, excluding cases no. 2 and 5, underwent radical excision of the tumor. The histologic analysis of the specimens revealed persistent malignant melanoma, with no significant alteration due to the carotid infusion. Only one patient (case no. 4) experienced local recurrence. However, all five patients died of disseminated disease within 3 years after DTIC infusion.

Discussion

This is the first report on intracarotid artery infusions using DTIC, and it indicates the good tolerability of the drug by the vessels, at doses two to three times higher than those used by other authors (Lejeune et al. 1972; Carter 1976). Another factor is the low toxicity encountered during and after this method of chemotherapy, as only two patients experienced bone marrow depression with total doses that reached 8 g. In case no. 4, blood values were restored to normal range after termination of the infusions, and surgery was performed with no difficulties 14 days later. The fact that we had objective responses and systemic toxicity indicate that the drug was active when infused over a 8-h period.

However, since it is now widely recognized that DTIC is very unstable, even when protected from light, it seems advisable to use several bolus DTIC infusions instead of continuous infusion.

With regard to the efficiency of the procedure, two of five patients experienced 50% tumor regression, but a second course of DTIC failed to modify the progression or recurrence of the disease. The question is raised as to whether such a high dose of DTIC would have induced the selection of the tumor cell populations. The same unexplained phenomenon occurred in our 4th case on the first attempt, and the tumor seemed stimulated during the therapy.

We question the value of intra-arterial infusion of DTIC as adjuvant treatment prior to surgery. Our series showed $\frac{1}{3}$ local recurrences, after remission of more than 6 months. However, since all subsequently died of disseminated disease, we can conclude either that they all had micrometastases or that the disease disseminated during the progression of the tumor during treatment. Therefore, efficient systemic treatment must be given after intra-arterial DTIC, regardless of whether this is followed by surgery.

We conclude that intra-arterial infusion of DTIC can be temporarily effective in selected cases of invasive and inoperable melanoma of the maxillofacial region.

Summary

Five inoperable invasive cases of malignant melanoma of the maxillofacial region were treated with seven intracarotid artery infusions of DTIC. Total doses of 3.5−9.5 g of DTIC were continuously administered for 15−25 days. Two of the five patients experienced transient objective regression after the first DTIC infusion but not after the second. Three patients were operated on after infusion and only one had recurrence. However, all patients died with disseminated disease within 3 years after DTIC infusion. Toxicity was encountered in two of seven infusions; it consisted in reversible leukopenia plus thrombopenia and leukopenia alone. These patients had received the highest doses, 9.5 g/25 days and 8 g/20 days respectively.

It is concluded that intra-arterial infusion of DTIC can be temporarily effective in the polydisciplinary treatment of invasive head and neck melanomas.

References

Carter SK (ed) (1976) Proceedings of the 6th New Drug Seminar on DTIC (Bethesda, April 25, 1975). Cancer Treat Rep 60: 123−214

Castermans A, Lejeune FJ, Matton G (1974) Le mélanome cutané. Acta Chir Belg 73: 89−299

Jortay AM (1975) Essae séquentiel sur la chimiothérapie intraartérielle dans les épithéliomas invasifs de la cavité buccale. Communication Assoc Belge de Carcinologie Cervico Faciale (Abstr) October 18, 1975

Joray AM, Lejeune FJ, Kenis Y (1977) Regional chemotherapy of maxillofacial malignant melanoma with intracarotid artery infusion of DTIC. Tumori 63: 299−302

Lejeune FJ, De Wasch G (1978) Malignant melanoma. In: Staquet M (ed) Randomized trials in cancer: a critical review by sites. Raven, New York, pp 339−357

Lejeune FJ, Smets W, Goffin JC (1972) Mélanomes malins cervicofaciaux. Revue de 78 cas. Bull Cancer 59: 255−268

Luce JK (1972) Chemotherapy of malignant melanoma. Cancer 30: 1604−1617

Savlov ED, Hall TC, Oberfield RA (1971) Intra-arterial therapy of melanoma with dimethyl triazeno imidazole carboxamide (NSS-45388). Cancer 28: 1161−1164

Combined Multimodality (Surgery, Radiotherapy, Intra-Arterial Chemotherapy) Treatment of Advanced Carcinoma of Paranasal Sinuses

M. Shafir and E. Raventos

Mount Sinai School of Medicine, City University of New York, New York, NY, USA

Cancer of the paranasal sinuses has attracted the attention of head and neck surgeons, otolaryngologists, plastic surgeons, radiotherapists, oncologists, due to its considerable local malignancy and to the major disfiguration is causes. Advanced carcinomas of the paranasal sinuses represent a particularly challenging problem because of the high rate of therapeutic failures.

Sato (1970) published a study of 68 patients with cancer of the paranasal sinuses treated by surgery, radiotherapy, and intra-arterial chemotherapy, in which he reported significant improvement in short-term survival, very satisfactory cosmetic results, and a short disability period.

Encouraged by these results, we treated a group of patients with advanced carcinomas of the paranasal sinuses; our protocol combined surgery, radiotherapy, and intra-arterial chemotherapy as well. The results, including 5-year follow-up, are presented here.

Material and Methods

The study included 12 patients with advanced squamous cell carcinomas of the paranasal sinuses. There were 11 men and one woman, ranging in age from 32 to 67 years. Five patients were classified T_3 and seven T_4; eight were classified N_0 and four N_1. Following histological confirmation, the extent of the disease was assessed by means of clinical and radiological examinations and a metastatic workup.

The patients were then subjected to retrograde catheterization of the external carotid artery through the superficial temporal artery; a round-tipped polyvinyl catheter with a lateral orifice was used, and its position confirmed by injection of diluted patient blue dye. The vascularity of the tumor was ascertained, and when the entire tumor area and normal surrounding tissue had been infused, the catheter was looped to the skin to avoid later displacement (Fig. 1).

The operative field of the catheterization was isolated and a "debulking" procedure performed, combining as necessary transcutaneous, transnasal, and large-antrostomy approaches in order to excise all gross tumor. The cavity was packed with iodine-vaseline gauze, which was changed daily.

On the first postoperative day intra-arterial chemotherapy and radiotherapy were simultaneously started. We infused 250 mg 5-fluorouracil (5-FU) in normal saline for 1 h, followed 1 h later with 200 rads through the ^{60}Co source, 5 days a week until total doses of

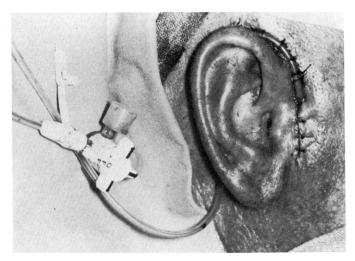

Fig. 1. Placement of external carotid artery catheter through the superficial temporal artery

5,000 mg 5-FU and 4,000 rads were reached. Radiotherapy was continued to tolerance, up to 8,000 rads, encompassing the original tumor volume and the pterigomaxillary fossa. Biopsies were taken from the operative cavity weekly during therapy, and at the end of the treatment. Cervical lymphadenectomy was performed by radical neck dissection 4–6 weeks after completion of this phase of the treatment in patients with clinically suspicious lymphadenopathies.

Results

All 12 patients had severe mucositis and dermatitis, requiring intensive supportive treatment. One developed severe systemic toxicity and died of sepsis shortly after completion of treatment (Figs. 2 and 3). He was the only patient in our series with a tumor extending across the midline, and was consequently treated on both sides.
Of 12 patients, 11 had negative biopsies at completion of the treatment. Two patients experienced recurrence in the pterigomaxillary fossa during the first year of follow-up. Three were still free of disease at the fifth year of follow-up, but the rest of the patients had loco-regional recurrence and developed lung metastases between the first and fifth years of follow-up.

Discussion

Treatment of advanced cancer of the paranasal sinuses is very difficult. Surgery and/or radiotherapy alone rarely achieve control of the disease. Jesse (1965) reported 30% survival at 3 years in a series of 87 patients with squamous cell carcinoma of the maxillary sinus who had received a combination of surgery and radiotherapy.
In recent years increasing interest has developed in a combined approach, utilizing chemotherapy, particularly intra-arterial, and radiotherapy. Donegan and Harris (1976) reported on 15 cases of recurrent advanced head and neck cancer (after surgery, of surgery

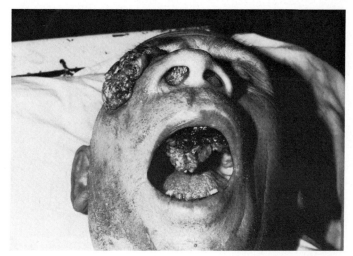

Fig. 2. Squamous cell carcinoma of both maxillary sinuses, fistulized through skin, nasal fossa, and oral cavity; pretreatment period is shown

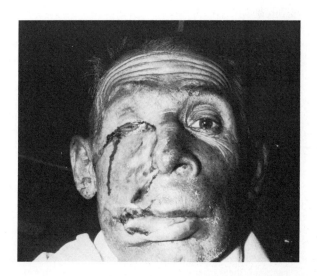

Fig. 3. Posttreatment appearance of same patient as shown in Fig. 2

plus radiotherapy) who were treated with intra-arterial 5-FU, methotrexate, and bleomycin; 87% objective response was obtained, with 20% complete regression. The regressions lasted for up to 13 months.

Auersperg et al. (1978) reported on 74 patients with advanced cancer of the oral cavity and oropharynx, treated by radiation, or intra-arterial chemotherapy, or a combination of the two. The highest response was observed in the group which received the combination therapy. Nervi et al. (1978) conducted a randomized study comparing radiotherapy alone with radiotherapy preceded by intra-arterial chemotherapy with methotrexate, in advanced carcinomas of the head and neck. Follow-up for 4 years showed a statistically significant better local control and survival rate for cancers of the oral cavity than obtained with other treatments.

Foye et al. (1960) showed a potentiation of radiation by 5-FU. In 1969, Jesse et al. reported on 46 patients with inoperable advanced cancers of the head and neck treated with intra-arterial 5-FU and radiotherapy; ten of these patients had a complete temporary regression of the tumor; eight of them remained free of disease for 18 months.

Our series demonstrates a multimodality approach which has a sound theoretical advantage − the surgery achieves an immediate reduction in the tumor load, thus allowing the radiotherapy a better chance of success. The 5-FU delivered intra-arterially immediately prior to the radiation achieves a high concentration in the involved area and, by the intense inflammation it produces, increases the vascularity and oxygenation, presumably rendering the radiotherapy more effective.

Conclusion

Our therapeutic regimen was well tolerated, and was cosmetically very acceptable. The survival rate for our series compares favorably with those reported for other forms of treatment. The positive results warrant further studies in this field.

References

Auersberg M, Furlan L, Marolt F, Jereg B (1978) Intra-arterial chemotherapy and radiotherapy in locally advanced cancer of the oral cavity and oropharynx. Int J Radiat Oncol Biol Phys 4: 273−277

Donegan L, Harris P (1976) Regional chemotherapy with combined drugs in cancer of the head and neck. Cancer 38: 1479−1483

Foye LV Jr, Willet FM, Hall B, Roth M (1960) Potentiation of radiation effects with 5-fluorouracil. Cancer Chemother Rep 6: 12−15

Jesse RH (1965) Pre-operative vs. post-operative radiation in the treatment of squamous carcinoma of the paranasal sinuses. Am J Surg 110: 552−556

Jesse RH, Goepfert H, Lindberg RD, Johnson RH (1969) Combined intra-arterial infusion and radiotherapy for the treatment of advanced cancer of the head and neck. Am J Roentgenol Radium Ther Nucl Med 105: 20−25

Nervi C, Arcangeli G, Badaracco G, Cortese M, Morelli M, Starace G (1978) The relevance of tumor size and cell kinetics as predictors of radiation response in head and neck cancer. Cancer 41: 900−906

Sato Y, Morita M, Takahashi H, Watanabe N, Kirikae I (1970) Combined surgery, radiotherapy, and regional chemotherapy in carcinoma of the paranasal sinuses. Cancer 25: 571−579

A Special Method of Intra-Arterial Infusion for Treatment of Head and Neck Cancer

J. v. Scheel, W. Krautzberger, B. Foth, and E.R. Kastenbauer

ENT-Abteilung, Klinikum Charlottenburg, Freie Universität Berlin,
Spandauer Damm 130, 1000 Berlin 19, FRG

Recent developments in head and neck oncology include an increase in the administration of chemotherapy in advanced, previously untreated tumors (Moore 1980; Schroeder and von Heyden 1981). The efficacy of chemotherapy can be improved considerably by using the intra-arterial (i.a.) infusion route originally proposed by Bierman et al. (1951) and Sullivan et al. (1953). The advantage of i.a. infusion can be further enhanced by a) infusing in an artery which receives a small fraction of the cardiac output (selective infusion), or b) by infusing a drug which has a low integral of recirculation (Eckman et al. 1974; Chen and Gross 1980). Moreover, prolonged infusion theoretically allows for exposure to a quantitatively greater number of cells during a sensitive phase of the cell cycle (Lokich 1980).

A critical evaluation of the most widely used methods of intra-arterial infusion – especially the Seldinger technique and cannulation of the superficial temporal artery – indicated comparatively narrow limits concerning selective and prolonged infusion which have previously been described in detail (von Scheel 1981). These findings culminated in the evolution of a new technique facilitating selective and prolonged intra-arterial infusion, in an attempt to increase the percentage of complete remissions.

Materials and Methods

The basic principle underlying the new method consists of the vascular-surgical construction of a subcutaneously palpable arterial blood vessel, which is easily punctured for i.a. infusion. The (inoperable) primary tumor is not removed by surgery, but rather treated by percutaneous, intra-arterial chemotherapy by intermittent cannulation of the vascular graft.

Surgical Technique

Immediately subsequent to radical neck dissection, the external carotid artery is severed at its origin from the common carotid artery. The latter is closed using a vein patch, or the stump of the external carotid artery is ligated if it is long enough. If the stump is too short, the external carotid artery may also be severed between the superior thyroid and the lingual artery. The proximal end of the external carotid artery is then sutured end-to-end to

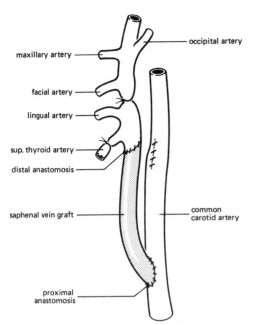

maxillary artery

occipital artery

facial artery

lingual artery

sup. thyroid artery

distal anastomosis

saphenal vein graft

common
carotid artery

proximal
anastomosis

Fig. 1. The anatomic situation after completion of the vascular anastomoses. Modification in patients with tumors supported by the left lingual artery. Cytostatic drugs infused to the subcutaneously palpable vein graft are supplied solely to the tumor region, since all branches of the external carotid artery not contributing to the blood supply in the tumor region are ligated during neck dissection

an autogenic saphenous vein graft taken from the thigh. The length of the graft should be 8–10 cm. The proximal end of the graft is connected end-to-side with the common carotid artery (Fig. 1). The proximal anastomosis should be performed initially, while retrograde blood supply of the internal carotid artery is maintained. Anticoagulation therapy with heparin should be performed immediately prior to the vascular-surgical procedure. All large branches of the external carotid artery not directly contributing to the blood supply in the tumor region must be ligated. This requires only two ligatures, for example, in patients with tumors of the tongue (Fig. 1).

Performance of Intra-arterial Chemotherapy

The skin sutures are removed on about the 7th postoperative day. Intra-arterial cytostatic drug therapy can be started on the 10th postoperative day. The vein graft is easily palpable due to its pulsation and to the removal of the sternocleidomastoid muscle during neck dissection. It can be punctured easily using a thin plastic cannula (Fig. 2) connected to a volumetric infusion pump. The correct positioning of the cannula is controlled fluoroscopically or by dye injection. Anticoagulation therapy with heparin or coumarin should be performed. The cannula may be removed during interruptions in therapy and is easily reinserted at the beginning of the next course of treatment. Intra-arterial chemotherapy is performed over several weeks or months in this way until complete remission is achieved. If early thrombosis of the vascular graft occurs, chemotherapy is continued intravenously. Subsequent irradiation therapy is mandatory in all cases.
The treatment schedule can be summarized as follows:

1. Neck dissection with vascular-surgical preparation of the neck arteries; primary tumor is not resected.
2. Intra-arterial chemotherapy.
3. Irradiation therapy.

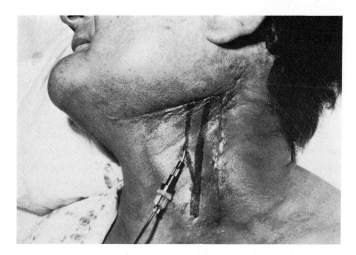

Fig. 2. The left side of the neck after neck dissection and vascular-surgical preparation for intra-arterial chemotherapy, which is to be initiated about 10 days postoperatively. The lines drawn on the skin indicate the position of the common carotid artery (*right*) and the saphenous vein graft (*left*)

Twelve patients have been treated so far according to this method. Two of them received methotrexate (MTX) with folinic acid rescue, and bleomycin (BLEO). In eight patients monotherapy with *cis*-diamminedichloroplatinum (DDP) was performed. Two patients had MTX/BLEO over a 4-week period, followed by DDP monotherapy, which was given intra-arterially as well. The daily dosage of DDP was 20 mg infused over 8 h, three times weekly. Anticoagulation consisted of low-dose heparin, thrombocyte aggregation inhibitors, or coumarin. Of the patients, 11 had squamous cell carcinoma and one, adenoid cystic carcinoma.

Results

Four of the patients had only partial remission because of early thrombosis of the artery infused. In these cases chemotherapy was continued intravenously. However, eight patients had complete remission, requiring i.a. treatment over a period of at least 4 weeks. The longest period of (intermittent) i.a. therapy was 10 weeks. Two patients exhibiting incomplete response after 4 weeks of treatment with MTX/BLEO achieved complete remission after additional i.a. infusion of DDP.

All patients with complete remission are now free of disease, the longest follow-up period being 22 months in two cases.

Comments

This new method has the following advantages over other intra-arterial infusion methods:

1. Regional chemotherapy may be performed over a prolonged period of time, i.e., several weeks or months. The Seldinger technique, by contrast, is limited to several hours and cannot be performed very frequently (Calvo et al. 1980).

2. Intra-arterial therapy can be repeated after interruptions during which the cannula has been removed. This is not possible in most cases involving cannulation of the superior temporal artery, because the cannulated vessel is usually obstructed by thrombosis after removal of the catheter.
3. A high degree of selectivity can be achieved by infusion into the artery feeding the tumor; selectivity of infusion is one of the prerequisites for increasing the concentration of drugs at the tumor site to an appreciable amount (Chen and Gross 1980).

Only advanced inoperable tumors in categories T_3 and T_4 (UICC) should be treated. Involvement of regional lymph nodes includes N_1, N_2 and also N_0, as a high percentage of clinically negative necks are found to be histologically positive (Kalnins et al. 1977). The tumors must be inoperable and/or located in a region where surgical destruction would lead to considerable functional deterioration in the patient. Primarily operable tumors with a better prognosis must be treated by surgery and irradiation. Further criteria are:

1. The patient should not be older than 65 years, as vascular surgery becomes more complex with increasing age.
2. There should have been no previous treatment.
3. Typical contraindications to chemotherapy and anticoagulation must be observed.
4. The tumor should be restricted to an area supplied by few but distinct branches of the external carotid artery.

The risk involved in this new method is not greater than that inherent in radical neck dissection itself. In no patient treated according to the method has a serious complication occurred to date. The vascular-surgical procedures (the preparation of the saphenous vein graft and its interposition to the neck arteries) require 1 h more than does conventional radical neck dissection.

The results obtained so far are encouraging, as a relatively high percentage of overall responses and complete remissions could be achieved. The complete remission of an adenoid cystic carcinoma, a type of tumor which is known to be particularly resistant to any kind of therapy, is especially noticeable. Thus, DDP has proved to be a very potent drug in i.a. therapy.

It is concluded that this new method facilitates reliably selective, percutaneous intra-arterial infusion over a prolonged period of time. It is possible, however, that the results may be further improved by the use of other drugs or schedules, or by the intensification of anticoagulation therapy.

Summary

Immediately after radical neck dissection the external carotid artery is lengthened by an autogenic saphenous vein graft and sutured more proximally to the common carotid artery. All branches of the external carotid artery not contributing to the blood supply in the tumor region are ligated. After the wound has healed, the vascular graft will be easily palpable and can be punctured repeatedly for *highly selective* intra-arterial chemotherapy of the inoperable primary tumor for a *prolonged period of time*. The method seems to be practicable, innocuous, and more effective than conventional methods of intra-arterial chemotherapy for head and neck cancer.

References

Bierman HR, Kelly KH, Byron RL, Dod KS, Shimkin MB (1951) Studies on the blood supply of tumours in man. II. Intra-arterial nitrogen mustard therapy of cutaneous lesion. J Natl Cancer Inst 11: 891−904

Calvo DB, Patt YZ, Wallace S, Chuang VP, Benjamin RS, Pritchard JD, Hersh EM, Bodey GP, Mavligit GM (1980) Phase I−II trial of percutanous intra-arterial cis-diamminedichloroplatinum (II) for regionally confined malignancy. Cancer 45: 1278−1283

Chen HSG, gross JF (1980) Intra-arterial infusion of anticancer drugs: Theoretic aspects of drug delivery and review of responses. Cancer Treat Rep 64: 31−40

Eckman WW, Patlak CS, Fenstermacher JD (1974) A critical evaluation of the principles governing the advantages of intra-arterial infusions. J Pharmacokinet Biopharm 2: 257−285

Kalnins IK, Leonard AG, Sako K, Razack MS, Shedd DP (1977) Correlations between prognosis and degree of lymph node involvement in carcinoma of the oral cavity. Am J Surg 134: 450−454

Lokich JJ (1980) Phase I study of cis-diamminedichloroplatinum (II) administered as a constant 5-day infusion. Cancer Treat Rep 94: 905−908

Moore C (1980) Changing concepts in head and neck surgical oncology. Am J Surg 140: 480−486

Schroeder M, von Heyden HW (1981) The role of chemotherapy in squamous cell cancer of the head and neck. HNO 29: 225−239

Sullivan RD, Jones R, Schnabel TG, Shorey J (1953) The treatment of human cancer with intra-arterial nitrogen mustard utilizing a simplified catheter technique. Cancer 6: 121−134

von Scheel J (1981) Methodical aspects of intra-arterial chemotherapy of malignant head und neck tumors. Laryngol Rhinol 60: 275−277

Indications and Counterindications
of Intra-Arterial Chemotherapy of Head and Neck Tumors

G. Szabó

Department of Oral- and Maxillofacial Surgery, Semmelweis University of Medicine,
1085 Budapest, Mária u. 52, Hungary

In a study of 373 patients with tumors of the head and neck area, we employed regional chemotherapy in over 200 cases and general chemotherapy in more than 300 (see Table 1). The main purpose of this study was to determine the area of indication for intra-arterial chemotherapy. Various examinations — patent blue staining of the eye fundus, xeroarteriography, and angioscintigraphy — were carried out in an effort to understand and explain the successes or failures of regional chemotherapy.

To avoid the most serious complication of intra-arterial treatment — thrombosis of the common or internal carotid artery — it is important that a fundus examination be performed after insertion of the indwelling catheter. If the blue dye passes into the common carotid artery, the arteries of the fundus will be stained blue 1—2 s after the injection, as will the veins of the fundus, 5—6 s later. After 10 s the arteries are again red, while the veins are still blue. After 15 s the dye can no longer be seen in the fundus. This is

Table 1. Distribution of tumors according to location

Tumors	Chemotherapy	
	i.a.	General
	(No. of cases)[a]	
Tongue	40	64
Floor of the mouth	31	66
Tonsil	14	13
Gingiva	10	16
Mandible	5	7
Palate	11	20
Parotid gland	28	16
Pterygoid area	8	10
Bucca	12	19
Skin of face	8	14
Cervical region	9	18
Lower and upper lip	5	14
Total	205	308

[a] There were 140 patients treated with both general and regional chemotherapy

Recent Results in Cancer Research, Vol. 86
© Springer-Verlag Berlin · Heidelberg 1983

of great importance, for the staining examination may be repeated immediately after retraction of the catheter, so that the new location can be checked.

Intra-arterial chemotherapy is *recommended* for *preoperative purposes* in cases of tumor situated in the parotid, maxillary, retromaxillary, and soft palatal regions; for *postoperative purposes* after removal of extensive or radiation-insensitive tumors (e.g., adenocarcinoma, cylindroma); for *palliative purposes* in the above mentioned cases, in the tonsillar region, and in those sarcomatous tumors which are well suppled with blood (Figs. 1–4).

It is *not recommended* in cases of radically operable carcinomas of the tongue, floor of the mouth, and lip.

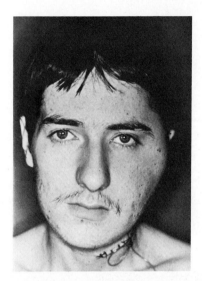

Fig. 1. Patient with sarcomatous lesion (round-cell sarcoma) in the left temporal and parotid region; before i.a. chemotherapy

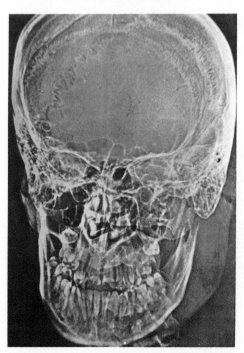

Fig. 2. Same patient as in Fig. 1; xeroradiography. The tumor has destroyed the left zygomatic arch and the temporomandibular joint

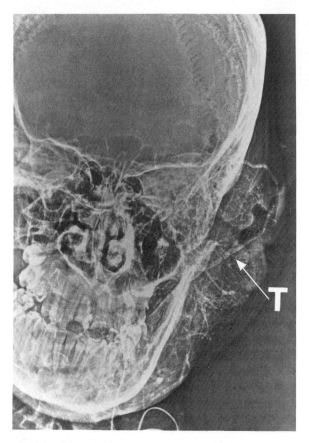 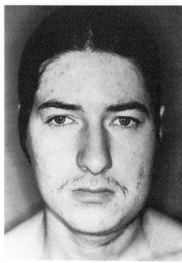

Fig. 3 *(Left)*. Same patient as in Figs. 1 and 2; xeroarteriography. The catheter was introduced via the superior thyroid artery. The tumorous lesion which is well supplied with blood is clearly visible. *T*, superficial temporal artery

Fig. 4 *(Right)*. Same patient as in Figs. 1–3; after the i.a. chemotherapy the tumorous lesion disappeared

Basic Principles in Hyperthermic Tumor Therapy

F. Dietzel

Strahlentherapeutische Abteilung, Städtische Krankenanstalten,
Kulmbacher Straße 23, 8580 Bayreuth, FRG

Introduction

The first report of heat being useful in cancer treatment is by Busch (1866), who noted the disappearance of a sarcoma after high fever caused by erysipelas. Bruns (1887) reviewed all cases of tumor regression after fever reported in literature. Coley (1893) injected patients with bacterial toxins deliberately to cause fever. There are many reports in the early 1900s of the use of applied hyperthermia in treating cancer. Interest declined during the 1930s, due in part to the advent of antibacterial agents; consequently, the number of studies diminished. There was then a period of renewed interest in hyperthermia, for example, in the possibility of combining heat with X-rays, but because heat application was technically difficult and therapeutic results of megavoltage radiotherapy by photons and electrons were excellent, hyperthermia disappeared again as a therapeutic agent.

During the past 10 years there has been an enormous increase in interest in the use of heat to treat cancer. The amount of literature on hyperthermic tumor therapy has grown exponentially. A review by Dietzel (1975) lists more than 900 references to papers published over a period of more than 100 years.

Three international symposia on cancer therapy by hyperthermia have been held, the first in 1975 in Washington, DC, the second in 1977 in Essen, FRG (Streffer et al. 1978), and the third in 1980 in Fort Collins, Colorado, USA. The proceedings of these three congresses give an exhaustive review on the present status of research in hpyerthermia as a cancer treatment modality.

Hyperthermia is of clinical interest in the temperature range of $40°-43°$ C. Higher temperatures of $44°-46°$ C are not feasible clinically. Whole-body hyperthermia in men is physiologically limited, because the rate of complications increases exponentially above $42°$ C. Only with local heat application is a higher elevation of tissue temperature possible and tolerable.

This paper focuses on six areas involved in principal hyperthermic effects on tumor cells in vitro and in vivo.

Hyperthermic Effects on Cellular Proliferation

Heat, itself, is a lethal agent to the cell in vitro. Survival of cells is dependant on both the temperature applied and the duration of exposure. Figure 1 shows the response of

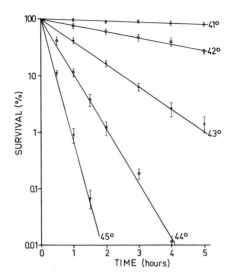

Fig. 1. Survival curves of HeLa cells exposed to elevated temperatures for different time periods

asynchronous HeLa cells in culture to different temperatures for varying time periods. Above 41° C, cell survival is seen to decrease exponentially as a function of exposure time.

Unlike cellular responses to X-rays, there is a markedly higher sensitivity of S-phase cells to heat (Westra and Dewey 1971). S-phase cells are relatively radioresistant. Also heat-sensitive is the M phase in which, the heat target is the spindle proteins; heating in the M phase produces polyploid cells. Synchronization of cell proliferation by heat shock is possible. The cytotoxic effects of hyperthermia and ionizing radiation complement each other during the cell cycle of exponentially growing cultures.

The synthesis of proteins, RNA, and DNA is inhibited after heat treatment (Mondovi et al. 1969a, b), but all three processes are not inhibited at the same time; RNA synthesis appears to be inhibited by less severe treatment than that required to inhibit DNA and protein synthesis (Dickson and Shah 1972). Some inhibitors of protein synthesis protect against the effects of heat, while all RNA-synthesis inhibitors increase the effects of heat (Palzer and Heidelberger 1973). From these results it can be concluded that primarily RNA synthesis is inhibited before DNA and protein synthesis decrease.

Hyperthermia, Oxygenation, pH-Value, Malnutrition

Hyperthermia above 41° C in mammalian cells causes decreased O_2 consumption. The aerobic glycolysis at higher temperatures decreases rapidly (Fig. 2), but anaerobic glycolysis is more resistant to higher temperature.

H. K. Kim et al. (1978) showed that an inhibitor of anaerobic glycolysis, 5-thio-D-glucose, can greatly increase the effect of hyperthermia on hypoxic cells in vitro. This observation seems to suggest that energy metabolism plays a role in heat-induced cell death.

The consequence of heating tissue to above 41° C is a decrease in pH-value. Figure 3, derived from data of Vaupel (1982), demonstrates this phenomenon in a typical manner.

The influence of nutritional factors was studied by Hahn (1974), who reported that the presence or absence of glucose, serum, and some other substances strongly influenced

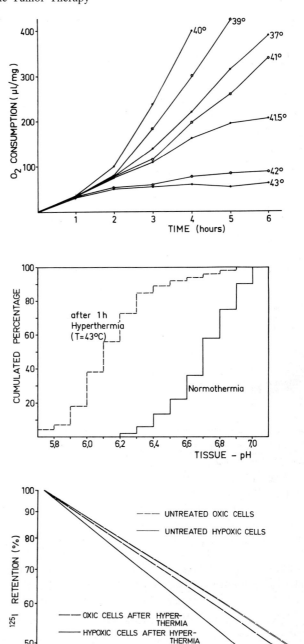

Fig. 2. O$_2$ consumption of mammalian cell population (SDB) under different temperatures (after Dickson and Shah 1972)

Fig. 3. Cumulative percentage of pH values in experimental tumors after hyperthermic treatment (after Vaupel 1982)

Fig. 4. Cell-loss rate in a tumor after hyperthermic treatment, measured by ^{125}I retention (after Dietzel et al. 1976)

chlonogenicity after hyperthermia. An even greater effect was observed when the pH of the surrounding cell-culture medium was low (Overgaard 1976; Freeman et al. 1977; Overgaard and Bichel 1977; Gerweck and Burlett 1978); a decrease in the pH from 4.7 to 6.4 dramatically increased the effect of hyperthermia.

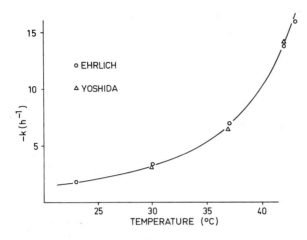

Fig. 5. Fluorescein-outflow rate at different temperature conditions in Ehrlich- (*O*) and Yoshida- (*A*) -ascites cells (after Strom et al. 1973)

Heat predominantly inactivates hypoxic cells in a tumor, as measurements of cell loss rate (Dietzel et al. 1978) demonstrate (Fig. 4). Solid experimental tumors show this response to heat, in the same way as do tumor cells in vitro under different oxygenation conditions, or spheroid tumors in vitro.

Hyperthermia and Membranes

Membranes have many important functions in the cell; in addition to the separation of several intracellular compartments, a role in many enzymatic processes has been reported (for a review see Harrison and Lunt 1975).

Wallach (1978) has reviewed reports on the possible involvement of membranes in the effects of hyperthermia. He suggests that the sudden change in slope of the Arrhenius curve which was found for heat-induced cell death (Dewey et al. 1977a, b) is probably caused by the influence of decreased viscosity of the lipid contents of the membrane on the stability of the protein content. A number of membrane-active agents may change the heat sensitivity of cells. Examples are procaine (Yatvin 1977), amphotericin B (Hahn 1978), and alcohol (Hahn et al. 1977).

Several membrane functions, such as the maintenance of membrane potential (Mikkelsen et al. 1978), adenylcyclase activity, the uptake and outflow of aminoisobutyrate, and the possibility of maintaining pH homeostasis inside cells (Haveman 1979), have also been shown to be influenced by hyperthermia. In addition, the capacity of cells to attach to culture vessels is decreased (Lin et al. 1978). This last observation may explain the increased rate of metastasis observed by Dickson and Ellis (1976) and Yerushalmi (1976a).

Cellular membranes consist of unsaturated lipid acids. At higher temperatures membrane function becomes insufficient, as the exponentially increasing outflow of fluorescein from Ehrlich-Ascites-Ca cells (O) and Yoshida-Ascites cells (A) demonstrates (Fig. 5).

Hyperthermia and Animal Tumors In Vivo

Crile (1963) described results of experiments designed to evaluate the effectiveness of hyperthermia, alone or combined with irradiation, in the treatment of S 180 sarcomas

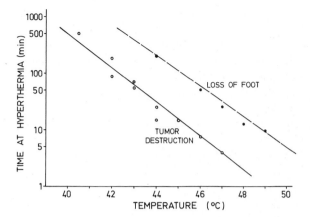

Fig. 6. Relationship between time at hyperthermia and level of hyperthermia to produce destruction of tumor in treated mice or loss of foot (after Crile 1963)

growing as transplants in the foot pads of mice. He found that 7-mm diameter tumors were readily destroyed by local hyperthermia applied by immersion of the tumor-bearing foot in a water bath. For example (Fig. 6), the majority of the treated animals were cured of their tumor by a 30-min treatment at 44° C. This was a clinically effective treatment since normal tissue damage was trivial; approximately 200 min more were required to cause loss of the foot in 50% of treated mice. Crile observed that the time required to produce a specified effect (eradication of tumor or loss of foot of the treated animal) was reduced by a factor of 2 for each rise of 1° C (Fig. 6).

Immunogenicity of Tumor Cells Following Inactivation by Moderate Levels of Hyperthermia. A report by Mondovi et al. (1972) suggests that Ehrlich-ascites cells exposed to 43.5° C for 3 h have greater immunogenicity than similar cells inactivated by x-irradiation. There are only a few reports published on this subject, and it clearly merits further attention.

Sensitivity of Hypoxic Tissues to Hyperthermia. Several studies on in vitro cell systems indicate that hypoxic cells are equally, or perhaps more, sensitive to the damaging effects of hyperthermia than are aerobic cells. Schulman and Hall (1974) determined hyperthermic cell survival curves for V79 Chinese hamster cells cultured under normal or hypoxic conditions; survival curves for aerobic cells at 43° C and hypoxic cells at 41° C, i.e., a 2° C difference, were of approximately the same slope.
Gerweck and Burlett (1978) found that inactivation of aerobic CHO cells increases dramatically as pH is reduced to below 6.9. The thermal sensitivity of tumor cells in vivo as a function of distance from capillary or as a function of pO_2 is an important subject for future experimentation.

Hyperthermia and Incidence of Metastases. A major concern regarding the response of tumor tissue to hyperthermia is the possible effect of such treatment on the stimulation of metastatic disease. Several authors (Dickson and Ellis 1974) examined the incidence of distant metastatic disease appearing in rats following treatment of Yoshida sarcoma transplants by whole-body or local hyperthermia. Hyperthermia in that system, when unsuccessful in achieving destruction of the transplanted tumor, was associated with an increased incidence of metastatic disease and a reduced survival time following both local and systemic hyperthermia (Dickson and Ellis 1976). However, this was contradicted by authors who found no increase in metastatic spread (Hahn et al. 1979).

Indications for the Influence of Immunological Factors. Several observations suggest that hyperthermia can also influence tumor growth through an immunological mechanism. Injection of heat-treated cells inhibited the percentage takes of transplanted tumor material much more strongly than did the injection of irradiated cells (Mondovi et al. 1972; Castillo and Goldsmith 1973).

Moreover, evidence has been reported that heat can change the function of the immune apparatus. In tumor-bearing rabbits several immunologic parameters were enhanced after local heat treatment (Dickson and Shah 1978). The effect of hyperthermia on tumors in mice and rats was increased by the administration of substances which potentiate immune defense (Szmigielski and Janiak 1978). In contrast, whole-body hyperthermia seemed to depress immunological reactions in rabbits (Dickson and Shah 1978), rats (Williams and Galt 1978), and man (Gee et al. 1978).

Hyperthermia and Cytotoxic Drugs

The thermodynamic inactivation of cells by hyperthermia may be expressed in the form of an Arrhenius plot, in which the inactivation rate determined from the exponential region of the survival curve $[k(min^{-1})]$ is determined as a function of the reciprocal of the exposure temperature. It is clear from Fig. 7, which shows several different cell lines from several laboratories, that there is a break in the inactivation curves, occurring at 43° C. The biological meaning of this inflection is not clear; however, 43° C seems to be a critical temperature. The mode of cell killing at temperatures above 43° C is similar, and independent of cell line (note that net sensitivities may differ by as much as a factor of 10), with activation energies in the range of 150 ± 25 kcal. Also at temperatures above 43° C, the biological response (inactivation rate) increases by a factor of 2 for each 1° C increase in the exposure temperature. At temperatures below 43° C, these generalities and multiple cell-line similarities no longer apply. This may reflect different targets for cytotoxicity above or below 43° C, or it may result from different inactivation rates of the same target(s). However, this could have important clinical implications if, for example, the malignant tissue to be treated is at 43° C or less compared to the surrounding normal tissue (or vice versa). The problem of local "hot spots" produced in some modes of heating is of particular concern in this regard. These data serve to emphasize the need for uniform temperature control and precise temperature measurements when hyperthermia is applied clinically.

Experiments to evaluate whole-body hyperthermia as an adjunct to chemotherapy in induced tumors in mice failed to demonstrate improved therapeutic response of different tumors to different drugs, such as cyclophosphamide, methyl-CCNU, vincristine, actinomycin D, adriamycin, and 5-fluorouracil (Rose et al. 1979).

In contrast, there have been encouraging reports on local hyperthermia by means of arterial limb or organ perfusion in the last few years. Combinations of hyperthermia and cytostatic drugs have been used clinically for more than 15 years. Regional arterial perfusion in the head (Woodhall et al. 1960) and extremities (Stehlin et al. 1975) was performed with heated perfusion fluid. The latter group reported important improvement in the cure rate, resulting from the addition of heat to regional chemotherapy for malignant melanomas.

Data from in vitro experiments on the interaction of heat and cytostatic drugs are rather scarce. They were reviewed by Hahn (1978). Three types of interaction between hyperthermia and drugs can be dinstinguished.

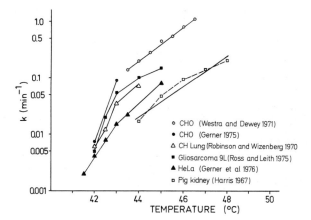

Fig. 7. Arrhenius plot for heat
inactivation of various cell lines

First, the activity of many drugs increases slightly with temperature. Arrhenius plots of these processes show only slight slopes, and activation energy is low, about 80 kJ · mole^{-1}. No special effects are observed above 42.0° C. Examples of drugs which show a similar pattern are the hypoxic sensitizer Ro-07-0582 (Stratford and Adams 1977) and the alkylating agents thio-TEPA (Johnson and Pavelec 1973), carmustine (BCNU), lomustine (CCNU), and methyl-CCNU (Hahn 1978).

A second type of mechanism is seen with cytotixic drugs which exhibit greatly increased effectiveness at temperatures above 42° C. For example, the uptake of adriamycin in the nucleus of cells was greater when hyperthermia was applied, while with bleomycin, heating inhibited the repair of potentially lethal damage (Hahn et al. 1975).

The third type of interaction involves drugs which are not active at normal temperatures, but become efficient once a temperature of 42.0° C is reached. Amphotericin B and various alcohols belong to this group. Their effect is attributed to an influence on the viscosity of the membranes.

The local application of heat may help to localize the field of action of drug. Shingleton (1962) cooled the major part of the bodies of dogs to about 32° C and heated the target areas to 41° C and 43° C; the uptake of labeled nitrogen mustard was much higher in the heated area. The same procedure was applied to patients (Shingleton 1962). A similar effect was reported by Overgaard (1976). Local heat after intraperitoneal injection of adriamycin increased the number of cures in tumor-bearing mice and decreased the side effects in the rest of the body. To date only local thermochemotherapy allows randomized phase-III studies in clinical application.

Hyperthermia and Radiation

The interest of the radiation therapist in hyperthermia as a possible, clinically important, antitumor-treatment modality, especially when combined with local irradiation, has been powerfully stimulated by several findings in thermobiological research. First, the hyperthermic sensitivity of mammalian cells is greatest in the S phase of the cell replication cycle, the phase of maximum resistance to X-radiation damage. Second, the oxygen enhancement ratio (OER) for thermal damage is apparently much less than the OER for radiation damage, and may be as low as 1. Third, radiation sensitivity of mammalian cells is increased by moderate and tolerable levels of hyperthermia. Fourth, these moderate and

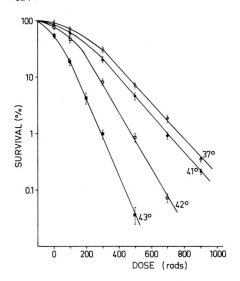

Fig. 8. Potentiation of radiation cell-killing by hyperthermic treatment. Cells (CHO) were pretreated prior to X-irradiation by exposure to different levels of hyperthermia (1 h for all exposures)

tolerable levels, when applied locally to tumors in experimental animals, have been shown in many instances to cause regression of the observed tumor mass, in some cases permanent and complete. Finally, the response of tumor and normal tissue to ionizing radiation is enhanced by concomitant administration of hyperthermia.

The combination of hyperthermia and ionizing radiation results in greater cytotoxicity than can be accounted for by addition of the cytotoxic effects of both agents when employed alone. This synergistic interaction is shown in Fig. 8, where cell survival has been normalized to show only the potentiation of radiation cell killing when combined with pre-irradiation hyperthermic doses (1 h) at temperatures from 41° C to 43° C. The survival-curve slopes increase with increasing temperature.

This potentiation of radiation response by hyperthermia is seen plotted in another manner in Fig. 9. Here cell survival, showing total cell killing due to both hyperthermia and X-irradiation, is graphed for a clinically pertinent dose (400 rad). This figure demonstrates that at 42° C and 43° C, a marked interaction is obtained for both pre- and post-irradiation 1-h thermal doses.

Since clinically useful doses are in the range of 100−600 rad per fraction, thermal enhancement ratio (TER) values in this region may be most important. It is clear that dramatic synergism occurs at temperatures of 42° C or more for doses as low as 200 rad.

The rationale for the combination of hyperthermia and ionizing radiation in radiation therapy stems from several factors. As previously discussed, the age-response functions (cell cycle specific survival responses) for these two modalities are complementary. When the two agents are combined, radioresistant S-phase cells are more sensitive to heat than G_1 phase cells.

Not only is hyperthermia complementary to radiation in its cell cycle specific killing response; it also acts to interfere with two different radiation damage recovery mechanisms.

Ben-Hur et al. (1974) have shown that a primary effect of hyperthermia is to inhibit cellular recovery from sublethal radiation damage. The interference of hyperthermia in these radiation repair systems may be a prime reason for the observed synergistic interaction of the two modalities.

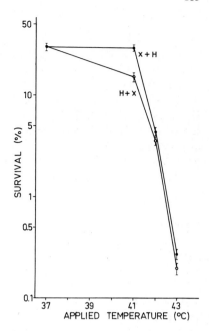

Fig. 9. Survival response of asynchronously growing CHO cells exposed to various temperatures for 1 h, and also given a radiation exposure of 400 rad either immediately prior to $(x + H)$, or immediately after $(H + x)$ the heat treatment

Fig. 10. The relevance of sequence and time interval between hyperthermia and irradiation on survival response; x, radiation exposure; H, heat treatment; □, 17.5 min/42.5° C; ●, 40 min/42.5° C (after Sapareto et al. 1978)

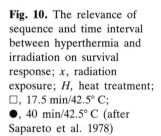

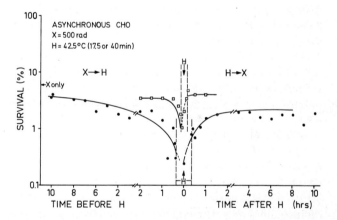

The effect of sequence on interaction of hyperthermia and radiation has been the subject of a number of studies. Many suggest that sequence is not important while an equal number indicate that either pre-, post-, or simultaneous application of heat with radiation results in greatest cytotoxicity. For practical clinical application it is important to combine hyperthermia and radiation at close intervals. The data of Sapareto et al. (1978) show very clearly that a superadditive enhancement effect is possible only if hyperthermia and radiation follow each other within 10 or 20 min (Fig. 10).

Not only the effect of radiation on tumors, but also the radiation-induced damage to normal tissues was increased by hyperthermia. The radiation reaction of human skin (Barth and Wachsmann 1948) and the radiation fibrosis of the bladder wall in dogs (Cockett et al. 1967) was increased by heat.

Quantitative information has been obtained in rodents. The skin reactions of mice (Robinson et al. 1974; Thrall et al. 1975; Stewart and Denekamp 1977), growth inhibition of the baby rat tail (Myers and Field 1977), mucosal damage of the intestine (Field et al. 1977), and effects on the central nervous system (Miller et al. 1976; Goffinet et al. 1977) were all enhanced by heating after irradiation.

There are also discrepancies with regard to therapeutic gain among reports in which the TER in mouse tumors and in mouse skin was compared. Some authors reported a distinct therapeutic gain by addition of hyperthermia to irradiation (Robinson et al. 1974). However, another group found no gain, as the TER for tumors in their experiments was similar to the TER for skin (Stewart and Denekamp 1978). One group noted a gain only under certain conditions (Thrall et al. 1975). Experiments by Dietzel et al. (1982) with solid neck tumors in mice showed a clear therapeutic gain regarding tumor control and survival on the one hand and, local skin reaction and radiogenic myelopathia on the other.

Summary

Literature on hyperthermic tumor therapy in the past 10 years has grown exponentially. Since 1975 three international symposia on cancer therapy by hyperthermia have been held. Hyperthermia is of clinical interest in the temperature range of $40°-43°$ C. Higher temperatures of $44°-46°$ C are not clinically realizable. With local heat application a higher elevation of tissue temperature is possible. Whole-body hyperthermia in men is limited physiologically, as the rate of complications increases exponentially above $42°$ C. The heat dose normally is defined by temperature degree and time of temperature elevation. Hyperthermia has several effects on tumor cells. It influences proliferation activity; whithin the mitotic cycle, preferentially the M-phase cells and S-phase cells are thermosensitive. It is possible to synchronize tumor proliferation by heat. Hyperthermia inactivates tumor cells in hypoxic condition as well. This was demonstrated in vitro with tumor cells under varying oxygenation and with spheroid experimental tumors. Experiments with solid tumors in animals had the same effect. Hyperthermia enhances the effect of radiation on tumors.

In solid human tumors only $3\%-5\%$ of cells are in growth fraction; 95% of tumor cells are hypoxic or prenecrobiotic. Only well-oxygenated cells are sensitive to a sparsely ionizing radiation and can be killed. This selective radiosensitivity is the reason why other radiation qualities for radiotherapy, which are also effective on hypoxic cells, are examined. Neutrons and heavy ions are densely ionizing radiations, which inactivate hypoxic radioresistant cells. Hyperthermia in combination with sparsely ionizing radiations − e.g., X-rays or gamma rays − could be an alternative to neutrons or heavy ions. The main problem with heat application in clinical radiotherapy is the lack of heating methods which are able to heat the entire volume of a large solid tumor homogeneously. In small experimental animals there is a TER of about $1.5-2.0$. The therapeutic gain of additional heat in radiotherapy is greatly dependent on localization of the tumor (skin, extremities) and on cooling of the skin.

Hyperthermia enhances cytostatic drugs. Many investigations have been done on the interaction of heat and cytostatics; in vitro experiments evaluated three types. First, the activity of many drugs increases slightly with temperature; no special effects are observed above $42°$ C. Examples of drugs of that pattern are the hypoxic sensitizer Ro-07-0582 and the alkylating agents thio-TEPA and CCNU. A second type of mechanism is seen with cytostatic drugs which exhibit greatly increased effectiveness at temperatures above $42°$ C; adriamycin and bleomycin belong to this type. The third type of interaction is with drugs which are not active at normal temperatures, but become efficient at $42°$ C, e.g., amphotericin B. To date only two clinical application modalities allow randomized phase-III studies: local thermoradiotherapy and local thermochemotherapy.

References

Barth G, Wachsmann F (1948) Über den Einfluß der Temperatur auf die Hautreaktion bei Röntgenbestrahlungen. Strahlentherapie 77: 87−90

Ben-Hur E, Elkind MM, Bronk BV (1974) Thermally enhanced radioresponse of cultured Chinese hamster cells − Inhibition of repair of sublethal damage and enhancement of lethal damage. Radiat Res 58: 38−51

Bruns P (1887) Die Heilwirkung des Erysipels auf Geschwülste. Beitr Klin Chir 3: 443−446

Busch W (1866) Über den Einfluß, welche heftigere Erysipeln zuweilen auf organisierte Neubildungen ausüben. Verh Naturforsch Preuss Rhein Westphal 23: 28−30

Castillo J, Goldsmith HS (1973) Immunological competence of heat-treated extracts of tumor or lymph nodes. Arch Surg 106: 322−324

Cavaliere R, Moricca G, Caputo A (1975) Regional hyperthermia by perfusion. Proceedings of the International Symposium on Cancer Therapy by Hyperthermia and Radiation, Washington DC, April 28−30, 1975. Americal College of Radiology, pp 251−265

Cockett ATK, Kazmin M, Nakamura R, Fingerhut A, Stein JJ (1967) Enhancement of regional bladder megavoltage irradiation in bladder cancer using local bladder hyperthermia. J Urol 97: 1034−1039

Coley WB (1893) The treatment of malignant tumors by repeated inoculation of erysipelas − with a report of ten original cures. Am J Med Sci 105: 487−511

Crile G Jr (1963) The effects of heat and radiation on cancers implanted in the feet of mice. Cancer Res 23: 372−380

Dewey WC, Hopwood LE, Sapareto SA, Gerweck LE (1977a) Cellular responses to combinations of hyperthermia and radiation. Radiology 123: 463−474

Dewey WC, Thrall DE, Gilette EL (1977b) Hyperthermia and radiation − a selective thermal effect on chronically hypoxic tumor cells in vivo. Int J Radiat Oncol Biol Phys 2: 99−103

Dickson JA, Ellis HA (1974) Stimulation of tumor cell dissemination by raised temperature (42° C) in rats with transplanted Yoshida tumors. Nature 248: 354−258

Dickson JA, Ellis HA (1976) The influence of tumor volume and the degree of heating on the response of the solid Yoshida sarcoma to hyperthermia. Cancer Res 36: 1188−1195

Dickson JA, Shah MD (1972) The effect of hyperthermia (42° C) on the biochemistry and growth of a malignant cell line. Eur J Cancer 8: 561−571

Dickson JA, Shah SA (1978) Stimulation of an anti-tumor immune response in VX2-bearing rabbits by curative hyperthermia. In: Streffer C, van Beuningen D, Dietzel E, Röttinger E, Robinson JE, Scherer E, Seeber S, Trott K-R (eds) Cancer therapy by hyperthermia and radiation. Proceedings of the 2nd International Symposium, Essen, June 2−4, 1977. Urban and Schwarzenberg, Baltimore, pp 294−296

Dietzel F (1975) Tumor und Temperatur. Aktuelle Probleme bei der Anwendung thermischer Verfahren in Onkologie und Strahlentherapie. Urban und Schwarzenberg, München

Dietzel F (1978) Thermo-Radio-Therapie. Tierexperimentelle Untersuchungen zur Kombinationsbehandlung mit Hochfrequenz und Röntgenbestrahlung am soliden Ehrlich-Karzinom der Maus. (Habil-Schrift Gießen 1977) Urban und Schwarzenberg, München

Dietzel F, Weber HJ, Porschen W, Feinendegen LE (1976) Zur Wärmeempfindlichkeit von oxischen und hypoxischen Zellen in einem Tumor. Naturwissenschaften 63: 585−586

Dietzel F, Linhart G, Bierbrauer J, Heil T (1978) Der Zellverlust nach kombinierter Thermo-Radio-Therapie − Bestimmung der Zellverlustrate bei euoxischen und hypoxischen Tumorzellen an Experimentaltumoren in vivo. Strahlentherapie 154: 564−570

Dietzel F, Linhart G, Grundei BR (1982) Fractionated radiotherapy and short-term microwave hyperthermia. Natl Cancer Inst Monogr 61: 267−269

Field SB, Hume SP, Law MP, Myers R (1977) The response of tissues to combined hyperthermia and X-rays. Br J Radiol 50: 129–134

Fowler JF, Adams GE, Denekamp J (1976) Radiosensitizer of hypoxic cells in solid tumors. Cancer Treat Rev 3: 227–256

Freeman ML, Dewey WC, Hopwood LE (1977) Effect of pH on hyperthermic cell survival. J Natl Cancer Inst 58: 1837–1839

Gee AP, Williams AE, Pettigrew RT, Smith AN (1978) The effect of whole-body hyperthermia therapy on the general immunocompetence of the advanced cancer patient. In: Streffer C, van Beuningen D, Dietzel F, Röttinger E, Robinson JE, Scherer E, Seeber S, Trott K-R (eds) Cancer therapy by hyperthermia and radiation. Proceedings of the 2nd International Symposium, Essen, June 2–4, 1977. Urban and Schwarzenberg, Baltimore, pp 312–315

Gerweck LE, Burlett PH (1978) Hypoxic and pH modificationof hyperthermic lethality. In: Streffer et al. (eds) Cancer therapy by hyperthermia and radiation. Proceedings of the 2nd International Symposium, Essen, June 2–4, 1977. Urban and Schwarzenberg, Baltimore, pp 178–180

Gerweck LE, Gilette EL, Dewey WC (1974) Killing of Chinese hamster cells in vitro by heating under hypoxic conditions. Eur J Cancer 10: 691–693

Gerweck LE, Gilette EL, Dewey WC (1975) Effect of heat and radiation on synchronous Chinese hamster cells: Killing and repair. Radiat Res 64: 611–623

Giovanella BC, Morgan AC, Stehlin JS, Williams LJ (1973) Selective lethal effect of supranormal temperatures on mouse sarcoma cells. Cancer Res 33: 2568–2578

Goffinet DR, Choi KY, Brown JM (1977) The combined effects of hyperthermia and ionizing radiation on the adult mouse spinal cord. Radiat Res 72: 238–245

Hahn EW, Alfieri AA, Kim JH (1979) The significance of loxal tumor hyperthermia/radiation onthe production of disseminated disease. Int J Radiat Oncol Biol Phys 5: 819–823

Hahn GM (1974) Metabolic aspects of the role of hyperthermia in mammalian cell inactivation and their possible role in cancer treatment. Cancer Res 34: 3117–3123

Hahn GM (1978) Interactions of drugs and hyperthermia in vitro and in vivo. In: Streffer C, van Beuningen D, Dietzel F, Röttinger E, Robinson JE, Scherer, E, Seeber S, Trott K-R (eds) Cancer therapy by hyperthermia and radiation. Proceedings of the 2nd International Symposium, Essen, June 2–4, 1977. Urban and Schwarzenberg, Baltimore, pp 72–79

Hahn GM, Braun I, Har-Kedar I (1975) Thermochemotherapy: Synergism between hyperthermia (42°–43°) and adriamycin (or bleomycin) in mammalian cell inactivation. Proc Natl Acad Sci USA 72: 937–940

Hahn GM, Li GC, Shiu E (1977) Interaction of amphotericin B and 43° C hyperthermia. Cancer Res 37: 761–764

Harrison R, Lunt GG (1975) Biological membranes, their structure and function. Wiley, New York

Haveman J (1979) The pH of the cytoplasm as an important factor in the survival of in vitro-cultured malignant cells after hyperthermia. Eur J Cancer 15: 1281–1288

Haveman J (1980) The influence of pH on the survival after X-irradiation of cultured malignant cells. Effects of carbonylcyanide-3-chlorophenylhydrazone. Int J Radiat Biol 37: 201–205

Johnson HA, Pavelec M (1973) Thermal enhancement of thioTEPA cytotoxicity. J Natl Cancer Inst 50: 903–908

Kim HK, Kim JH, Hahn EW (1978) Selective potentiation of hyperthermic killing of hypoxic cells by 5-thio-D-glucose. Cancer Res 38: 2935–2938

Kim JH, Kim SH, Hahn EW (1975) Enhanced killing of hypoxic tumor cells by hyperthermia. Br J Radiol 48: 873–874

Kim JH, Hahn EW, Tohita N (1978) Combination hyperthermia and radiation therapy for cutaneous malignant melanoma. Cancer 41: 2143–2148

Kim SH, Kim JH, Hahn EW (1975) The radiosensitization of hypoxic tumor cells by hyperthermia. Radiology 114: 727–728

Kim SH, Kim JH, Hahn WE (1976) The enhanced killing of irradiated HeLa cells insynchronous culture by hyperthermia. Radiat Res 66: 337–345

Lin PS, Kwock L, Hefter K, Wallach DFH (1978) Modification of rat thymocyte membrane properties by hyperthermia and ionizing radiation. Int J Radiat Biol 33: 371–382

Mikkelsen RB, Verma SP, Wallach DFH (1978) Hyperthermia and the membrane potential of erythrocyte membranes as studied by Raman spectroscopy. In: Streffer C, van Beuningen D, Dietzel F, Röttinger E, Robinson JE, Scherer E, Seeber S, Trott K-R (eds) Cancer therapy by hyperthermia and radiation. Proceedings of the 2nd International Symposium, Essen, June 2–4, 1977. Urban and Schwarzenberg, Baltimore, pp 160–162

Miller RC, Leith JT, Veomett RC, Gerner EW (1976) Potentiation of radiation myelitis in rats by hyperthermia. Br J Radiol 49: 895–896

Mondovi B, Strom R, Rotilio G, Finazzi Agro A, Cavaliere R, Rossi Fanelli A (1969a) The biochemical mechanism of selective heat sensitivity of cancer cells I. Studies on cellular respiration. Eur J Cancer 5: 129–136

Mondovi B, Finazzo Agro A, Rotilio G, Strom R, Moricca G, Rossi Fanelli A (1969b) The biochemical mechanism of selective heat sensitivity of cancer cells II. Studies on nucleic acids and protein synthesis. Eur J Cancer 5: 137–146

Mondovi B, Santoro AS, Strom R et al. (1972) Increased immunogenicity of Ehrlich-ascites cells after heat treatment. Cancer 30: 885–888

Myers R, Field SB (1977) The response of the rat tail to combined heat and X-rays. Br J Radiol 50: 581–586

Overgaard J (1976) Influence of extracellular pH on the viability and morphology of tumor cells exposed to hyperthermia. J Natl Cancer Inst 56: 1243–1250

Overgaard J (1977a) The effect of sequence and time intervals of a solid mouse mammary adenocarcinoma in vitro. Br J Radiol 50: 763–765

Overgaard J (1977b) Effect of hyperthermia on malignant cells in vivo. A review and hypothesis. Cancer 39: 2637–2646

Overgaard J (1977c) Combined adriamycin and hyperthermia treatment of a murine mammary carcinoma. Cancer Res 36: 3077–3081

Overgaard J, Bichel P (1977) The influence of hypoxia and acidity on the hyperthermic response of malignant cells in vitro. Radiology 123: 511–514

Palzer RJ, Heidelberger C (1973) Influence of drugs and synchrony on the hyperthermic killing of HeLa cells. Cancer res 33: 422–427

Robinson JE, Wizenberg M, McCready WA (1974) Radiation and hyperthermial response of normal tissue in situ. Radiology 113: 195–198

Rose WC, Veras GH, Laster WR, Schabel FM (1979) Evaluation of whole-body hyperthermia as an adjunct to chemotherapy in murine tumors. Cancer Treat Rep 63: 1311–1325

Sapareto SA, Hopwood LE, Dewey WC (1978) Combined effects of x-irradiation and hyperthermia on CHO cells for various temperatures and orders of application. Radiat Res 73: 221–223

Schulman N, Hall EJ (1974) Hyperthermia: its effect on proliferative and plateau phase cell cultures. Radiology 113: 209–211

Shingleton WW (1962) Selective heating and cooling of tissue in cancer chemotherapy. Ann Surg 156: 408–416

Stehlin JS, Giovanella BC, De Ipolyi PD, Muenz LR, Anderson R (1975) Results of hyperthermic perfusion for melanoma of the extremities. Surg Gynecol Obstet 140: 338–348

Stewart FA, Denekamp J (1977) Sensitization of mouse skin to x-irradiation by moderate heating. Radiology 123: 195–200

Stewart FA, Denekamp J (1978) The therapeutic advantage of combined heat and X-rays on a mouse fibrosarcoma. Br J Radiol 51: 307–316

Stratford IJ, Adams GE (1977) Effect of hyperthermia on differential cytotoxicity of a hypoxic cell radiosensitizer. Ro-07-0582, on mammalian cells in vitro. Br J Cancer 35: 307–313

Streffer C, van Beuningen D, Dietzel F, Röttinger E, Robinson JE, Scherer E, Seeber S, Trott K-R (eds) (1978) Cancer therapy by hyperthermia and radiation. Proceedings of the 2nd International Symposium, Essen, June 2–4, 1977. Urban and Schwarzenberg, Baltimore

Strom R, Sciosca Santoro A, Crifo C, Bozzi A, Mondovi B, Rossi Fanelli A (1973) The biochemical mechanism of selective heat sensitivity of cancer cells IV. Inhibition of RNA synthesis. Eur J Cancer 9: 103–112

Szmigielkski S, Janiak M (1978) Reaction of cell-mediated immunity to local hyperthermia of tumors and its potentiation by immunostimulation – a review. In: Streffer C, van Beuningen D, Dietzel F, Röttinger E, Robinson JE, Scherer E, Seeber S, Trott K-R (eds) Cancer therapy by hyperthermia and radiation. Proceedings of the 2nd International Symposium, Essen, June 2–4, 1977. Urban and Schwarzenberg, Baltimore, pp 80–88

Thrall DE, Gilette EL, Dewey WC (1975) Effect of heat and ionizing radiation on normal and neoplastic tissue of the C3H mouse. Radiat Res 63: 363–377

Vaupel P (1982) Einfluß einer lokalisierten Mikrowellen-Hyperthermie auf die pH-Verteilung in bösartigen Tumoren. Strahlentherapie 158: 168–172

Wallach DFH (1978) Action of hyperthermia and ionizing radiation on plasma membranes. In: van Beuningen D, Dietzel F, Röttinger E, Robinson JE, Scherer E, Seeber S, Trott K-R (eds) Cancer therapy by hyperthermia and radiation. Proceedings of the 2nd International Symposium, Essen, June 2–4, 1977. Urban and Schwarzenberg, Baltimore, pp 19–28

Westra A, Dewey WC (1971) Variation in sensitivity to heat shock during the cell cycle of Chinese hamster cells in vitro. Int J Radiat Biol 19: 467–477

Williams AE, Galt JM (1978) The effects of whole-body hyperthermia on immunological function in rats (Abstr). In: Streffer C, van Beuningen D, Dietzel F, Röttinger E, Robinson JE, Scherer E, Seeber S, Trott K-R (eds) Cancer therapy by hyperthermia and radiation. Proceedings of the 2nd International Symposium, Essen, June 2–4, 1977. Urban and Schwarzenberg, Baltimore, pp 312–315

Woodhall B, Pickerell KL, Georgiade NG, Mahaley MS, Dukes HT (1960) Effect of hyperthermia upon cancer chemotherapy: Application to external cancers of head and face structures. Ann Surg 151: 750–759

Yatvin MB (1977) The influence of membrane lipid composition and procaine on hyperthermic death of cells. Int J Radiat Biol 32: 513–521

Yerushalmi A (1976a) Influence of metastatic spread of whole-body or local tumor hyperthermia. Eur J Cancer 12: 455–463

Yerushalmi A (1976b) Treatment of a solid tumor by local simultaneous hyperthermia and ionizing radiation: dependence on temperature and dose. Eur J Cancer 12: 807–813

Therapy of Fibrosarcoma in the Rectum of Rats by Selective Hyperthermia

D. Braasch

Institut für Physiologie, Philips-Universität, Deutschhausstrasse 2 3550 Marburg, FRG

It is known that the difference in heat tolerance between normal and malignant tissues is rather small, approximately in the range of $0.2°-0.4°$ C. Nevertheless, numerous attempts have been made to use this small difference for tumor therapy. The methods tried were whole-body hyperthermia, local heating with high-frequency diathermia, or selective perfusion with heated blood; most of these experiments failed. It appears that the main difficulty is to establish an effective temperature of $44.0°$ C with the needed accuracy of $\pm 0.1°$ C in a tissue in which arterial inflow is $37°$ C, i.e., $7°$ C below the curative temperature.

So far the only mode of therapy which allows a sufficiently accurate application of heat is the long-known immersion of the tumor-bearing extremity in heated water. Numerous successful treatments of experimental tumors by this method have been described.

It appears that the immersion method, which is as simple as it is effective, can be easily adapted to the rectum.

Material

Fibrosarcomas were induced in male Lewis/han rats, 200−400 g, by Methylcholanthrene. The tumors were in the 90−95 transplant generation. Transplanted into the rectum wall, the tumor was 100% retransplantable and lethal within 6−8 weeks.

Hyperthermia

After a midline incision of the skin of the scrotum, the rectal tube was freed, a free gap thus forming between the surrounding connective tissues, or more cranialy, between the muscles of the pelvis and the rectal tube. By means of ten thin perforated tubes, this gap was perfused for 60 min with isotonic NaCl heated to $44°$ C; thus, the rectal wall and the tumor were surrounded by a layer of heated water in turbulent flow. In addition to the external gap heating, the rectum and the lower colon descendens were perfused by means of a perforated Plexiglass tube, i.e., the rectum wall was placed like a sandwich between two layers of hot water. This helps to keep the temperature of the wall constant within $\pm 0.1°$ C.

Recent Results in Cancer Research, Vol. 86
© Springer-Verlag Berlin · Heidelberg 1983

Results

The rectum of a rat tolerates heating to 44.0° C for 60 min, provided the bacterial contamination of the gut is kept low by means of a nonresorbable antibiotic, for instance, neomycin plus bacitracin. Rats not protected will die within 3 days after heating.

The muscles of the rectum are relatively resistant to hyperthermia, whereas the typical structure of the mucosa becomes replaced by a nonstructural thick layer of cells. This change in structure is probably reversible, since the mucosa may recover to normal within 2 months. Defecation is not impaired by this change in structure.

The tumor disappears within 4 weeks and in series of four rats, three may be cured, provided their immune reaction is not impaired. For instance, if the immune system becomes suppressed by an additional tumor growing in the neck with a diameter of more than 5 mm, the heated tumor in the rectum may resist the otherwise curative hyperthermic treatment.

Though the number of reliable experiments to date is too small to allow final conclusions to be drawn, it appears that heat per se is not the only effective mechanism; hyperthermia may also render the heated tumor cell more susceptible to the attacks of the immune system.

Chemotherapy by Isolated Regional Perfusion for Melanoma of the Limbs*

E. T. Krementz**

Department of Surgery, Tulane University, School of Medicine,
1430 Tulane Avenue, New Orleans, LA 70112, USA

The original work with chemotherapy by regional perfusion began at Tulane University in 1957 (Creech et al. 1958; Ryan et al. 1958). Based on previous work using indwelling arterial catheters to deliver chemotherapy directly into tumor-bearing regions (Bierman et al. 1950; Klopp et al. 1950; Sullivan et al. 1953), the use of an extracorporeal oxygenated circuit was adapted to maintain and deliver a chemotherapeutic agent to the isolated tumor-bearing region, obtaining high-dose tumor exposure, with minimal systemic effects. Drug dosages were limited only by the local tissue tolerance. The technique was applied to a variety of tumor types, and in most areas of the body, but the most dramatic responses were seen in melanoma of the extremities, for which no good systemic agents existed at that time. Objective responses were seen in more than 50% of melanoma patients following limb perfusions, a response rate still unequaled by any systemic agent or combination of agents.

This operative method of regional chemotherapy opened a new field of stimulating clinical research. The project started in the surgical laboratories at Tulane, and in the operating rooms at Charity Hospital of Lousiana in New Orleans, and was expanded and studied in major medical centers throughout the world. As with many techniques requiring expertise, some groups began utilizing the method on a casual basis; poor selection of cases and increased technical complications produced some unsatisfactory results, and the widespread use of perfusion diminished. In those centers with sufficient numbers of patients and continuing interest, the method has been used effectively for treatment of melanoma and soft tissue sarcomas of the limbs, and occasionally for other cancers of the pelvis (McBride et al. 1978; Stehlin 1969; Wagner 1976). In recent years a rebirth of interest in the method has occurred, and the number of centers using perfusion has expanded in this country and abroad (Aigner et al., Regional Perfusion with cis-Platinum and Dacarbazine, this volume; Bulman and Jamieson 1980; Janoff et al., to be published; Koops et al. 1975).

* This investigation was supported in part by grant number CA 18007, awarded by the National Cancer Institute DHEW, and in part by the Ladies Auxiliary of the Veterans of Foreign Wars

** The author wishes to express his appreciation to Maria O. Hornung, PhD, for her assistance in the preparation and editing of the manuscript; to Marilyn Campbell, BS, RN, for collection and analysis of the regional chemotherapy data; to Marcia Case for the preparation of the manuscript; and to the many members of the Tulane faculty, the surgical residents, and staff for their participation in and contributions to this project

Technique

The general technique for hyperthermic perfusion of the upper and lower limbs has been described elsewhere (Creech et al. 1958, Krementz et al. 1979). Certain features which we consider important are referred to here.

In upper-extremity perfusions, the first portions of the axillary artery and vein are the vessels of choice for cannulation (Fig. 1). This permits good distribution of drugs throughout the axilla, the distal shoulder, and the entire upper extremity. For lesions in the proximal shoulder, or high in the axilla, it is possible to cannulate the subclavian vessels using a sternal splitting procedure or by dividing the clavicle and exposing and occluding the subclavian vessel just distal to the vertebral vessels. When this technique is used, small catheters are inserted in retrograde fashion into the brachial artery and vein, the tip being placed at the level of the occluding tape on the vessels (Fig. 2). This permits retrograde perfusion of the extremity, with the perfusate returning from the level of the subclavian tapes. Small catheters must be used so that the flow in the axillary vein is not obstructed.

In the lower extremity, the common femoral vessels are usually used for lesions at the mid-thigh level or below (Fig. 3). For lesions in the upper thigh or groin the external iliac vessels are used; these are approached through a lower quadrant, retroperitoneal muscle-splitting incision. Experience has shown that fewer vascular complications follow more proximal placement of the perfusion catheters. This is due partly to the increased mechanical problems of working with the smaller distal vessels, and partly to the fact that fewer residual complications follow the use of larger vessels. In addition, the more proximal the site of cannulation is, the greater the loss of perfusate will be. Moreover, with more proximal perfusion, high flow rates can be obtained; these are useful in maintaining optimum oxygenation and better tissue diffusion of the agent into the tumor areas. However, the higher the flow rate, and the more proximal the cannulation, the greater is the escape of drug and the poorer the isolation.

For femoral artery perfusions (Fig. 4), the incision is made overlying a point just above the inguinal ligaments to the apex of the femoral triangle. The deep fascia is incised and the common femoral vessels are identified and dissected free, from the point where they emerge from beneath the inguinal ligament down to the level where the first profunda

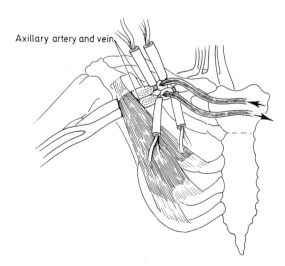

Axillary artery and vein

Fig. 1. Point of catheterization of the first portion of the axillary artery and vein for upper limb perfusion

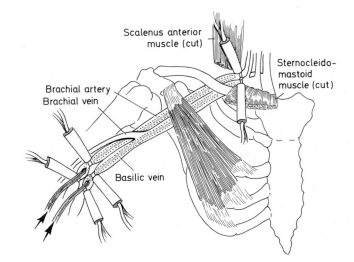

Fig. 2. Placement of catheters retrograde through the brachial vessels up to snares around the subclavian vessels to permit a more proximal perfusion, in order to include the shoulder and upper axilla

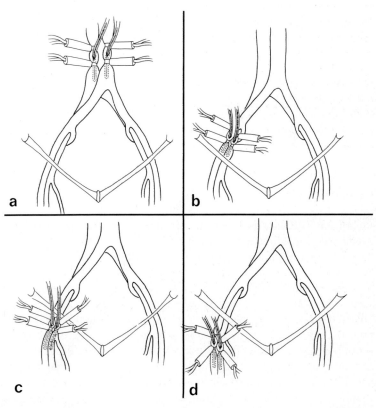

Fig. 3. Catheter placement for pelvic (**a**), external iliac (**b**), common femoral (**c**), and superficial femoral (**d**) perfusions

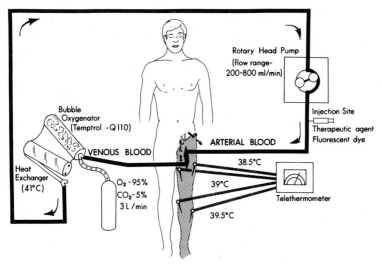

Fig. 4. Flow scheme for a lower-limb hyperthermic regional perfusion. Perfusate consists of 500–600 ml Ringer's lactate, 200 ml whole blood, and 3,000 units heparin

branch can be identified. Lymph nodes present along the femoral vessels are removed and sent for frozen section. Vessels are cannulated at a point superior to the bifurcation of the femoral vessels, and the catheter positioned so that the perfusate enters both vessels. The catheters are usually somewhat larger than those used for arm perfusion, but in all cases are selected to accomodate the vessel lumen.

For external iliac perfusions, the incision is made parallel to the inguinal ligament. Retroperitoneal exposure is carried out, and suspicious lymph nodes from the iliac area are removed. The vessels are cannulated at the level of the external iliac artery and vein. The inferior epigastric vessels are occluded and the obturator vessel may be temporarily occluded to obtain better isolation.

Chemotherapeutic Agents

Melphalan (l-PAM) is the drug of choice for regional perfusion. It is used almost exclusively for adjuvant perfusion and is included in most combinations for advanced disease. In early studies it was shown by Luck (1956) to be effective in melanoma. It also has the advantages of an alkylating agent, but without the marked vesicant properties of nitrogen mustard (HN_2). In 1969 melphalan began to be supplied with an acid/alcohol solvent in which it is dissolved before use. It is necessary to adjust the low pH with a buffered propylene glycol diluent. Total doses were modified downward in the late 1960s with the addition of hyperthermia, which was shown to enhance chemical action and produced unacceptable tissue toxicity when combined with high drug doses. Other alkylating agents which have been found useful are triethylenethiophosphoramide (TSPA) and HN_2. TSPA has not been shown to produce better responses than melphalan and is therefore reserved for use in combinations, or alone if l-PAM is not available. HN_2 is a highly reactive agent and is used alone or in combination for regional satellitosis. Actinomycin D has also shown some activity against melanoma, but is used only in

Table 1. Drugs used in 942 perfusions for melanoma of the limbs

Drug	First perfusion	Subsequent perfusions	Total
Melphalan	602	53	655
Nitrogen mustard	11	42	53
Melphalan, thiotepa	142	33	175
Melphalan, actinomycin D, nitrogen mustard	17	7	24
Other combinations and agents	25	9	32

Table 2. Safe range of drug doses for perfusion of the limbs in mg/kg body wt., based on actual or ideal weight, whichever is less

Drug	Upper limb	Lower limb
Single agents		
Melphalan	0.6 − 1.0	0.8 − 1.4
Thiotepa	0.6 − 1.0	0.8 − 1.4
Nitrogen mustard	0.3 − 0.6	0.4 − 0.7
Multiple agents		
Melphalan and	0.4 − 0.6	0.05 − 0.8
Thiotepa	0.3 − 0.5	0.4 − 0.7
Melpalan and	0.5 − 0.8	0.7 − 1.2
Actinomycin D	0.005 − 0.008	0.007 − 0.012
Melphalan and	0.5 − 0.7	0.6 − 0.9
Nitrogen mustard	0.09 − 0.14	0.11 − 0.16
Melphalan,	0.5 − 0.7	0.6 − 0.9
Actinomycin D and	0.006 − 0.01	0.008 − 0.012
Nitrogen mustard	0.07 − 0.11	0.08 − 0.15

combination with alkylating agents. The agents, combinations, and drugs used in 942 perfusions are shown in Table 1. Antimetabolities have no demonstrated place in short-term chemotherapy and have not been used. All agents are administered directly into the arterial line, but never in a single bolus injection. Melphalan is given in three to five aliquots, never more than 20 mg each, at intervals of 3 min. TSPA is given in the same manner. HN_2 is usually administered at the rate of $1-2$ mg/min; a single dose should never exceed 2 mg since, if HN_2 is given in large amounts, the potential for injury to nerves is high, resulting in increased incidence of arteritis, thrombosis, neuralgia, or even paralysis. The dose ranges for agents used are given in Table 2.

Newer agents effective in the treatment of melanoma may also be suitable for regional perfusion therapy. We have not used dacarbazine (DTIC), reserving it for systemic or long-term intra-arterial administration. Our experience with *cis*-platinum and adriamycin is limited, as we have carried out only a few preliminary perfusions recently. *cis*-Platinum seems to be effective and well tolerated at high dose levels but adriamycin is precipitated in the presence of heparin.

Clinical Material

From 1957 through 1980, 845 patients with invasive malignant melanoma underwent 942 regional perfusions. The clinical material is limited to those patients with malignant melanoma in an extremity, for the technique is most effective when the treated area can be isolated. There were 797 patients with extremity perfusions; 105 of them underwent additional perfusions, with 26 having more than two. Two patients have each had five perfusions. It should be noted that multiple perfusions are no longer carried out, except in unusual circumstances. Only 18 patients have had a second perfusion since 1970.

The clinical staging system used for this report is shown in Table 3. Stage I includes localized disease only; stage II disease includes local recurrence or a primary with satellites within 3 cm of the primary; stage III includes regional disease up to and including the first-station nodes. (Axillary and femoral/inguinal nodes, rather than epitrochlear or popliteal nodes, are considered to be first-station nodes.) Stage IV includes patients with systemic disease; patients with positive supraclavicular or iliac nodes are included in this stage. Of the 797 patients reported here, 5% were black and 60% were female; the lower limb was more frequently involved (60%). Approximately 50% of the total number had disease at stages III and IV.

There were 281 patients with stage-III disease. Of these, 80 had metastatic disease at the time of diagnosis and perfusion constituted part of their initial therapy. Another 127 patients had had prior surgical treatment of the primary lesions and underwent perfusion at the time of the first recurrence of metastatic disease. The remaining 74 patients had had one or more surgical procedures or other therapeutic measures for metastases prior to referral and were perfused relatively late in the course of their disease.

Table 3. Number of patients and stage of disease treated by regional perfusion for melanoma of the limb between 1957 and 1980

Stage of disease	Number treated
I Localized, primary lesions	
Level II	18
Levels III−IV	320
II Metastases within 3 cm of primary	
Primary with local satellites	9
Local recurrence	11
III Regional metastases	
A In-transit, skin or soft tissue	71
B Regional lymph nodes	124
AB Lymph nodes, skin and soft tissue	86
Limb metastases from unknown primary	28
IV Extraregional disease	
Primary in trunk with metastases to limb	46
Primary in limb	
With positive iliac nodes	40
With systemic metastases	44
Total	797

There were 28 patients perfused for metastatic disease in an extremity from an unknown primary site. They are considered separately in calculating survival rates, but are clinically comparable with other patients with stage-III disease.

There were 129 patients with stage-IV disease. There are times when perfusion is employed to control unmanageable regional disease if amputation is not advisable or not permitted, and there is no doubt that the preservation of a functional extremity, especially a leg, is of great importance to the patient.

Of the 40 patients with metastases to the iliac nodes, nine were found positive at diagnosis and perfused for primary disease. Multiple cutaneous or subcutaneous metastatic lesions were also present in 23 of these 40 patients. The remaining eight patients were perfused for metastases to regional nodes, and were found to have positive iliac nodes as well.

There were 44 patients with systemic disease at the time of perfusion, and perfusion was performed to relieve symptoms or to save the extremity. The introduction of better chemotherapeutic agents such as DTIC, the nitrosoureas, and *cis*-platinum in the late 1960s and thereafter, and of combinations of agents administered either intra-arterially by continuous infusion or systemically, have improved responses so that perfusion in the face of systemic disease is now rarely performed. Since 1970 only eight patients have had regional perfusions in spite of systemic metastases, and all have received intensive systemic therapy as well.

There were 45 patients who were perfused for axillary or inguinal regional lymph-node metastases from primary lesions on the trunk, 87% of whom had involvement of the upper extremity.

Pathology and Staging

The pathologic evaluation for all patients in this series is currently carried out by Dr. Richard J. Reed, Professor of Pathology; it was previously done by Dr. Wallace H. Clark when he was a member of the Department of Pathology at Tulane School of Medicine. Since specific prognostic characteristics of primary melanoma lesions have become better defined, those patients who underwent regional perfusions for invasive primary lesions which would now be identified as good risk lesions, i.e., Clark's level II (Clark et al. 1969), or less than 0.75 mm thick (Breslow 1970), have been excluded from the survival table. Only those patients with extremity lesions having histologic characteristics associated with a moderate-to-high potential for metastases are considered candidates for perfusion, i.e., Clark's level III, IV, and V, or lesions thicker than 0.76 mm. Most patients who undergo regional perfusion have had pathologic sampling of regional lymph nodes at the area adjacent to the insertion of the catheters. Prophylactic regional lymph node dissection was done on the majority of stage-I patients treated from 1957 to 1977, although these dissections were often not radical in the classic sense, and would be most accurately described as a superficial groin dissection or lymphadenectomy. In axillary perfusions, the highest axillary nodes are removed at the time of catheter insertion. Selection of patients having either lymph node excision or more radical lymph node dissection was always based on the risk assessment of the primary lesions, recognized by experienced pathologists and clinicians long before the current microstaging system evolved. In addition to the evaluation of level, thickness, and clinical stage, we also consider the sex of the patient and the histologic type of the melanoma — i.e., lentigo maligna melanoma, superficial spreading melanoma, nodular, acral, or lentiginous melanoma (Krementz et al. 1982; Reed 1976) in planning treatment.

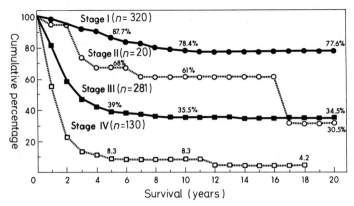

Fig. 5. Results of treatment in 751 patients with invasive malignant melanoma of the limbs by chemotherapy, by perfusion, and by surgical excision, according to stage. 1957–1980 (compare with Table 4)

Table 4. Results of chemotherapy by perfusion and exision of malignant melanoma of the limbs, in cumulative (%), at 5, 10, 15, and 20 years for 751 patients as of 1980

	Years			
	5	10	15	20
Stage I – 320 patients	87.7	78.4	77.6	77.6
Male – 112	79.7	66.1	66.1	66.1
Upper limb – 45	91.8	83.1	83.1	83.1
Lower limb – 67	70.8	53.7	53.7	53.7
Female – 208	91.6	84.6	83.4	83.4
Upper limb – 74	88.3	83.0	79.1	79.1
Lower limb – 34	93.3	85.1	85.1	85.1
All upper – 119	89.6	82.9	80.7	80.7
All lower – 201	86.5	75.7	75.7	75.7
Stage II – 20 patients	67.7	60.9	60.9	30.5
Stage III – 281 patients	38.9	35.5	34.5	34.5
A (In-transit) – 71[a]	35.6	28.4	28.4	28.4
B (Nodes) – 124	45.2	44	41.9	41.9
Single – 55	65.9	65.9	62.3	62.3
Multiple – 69	25.8	23.4	23.4	23.4
AB 86[b]	32.1	28	28	28
Primary unkown – 28	52.9	52.9	52.9	52.9
Stage IV – 130 patients	8.3	8.3	4.2	4.2
Primary outside – 46	7.2	7.2	0	NS
With iliac nodes – 40	16.2	16.2	NS	NS
Systemic – 44	5.2	5.2	5.2	NS

NS, no sample
[a] Of 71, 41 advanced and nonresectable
[b] Of 86, 38 advanced and nonresectable

Results

The results of chemotherapy by regional perfusion alone or in combination with excisional surgery in 751 patients with invasive melanoma of the limbs are shown in Fig. 5, plotted according to stage. Survival is calculated by the life-table method of Cutler and Ederer (1968). Most of the curves reflect a follow-up period of 20 years. Only 6 of 797 patients treated over the 20-year period have been lost to follow-up. If no patients remain in specific categories, the curve is discontinued at the appropriate year.

All patients in stages I and II underwent excisional surgery. The majority of patients in stage III had additional excisional surgery whenever removal of all tumor was feasible; however, most patients with satellitosis were treated by perfusion alone. In all cases where regional lymph node dissection (RLND) was indicated, it was performed at the time of perfusion. The 10-year survival rates in stages I through IV are 78.4%, 61%, 35.5%, and 8.3% respectively (Table 4).

Discussion

Malignant melanoma is a challenging and provocative neoplasm to study and treat. It is a viable and accessible tumor that has a reputation for erratic behavior associated with a bad prognosis. In recent years, however, new therapeutic approaches have resulted in an improved prognosis, far better than that for cancer of the lung or stomach, and equal to or better than those for breast and colon cancers.

The correlation of clinopathologic stages with prognosis has done much to enable the selection of optimum therapy for potentially curable patients. Still, in spite of our advances, more than 50% of patients die within 10 years of diagnosis with disseminated disease (National Cancer Institute 1976). This may be due in part to the failure of clinicians everywhere to consistently apply the knowledge available to them. The report of the Cancer Surveillance, Epidemiology and End Results (SEER) Program, N.C.I., indicates that approximately 80% of patients have localized disease at diagnosis, and it is to this majority that our best efforts should be directed.

Surgical therapy is the treatment of choice for melanoma, but even when applied by knowledgeable clinicians, 5-year control of localized invasive disease is achieved in approximately 50%−80% of cases, and when regional metastases are present the survival rates fall to 15%−40% (Lee 1980). For patients with in-transit metastases (satellitosis) − a circumstance which follows radical surgery for lower-extremity lesions in approximately 20% of cases (McCarthy et al. 1974; Moore and Gerner 1971) − the survival rate is approximately 10%−20% (Lee 1980).

Effective systemic chemotherapy, using DTIC alone or in combinations, has proven to be our most effective agent for disseminated disease, resulting in a few cures, and objective response rates of 20%−30%. But systemic chemotherapy has not been of proven benefit when used adjunctly. Immunotherapy, as presently understood, produces occasional dramatic responses, and can be a useful, but undependable, adjunct to other forms of therapy. Basic research hopefully will unravel the secrets of the immune system, and more effective therapy will be designed for the future.

We advocate the addition of adjuvant regional chemotherapy by perfusion for stage-I extremity lesions, which, by current clinicopathologic staging criteria, correlate with a moderate-to-high incidence of regional metastases, specifically Clark's levels III, IV, and V, which are 0.76 mm or greater in thickness. The exceptions to this rule are lesions classified as lentigo maligna melanoma less than 1.5 mm in thickness (regardless of level), and, in some cases, superficial spreading melanomas less than 1.0 mm thick. Adequate surgical excision of the primary is essential but the addition of local chemotherapy makes radical local surgery unnecessary. Only 10 of 320 (3.2%) stage-I patients in the perfusion series developed local recurrence.

Regional lymph node dissection is not performed in all cases of clinical stage-I disease, but it is recommended for patients with nodular or acral lentiginous melanomas thicker than 1.5 mm, and for any type of melanoma more than 2 mm thick. Even though many patients in the series were treated before level and thickness were specifically evaluated, the incidence of subsequent regional lymph node metastasis was only 5.9% and only 15 patients (4.6%) developed in-transit metastases following surgery and perfusion. In a series of 197 perfused patients at M.D. Anderson Hospital, Houston TX (Sugarbaker and McBride 1976), of whom only 14 had RLND, only 4% developed satellitosis. The total incidence of regional recurrence of any kind in our series was 11.2%, and it was associated with the simultaneous appearance of distant metastases in one third of the cases. We conclude that chemotherapy by extremity perfusion as an adjunct to surgical therapy is of definite benefit in achieving maximum control of regional disease.

It is acknowledged that a randomized trial comparing optimum surgery with and without perfusion in stage-I melanoma is needed, and several attempts to conduct such a trial have been made. However, advocates of perfusion feel that randomization would compromise their commitment to provide optimum therapy, and other potential investigators are often reluctant to invest the time and effort required to establish a perfusion program.

There is considerably more agreement among clinicians as to the value of chemotherapy by perfusion in recurrent or metastatic regional disease, where objective response rates of more than 50% are the rule and not the exception. The 5-year survival rates for all patients with stage-III disease is 39%. Of even greater significance is the stabilization in survival rates after 8 years, as the 15 and 20 year survivals are 34.5%. In even the most advanced cases (those with both in-transit and regional node metastasis), the 5-year survival is 32.1% and the 10, 15, and 20 year survivals are 28%. The results of treatment in all stages are summarized in Table 4).

The judicious administration of chemotherapy by perfusion, with its unique advantages of isolation and hyperthermia, combined with surgery, offers the patient with primary malignant melanoma on an extremity an excellent chance for recurrence-free survival, and the patient who has already developed regional metastasis a reasonable hope of control.

References

Bierman HR, Shimkin MB, Byron RL Jr et al. (1950) The effects of intra-arterial administration of nitrogen mustard. Fifth International Cancer Congress, Paris, 1950, pp 187–188

Breslow A (1970) Thickness, cross-sectional areas and depth of invasion in the prognosis of cutaneous melanoma. Ann Surg 171: 902

Bulman AS, Jamieson CW (1980) Isolated limb perfusion with melphalan in the treatment of malignant melanoma. Br J Surg 67: 660

Clark WH Jr, From L, Bernardeno SA et al. (1969) The histogenesis and biologic behavior of primary melanoma of the skin. Cancer Res 29: 705

Creech O Jr, Krementz ET, Ryan RT, Winblad JN (1958) Chemotherapy of cancer: Regional perfusion utilizing an extracorporeal circuit. Ann Surg 148: 616

Cutler SJ, Ederer F (1968) Maximum utilization of the life-table method in analyzing survival. J Chronic Dis 8: 699

Janoff K, Moseson D, Nohlgren J, Fletcher W et al. (to be published) The treatment of stage I melanoma of the extremities with regional hyperthermic isolation perfusion. Ann Surg

Klopp CT, Alford TC, Bateman J et al. (1950) Fractional intra-arterial cancer chemotherapy with methyl-bisamine hydrochloride. A preliminary report. Ann Surg 132: 811

Koops HS, Oldhoff J, van der Ploeg E et al. (1975) Isolated regional perfusion in the treatment of malignant melanomas of the extremities. Archivum Chir Neerl 17: 237

Krementz ET, Carter D, Sutherland CM, Campbell M (1979) The use of regional chemotherapy in the management of malignant melanoma. World J Surg 3: 289–304

Krementz E, Reed J, Coleman W et al. (1982) Acral lentiginous melanoma: A clinocopathologic entity. Ann Surgery 195: 632

Lee M (1980) Loco-regional recurrent melanoma: I. Natural history. Cancer Treat Rev 7: 59

Luck JM (1956) Action of p-[di(2-chloroethyl)]-amino-1-phenylalanine on Harding-Passey mouse melanoma. Science 123: 984

McBride CM, McMurtrey MJ, Copeland E, Hickey RC (1978) Regional chemotherapy by isolation perfusion. Int Adv Surg Oncol 1: 1

McCarthy JG, Haagensen CD, Herter FP (1974) The role of groin dissection in the management of melanoma of the lower extremity. Ann Surg 179: 156

Moore GE, Gerner RE (1971) Malignant melanoma. Surg Gynecol Obstet 132: 1971

National Cancer Institute (1976) Cancer Patient Survival. Report Number 5 Available from End Results Section, Biometry Branch, Division of Cancer Cause and Prevention, National Cancer Institute

Reed RJ (1976) Cutaneous malignant melanoma. In: Hartmann W (ed) New concepts in surgical pathology of the skin. Wiley, New York, pp 73–96

Ryan RT, Krementz ET, Creech O Jr et al. (1958) Selected perfusion of isolated viscera with chemotherapeutical agents. Surg Forum 8: 158

Stehlin JR Jr (1969) Hyperthermic perfusion with chemotherapy for cancers of the extremities. Surg Gynecol Obstet 129: 305

Sugarbaker EV, McBride CM (1976) The results of isolation-perfusion for invasive stage-I melanomas of the extremities. Cancer 37: 188

Sullivan RD, Jones R Jr, Schnabel TG Jr et al. (1953) The treatment of human cancer with intra-arterial nitrogen mustard uitlizing a simplified catheter technique. Cancer 6: 121

Wagner DE (1976) A retrospective study of regional perfusion for melanoma. Arch Surg 111: 410

Intra-Arterial Infusion of Bromodeoxyuridine and Radiotherapy in Osteosarcoma and Other Bone Malignancies*

F. J. Lejeune, R. Regnier, J.-M. Nogaret, and M. Jabri

Institut Jules Bordet, Centre des Tumeurs de l'Université Libre de Bruxelles, Service de Chirurgie, Rue Héger-Bordet 1, 1000 Bruxelles, Belgium

Introduction

Amputation of a limb does not seem to improve survival in osteosarcoma (Huvos 1979; Lejeune et al. 1972). About 80% of patients referred for primary osteosarcoma are expected to die, mostly of lung metastases, within 5 years (Prise and Jeffrey 1973). It is commonly accepted that most osteosarcoma metastases are present at the time of primary tumor diagnosis in the form of undetectable micrometastases. In recent years several adjuvant regimens of chemotherapy have been proposed for treating lung micrometastases, mainly using high doses of methotrexate and adriamycin (Huvos 1979). Accordingly, the extent of the surgical procedure has been reduced, especially for primary limb tumors, without diminishing local control of the tumor (Rosen et al. 1976).

For osteosarcoma of the limbs, the most commonly used limb-preservation technique has been the "en bloc" bone dissection, immediately followed by inner prosthetic replacement (Marcove 1977). However, the latter procedure is indicated only for "mini-osteosarcoma", where the soft tissues surrounding the bone are not invaded. This limitation is due to the fact that invaded soft tissue may be left behind and be responsible for resulting regional recurrence and for distant dissemination. Therefore, when we started the present pilot study, there was no alternative to amputation for "maxi-osteosarcoma", which spreads into the surrounding muscles.

Goffinet et al. (1975) proposed the use of intra-arterial radiosensitization and irradiation for patients with osteosarcoma who refused limb amputation. They reported two of three cases with complete local control of the sarcoma using bromodeoxyuridine (BUDR) as a radiosensitizer, and "flash irradiation". We decided to use this method to treat "maxi-osteosarcoma" and bone metastases. We report here on a prospective pilot trial on this method.

The purpose of this trial was to ascertain whether local control of the tumor – either primary osteosarcoma or any bone metastasis – can be achieved without amputation, with pain relief and acceptable limb function.

---

* Doctor J. Frühling, of the Radiotherapy Department, is acknowledged for having performed the bone scintigraphy program

Patients, Materials and Methods

Patient Eligibility

Patients with osteosarcoma with overt soft-tissue involvement and patients with single bone metastases from any other treated primary were admitted to the study. They could have no sign of arteritis. The tumor area had to be vascularized by arterial branches from a catheterizable artery.

Bone Tumor Workup

After physical examination, all patients were subjected to complete blood tests, including blood count and biochemical measurements. All underwent conventional X-rays, tomography, and CT scanning of the tumor area, as well as tomography of the lungs and bone scintigraphy, including dynamic study.

Histological evidence of the tumor was always obtained by means of an arteriography-guided drill biopsy according to a previously described method (Ballaux et al. 1980), which avoids unnecessary open-air biopsy.

Techniques

A PVC catheter was inserted into a peripheral, main artery − in most cases the superficial femoral artery − for infusion of the entire tumor area. This was done surgically through a Dacron patch securing the catheter. The catheter was connected to an Ivac pump through an anti-efflux valve. BUDR model 601 (IVAC, San Diego) was dissolved in 250 ml 5%-dextrose solution and administered at a dose of 15 mg/kg per day on days 1 and 2 continuously. For the following 3 days, neither radiosensitizer nor heparin was infused, the permeability of the catheter being guaranteed by a continuous dextrose infusion. When necessary, the correct position of the catheter was checked on a gamma camera after injection of ^{99m}Tc as a marker.

Radiotherapy was given by a single flash on day 3, just after the end of BUDR infusion. The flash consisted of 600 rads in the form of photons delivered by a Saturne Linear Accelerator. Eight courses of the above-described 5-day cycle were administered. After completion of the treatment arteriography was performed through the catheter, which was then pulled out. In six cases, lung irradiation was performed at a total dose of 1200 rads within eight courses. In five cases, high-dose methotrexate and citrovorum factor rescue, vincristine, and adriamycin were given in combination, according to the Jaffe "II" schedule (Jaffe et al. 1977).

Assessment of Response

At the end of the eight courses of treatment, and every 6 months, elective angiographies were made. Reduction of tumor hypervascularization was the main sign of tumor regression. In addition, this was semiquantitatively assessed by comparing dynamic bone scintigraphies. A histological study of the treated tumor area was made when possible, either by arteriography-guided drill biopsy or by extensive sampling at autopsy or after amputation. The function of the treated limb was regularly observed and the intensity of pain recorded.

Results

Characteristics of Patients

Of 17 cases in our study, 11 were osteosarcomas. The majority of these (nine) were located in the lower limbs, six in the distal femur and three in the proximal tibia; in most cases soft tissue involvement was obvious, with a tumor clinically visible. There was one small tumor on the iliopubic branch, accompanied by a pathological fracture, and there was a large skull osteosarcoma, 15 cm in diameter. In this case the catheter was inserter into the external carotid artery via the temporal artery.

Of six other bone malignancies, four were primary sarcomas of the bone other than osteosarcomas − two fibrosarcomas, one of the proximal femur and one of the femur shaft; two chondrosarcomas, one ischiopubic, the other iliac. The remaining two were an iliac neurofibrosarcoma metastasis and an unclassifiable tumor of the distal femur.

The patients with osteosarcomas with soft tissue involvement were between 10 and 75 years of age (median: 18.5); eight were male and three female. Those in the second group were between 13 and 70 years (median 45.5); two were male and four female.

Local Response to Intra-Arterial BUDR and Irradiation

Ten of the 11 osteosarcoma cases are available for evaluation. Median follow up time has been 3 years and median survival has been 1 year. Primary tumour control of osteosarcoma was achieved in nine of ten cases, i.e., in all lower limb osteosarcomas. The only failure was the skull osteosarcoma. Histological evidence of tumor lysis was obtained in all of the six cases studied. Of the six nonosteosarcoma tumors, control was obtained in three cases, with histological evidence in two. The overall results show bone tumor control in 12 of 16 cases after intra-arterial BUDR and irradiation, which is about 75%. Pain relief was obtained in all limb tumors, whether they were osteosarcoma or not, after four courses of treatment. In other localizations pain was reduced, but still present.

Side Effects

Mild, reversible leukopenia with more than 2,000 WBC/mm^3 was encountered in 16 of 17 cases. Three young patients (10, 12, and 13 years) experienced arterial thrombosis, and two required amputation. Two patients experienced skin toxicity, and late toxicity consisting in severe fibrosis appeared in ten of 12 evaluated lower limb cases. An irreversibly flexed knee was observed in six of nine evaluated lower limb cases despite intensive physiotherapy.

Local Recurrence and Progression

To date, two patients have experienced recurrence of progression of disease in the treated bone. One woman, aged 48, with distal femur telangiectatic osteosarcoma, had to have hip disarticulation for a recurrence in the proximal part of the femur 11 months later, after which she received half the HD of methotrexate for 1 year. She is still alive with no evidence of disease $4\frac{1}{2}$ years later.

A man with skull osteosarcoma did not receive full treatment for catheter dislodgement, and refused further treatment when the tumor progressed.

Discussion

The preliminary results of this pilot study clearly show that in most cases local control of bone osteosarcoma with pain relief can be achieved. This confirms the rationale of using an intra-arterial radiosensitizer (Goffinet et al. 1975). Since the drug was administered through a regional artery, there was heavy perfusion of the hypervascularized tumors with less systemic toxicity. Poor results with tumors localized on central parts of the skeleton indicate that drug perfusion was less elective. There was almost no detectable fibrosis in these body areas.

Intraarterial BUDR followed by flash irradiation produced much more local control of the bone tumor than is expected from irradiation alone (Dahlin and Coventry 1967; Huvos 1979; Lejeune et al. 1972) or combined with chemotherapy (Huvos 1979). However, strong fibrosis appeared gradually during at least the first 12 months after treatment. This was the most obvious for knee lesions. Intensive physiotherapy was planned for at least 1 year but most patients were reluctant to continue for such a long period. We found it difficult to convince the patients and their families that after such treatment fibrosis is very slow, but long lasting and progressive. On the whole, seven of the nine patients with tumors in the knee recovered some walking ability with the aid of crutches. Three of them have been found to walk almost normally without crutches. Thus, the functional results appear acceptable.

In contrast, the preliminary assessment of the survival of the osteosarcoma patients seems to be poor. It is similar to that figures for any other kind of treatment found in the literature (Dahlin and Coventry 1967; Huvos 1979).

Our study demonstrates that a limb-salvage procedure in osteosarcoma is justified, since death will occur in 80% of cases with in a short period of time, whether or not amputation has been performed. Since only local control has been achieved in osteosarcoma of the extremities, we are continuing our study of lower limb osteosarcoma with extensive soft tissue involvement.

Summary

In order to avoid amputation, which does not seem to improve survival in osteosarcoma, we have initiated a limb-preservation program using intra-arterial radiosensitization. Eleven osteosarcomas with soft tissue involvement and six other bone malignancies were prospectively treated according to the following protocol: (a) surgical insertion of an intra-arterial catheter through a Dacron patch, (b) intra-arterial infusion of 15 mg/kg BUDR on days 1–2 every 5 days for 40 days, (c) 600 rads flash irradiation on day 3 every 5 days, × 8. Median follow-up time has been 36 months.

In the osteosarcoma group, median survival has been 12 months. Four of the five osteosarcoma patients who died had received prophylactic HD methotrexate-vincristine-adriamycin systemic chemotherapy; one patient refused.

Local control of tumor has been obtained in ten of 17 cases: in seven of 11 osteosarcomas and in three of six other malignancies. Histological evidence of tumor destruction was obtained in five of seven osteosarcomas studied and in two of three other bone malignancies.

Side effects were acceptable: three cases with thrombosis, followed in two cases by amputation, and two cases of skin toxicity. Late toxicity consisted in severe fibrosis in all cases, with permanent flexion of the knee in six of nine cases. These results justify continuation of the study.

References

Ballaux JM, Schils C, Frühling J, Osteaux M, Heimann R, Lejeune FJ (1980) Diagnosis of bone tumours by arteriography-guided drill biopsy. Tum Diagn 2:96−100

Dahlin DC, Coventry MB (1967) Osteogenic sarcoma. A study of 600 cases. J Bone Joint Surg [Am] 49:101−110

Goffinet RD, Kaplan HS, Donaldson SS, Bagshaw AM, Wilbur JR (1975) Combined radiosensitizer infusion and irradiation of osteogenic sarcomas. Radiology 117:211−214

Huvos AG (1979) Bone tumors. Diagnosis, treatment and prognosis. Saunders, Philadelphia

Jaffe N, Traggis D, Cassady JR, Filler RM, Watts H, Frei E 3rd (1977) The role of high-dose methotrexate with citrovorum "rescue" in the treatment of osteogenic sarcoma. Int J Radiat Oncol Biol Phys 2:261−266

Lejeune F, Regnier R, Lustman-Marechal J, Mattheiem W, Henry J, Smets W (1972) Revue de 70 cas de sarcomes de la lignée osteogenique. Acta Chir Belg 71:321−398

Marcove RC (1977) En bloc resection for osteogenic sarcoma. Can J Surg 20:521−528

Price CHG, Jeffree GM (1973) Metastatic spread of osteosarcoma. Br J Cancer 28:515−524

Rosen G, Murphy ML, Huvos AG, Gutierrez M, Marcove RC (1976) Chemotherapy, en bloc resection, and prosthetic bone replacement in the treatment of osteogenic sarcoma. Cancer 37:1−11

Super-Selective Cytostatic Treatment of Malignant Tumors of the Soft Tissue and Bone

P. Schepke

Röntgenabteilung, Chirurgische Universitätsklinik Erlangen, Krankenhausstraße 12, 8520 Erlangen, FRG

From July, 1980 to February, 1982, ten patients (age ranging from 14 to 57 years) with malignant tumors of the soft tissues and bones were treated by arterial cytostasis at the Radiologic Department of Surgery, University of Erlangen.

The tumors were considered inoperable due to their size and extent or treatable only by extended radical surgery.

All patients with osteogenic sarcoma were treated, in addition, according to the T 9 protocol of Rosen (1979; see Table 1).

Our aim in applying super-selective arterial tumor cytostasis was to increase the concentration at the tumor site in order to obtain a better response. A special advantage seems to be the concentration of the cytostatic agent in the arterial influx and venous efflux areas.

After a survey angiography (Fig. 1), the various tumor vessels were probed super-selectively. In single-vessel supply the cytostatic agent was given over 24 h, in multiple-vessel supply − in our patients up to eight vessels − the cytostatic drug was administered as a short-term perfusion using these vessels according to their fraction of the total blood supply of the tumor.

It is very important to check the exact position of the catheter, since different tumor vessels supply different tumor areas and therefore, only parts of the tumor would be perfused if the position of the catheter were incorrect.

After the second selective cytostatic treatment cycle the tumor should be almost totally devitalized (Fig. 3). In seven of the ten patients reduction of the tumor was observed as shown. Seven patients also underwent surgery following the super-selective chemotherapy; the specimens obtained were examined histologically, and the results correlated with those of clinical and angiographic examinations.

Complications which developed were considered acceptable, and were of short duration. Eight in ten patients experienced local erythema; two had locally superficial necrosis of the skin and two locally deep necrosis; two had ulcerations; nine reported local pain. There was no necrosis of the soft tissue observed. These complications caused no delay, and the planned extremity-saving operation could be performed in every case.

This operation to save the limb is illustrated by one particular case of a woman suffering from a primarily inoperable telangiectatic osteosarcoma of the iliac bone, with massive soft tissue infiltration and involvement of the sacrum. After 6 months of systemic chemotherapy a large part of the tumor remained (Fig. 4). However, after two cycles of super-selective chemotherapy infused via the cranial gluteal artery, and continued systemic cytostasis for 3

Recent Results in Cancer Research, Vol. 86
© Springer-Verlag Berlin · Heidelberg 1983

Table 1. Data on ten patients treated by super-selective arterial chemotherapy from July, 1980 to February, 1982

Patient	Sex	Age	Histology	Localization	Medication (dose and no. of cycles)	Period of observation (months)
MB	Female	20	Osteosarcoma	Ileum and sacro-iliac joint; infiltration of the abdominal wall	ADB 3 × 100 mg	36
WW	Male	14	Nondifferentiated soft tissue sarcoma	Right scapula	ADB 3 × 70 mg	9
PSch	Male	19	Osteosarcoma	Right distal femur	ADB 3 × 120 mg	9
RR	Male	23	Malignant fibrohistiocytoma	Proximal humerus	ADB 1 × 150 mg	8
EJ	Female	14	Osteosarcoma	Distal femur	ADB 1 × 90 mg	7
HK	Male	44	Malignant melanoma with metastases	Axilla	DTIC 1 × 120 mg	3
PW	Male	42	Fibrosarcoma	Proximal tibia	ADB 1 × 170 mg 1 × 100 mg	3
WSch	Male	39	Recurrent synovial cell sarcoma	Femur	ADB 2 × 100 mg	3
KSchu	Female	28	Synovial cell sarcoma	Proximal femur	ADB 2 × 140 mg	2
OK	Male	57	Synovial cell sarcoma	Distal femur	ADB 2 × 190 mg	2

ADB, adriamycin; *DTIC*, dacarbazine

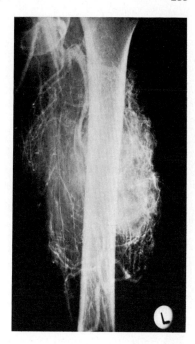

Fig. 1. Angiograph showing staining of tumor and selective visualization of various vessels in a synovial cell sarcoma

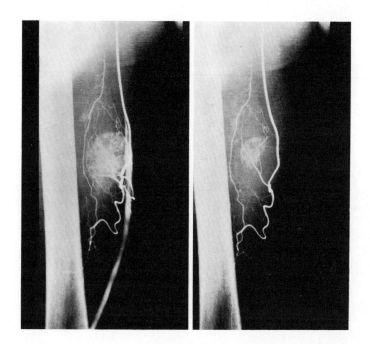

Fig. 2 (*Left*). Localization of the catheter for super-selective cytostasis; angiograph

Fig. 3 (*Right*). Angiograph showing small amount of tumor remaining after the second cytostatic treatment cycle. Tumor is almost totally devitalized

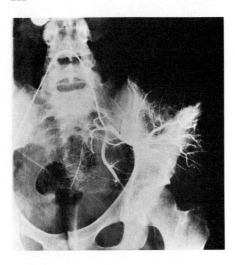

Fig. 4. Angiograph of telangiectatic osteosarcoma of the iliac bone after 6 months of systemic chemotherapy. A large part of the tumor is still visible

months, the patient was able to undergo local radical surgery. She has now been free of recurrent tumor and metastases for 36 months, dating from the start of therapy.

Histological examinations of seven cases showed 90%–100% tumor regression in three, 70%–90% regression in three, and no regression in only one, as a result of intra-arterial chemotherapy.

The results seem to confirm our concept of super-selective arterial cytostasis as a support for systemic chemotherapy and as a preoperative treatment alone, and to indicate continued use of the method.

Reference

Rosen G, Marcove RC, Caparros B, Nirenderg A, Cosloff C, Huvos AG (1979) Primary osteogenic sarcoma. Cancer 43: 2163–2177

Tourniquet Infusion with DTIC in Therapy-Resistant Melanoma on the Extremities: A Pilot Study

P.-E. Jönsson, C. Ingvar, and H. Stridbeck

Departments of Surgery and Diagnostic Radiology, University of Lund, 221 85 Lund, Sweden

Introduction

For three decades regional chemotherapy has been given by intra-arterial infusion or isolated perfusion techniques (Creech et al. 1958; Klopp et al. 1950). The isolation perfusion technique was altered to include heat after Cavaliere et al. (1967) reported their results of hyperthermic perfusions without anticancer drugs. Stehlin et al. (1979) have reported especially improved results in patients with in-transit melanoma metastases. The ultimate aim of isolation perfusion is to maintain a high level of the anticancer drug in the tissue of the tumor-bearing area with minimal leakage to other parts of the body. The technique is an extensive procedure including general anesthesia and surgery, and an extracorporeal circulation, which is not so easily reproduced. In 1979 Karakousis et al. (1979a, b) described a modification of regional intra-arterial infusion chemotherapy – tourniquet infusion – which achieved tissue levels of different anticancer drugs comparable to those attained with hyperthermic perfusion. A catheter is placed percutaneously with its tip in the main artery of the extremity, and a pneumatic tourniquet is applied to the extremity above the level of the catheter tip. The preliminary results in a restricted series of patients with various malignant tumors on the lower extremities showed good tumor response with moderate toxicity.

With the data given as background, we decided to use tourniquet infusion with dacarbazine (DTIC) in patients with unsatisfactory tumor response after hyperthermic perfusion with melphalan (Alkeran). Our experience with the first three patients is here reported.

Material and Methods

Three patients (one man, two women, 50, 64, and 71 years old) with recurrent melanoma on the lower extremities were treated. The diagnosis was established by fine-needle biopsies. All three patients had earlier been subjected to hyperthermic melphalan perfusion and/or surgery (Table 1).

The pretreatment evaluation included physical examination, laboratory tests, and chest X-rays. Liver scans and computer tomography of the brain were also performed then, or between the first courses of therapy. Regular checks were performed during therapy and follow-up.

Table 1. Patient data and results of therapy

Patients	Tumor site	Prior therapy	Results of prior therapy	Number of tourniquet infusions	Tumor response	Duration[a] (months)
Male, 50	Right calf	Two regional perfusions	No tumor response Tumor progression	5	Partial	5
Female, 64	Left leg	Regional perfusion and surgery	Tumor progression	5	Partial	6
Female, 70	Right leg	Two regional perfusions	No tumor response Tumor progression	4	Partial	5

[a] Duration equal to follow-up time

Tumor response was classified as follows: complete tumor response — 100% regression of objectively measurable tumor persisting for a minimum of 1 month; partial tumor response — 50% or more regression of objectively measurable tumor, also persisting for a minimum of 1 month.

Tourniquet Infusion Technique

Under local anesthesia a catheter was inserted percutaneously through the femoral artery or the left brachial artery with the tip of the catheter in the superficial femoral artery of the tumor-bearing extremity. The position was checked by fluoroscopy daily during the infusion period.

A rubber Esmarch bandage was applied as tourniquet on the proximal thigh. The arterial blood flow was decreased by about half, and the venous outflow completely. Blood flow was checked by ultrasonography.

The daily dose of 250 mg/m^2 DTIC was given for days, repeated after a 3- to 4-week interval. The drug was administered by manual injection over 5 min synchronously with a saline infusion at higher than systolic pressure. The saline infusion was continued for some minutes after the injection of the drug was completed. The tourniquet was released after 25 min. No sedation was given to the patients during the procedure. Thrombosis prophylaxis was given in the form of 5,000 U heparin subcutaneously every 6 h. The catheter was infused with saline during the period of time between DTIC injections.

Results

Complications

All patients complained of slight vascular pain during the start of injection. The first day gastrointestinal intolerance, nausea and vomiting occurred in all patients. No catheter complications or bone marrow toxicity were registered.

Tumor Response

All patients had tumor response greater than 50%. The drug effect on the tumors was obvious already after the first course of therapy with tourniquet. One patient received the first course without tourniquet because of extreme vascular pain. After this course there was no sign of tumor response. The next course was given with tourniquet, after which partial tumor response occurred. The duration of tumor response was 5, 5, and 6 months, respectively, which is the same as the follow-up time.

Discussion

The drug most consistently used for isolation perfusion in patients with malignant melanoma is melphalan. Its use is based on experimental studies in rats with transplanted melanoma (Luck 1956). The rationale is that melphalan carries cytotoxic radicals into the melanin metabolism of the tumor cells. When administered systemically to melanoma patients melphalan has a low tumor-response rate and has not proved to be of any major benefit (Comis and Carter 1974). In contrast several studies, controlled and uncontrolled, have indicated an overall tumor response for DTIC on the order of 20%−30% (Costanzi 1976).

An important concept of chemotherapy is that most drugs are phase-dependent, and therefore need to be administered at intervals, over a longer period of time, to give optimal results. Isolation perfusion is a single treatment which is not usually repeated so frequently. Systemic leakage of the drug may be critical in isolation perfusion, when potent drugs are used at high concentrations, but leakage is not a major problem in tourniquet infusion, as the drug dose is the same as that for systemic administration. The simplicity of tourniquet infusion is an advantage. It enables daily drug administration continuing for days to weeks, with shorter and longer intervals between. Karakousis et al. (1979b) used a pneumatic tourniquet which was inflated above the systolic pressure for 5 min when the drug was given. We tried to decrease the arterial blood flow rather than interrupt it, which may lead to a more even distribution of the drug in the extremity. Drug distribution, however, was judged to be fairly uniform in animal experiments (Karakousis et al. 1979a). The tissue drug levels were comparable when a tight or loose tourniquet was used, but the leakage to the systmic circulation was greater when the tourniquet was applied loosely (Karakousis et al. 1979a). When tissue concentrations of melphalan were measured in the extremity after tourniquet infusion they were comparable to or higher than those measured after hyperthermic perfusions. Perhaps the use of Ringer solution instead of blood as perfusate in these experiments may influence the results. There are no comparable data available for DTIC.

The great difference between the immediate tumor response in our patients after tourniquet infusion compared with prior therapy by hyperthermic perfusion may emphasize the importance of different drug sensitivities. Another advantage of tourniquet infusion is that several drugs can easily be tested on the patient.

The surprisingly good results may also depend on the higher level of DTIC in tissue achieved by tourniquet infusion as compared with that reached in systemic administration. Our earlier experience with treatment of patients by intra-arterial infusion of DTIC has not been impressive (Jönsson 1980). As expected, toxicity was comparable to that with systemic administration.

Even though this pilot study of three patients is too small to permit any conclusions as to the long-range results of tourniquet infusion with DTIC in melanoma patients, the fact remains that the treatment in these patients, was highly effective. The study should lead to further evaluation of the technique. It is important that this be combined with basic work on the pharmacokinetics of DTIC as well as of other drugs in relation to the blood flow. The possibility of using other treatments at the same time, e.g., hyperthermia and radiotherapy, is another advantage.

References

Cavaliere R, Ciogatto EG, Giovanella BC, Heidelberger C, Johnsson RO, Margottino M, Mondovi B, Moricca G, Rossi-Fanelli A (1967) Selective heat sensitivity of cancer cells. Cancer 20: 1351

Comis RL, Carter SK (1974) Integration of chemotherapy into combined modality therapy of solid tumors. IV. Malignant melanoma. Cancer Treat Rev 1: 285

Costanzi JJ (1976) DTIC. Studies in the Southwest oncology group. Cancer Treat Rep 60: 189

Creech O Jr, Krementz ET, Ryan RF, Winblad JN (1958) Regional perfusion utilizing an extracorporeal circuit. Ann Surg 148: 616

Jönsson P-E (1980) Metastatic malignant melanoma. Diagnosis and therapy. Thesis, University of Lund, Sweden

Karakousis CP, Kanter PM, Lopez RE, Moore R, Holyoke ED (1979a) Modes of regional chemotherapy. J Surg Res 26: 134

Karakousis CP, Rao V, Holtermann OA, Kanter PM, Holyoke ED (1979b) Tourniquet infusion chemotherapy in extremities with malignant lesions. Surg Gynecol Obstet 149: 481

Klopp CT, Bateman JC, Bery N, Alford C, Winship J (1950) Fractionated regional cancer chemotherapy. Cancer Res 10: 229

Luck JM (1956) Action of p-di(2-chloro-ethyl)-amino-L-phenylalanine on Harding-Passey mouse melanoma. Science 123: 984

Stehlin JS Jr, Giovanella BC, de Ipolyi PD, Andersson RF (1979) Eleven years' experience with hyperthermic perfusion for melanoma of the extremities. World J Surg 3: 305

Intra-Arterial Adriamycin for Limb Sarcomas

A. Azzarelli, L. Gennari, G. Bonfanti, R. Audisio, and V. Quagliuolo*

Istituto Nazionale Tumori, Via Venezian 1, 20133 Milano, Italy

In the majority of cases, despite increased efforts to perform adequate surgery, even with amputation, the outcome for patients with soft tissue limb sarcomas is unhappy, mainly due to local relapses and pulmonary metastases.

With the major aims of achieving tumor shrinkage thus improving the surgical approach in terms of limb-sparing treatment, of reducing the theoretical risk of spreading metastases during surgical manipulation, and of evaluating possible tumor tissue chemosensitivity, a new therapeutic policy has been outlined at our institute and employed for operable soft tissue sarcomas of the limbs: intra-arterial chemotherapy followed by radical surgery and possible radiotherapy.

Material and Methods

The treatment schedule provides for preoperative infusion therapy with adriamycin delivered by continuous intra-arterial infusion for 8 consecutive days, up to a total dose of 100 mg/m². A polyethylene catheter was inserted into the homolateral external iliac artery through the homolateral femoral artery (anti-blood stream) according to accessibility and angiograms; in two cases of buttock lesions the catheter was inserted into the common iliac artery. The only patient with a tumor of the upper third of the arm was cannulated through the homolateral brachial artery. The drug was given by means of a suitable infusion pump. This treatment was followed by radical surgery within 6 days after the end of infusion chemotherapy. When the surgery was considered inadequate, facultative radiotherapy was also employed, i.e., in cases of marginal, nonradical, or contaminated operations.

Eligible patients had histologically proven operable soft tissue sarcomas of the limbs, larger than 8 cm in diameter, and had had no prior chemo- or radiotherapy. Patients who had relapsed after nonradical surgery were also candidates.

Results and Discussion

Our small series comprised 13 patients during the period from January 1981 to April 1982. Their ages ranged from 13 to 57 years (mean: 38.5), and there was no significant difference

* We thank Dr. Bruno Damascelli and his staff for providing the angiograms and inserting the catheters

Table 1. Characteristics of patients, therapy performed, and results

Pat. no.	Sex	Age	Histology	Site of tumor	Total dose (mg ADM)	Clinical response	Type of surgery	Radical	Histologic necrosis (%)	Postop. RT	Follow-up (months)
1	F	43	Mixoid liposarcoma	Midthigh	176	<50%	Wide excision	Yes	>90	No	16 living NED
2	F	57	Polimorphous liposarcoma	Upper thigh	160	<50%	Disarticulation	Yes	>90	No	16 living NED
3	F	43	Malignant fibrous histiocytoma	Midthigh	116	NC	Wide excision	Yes	>90	No	15 living NED
4	F	30	Malignant fibrous histiocytoma	Buttock	160	NC	Wide escision	Yes	>90	No	12 living M+ (lung)
5	M	23	Undifferentiated sarcoma	Buttock	170	<50%	Marginal excision	Dubious	>90	Yes	12 living M+ (lung)
6	M	35	Malignant fibrous histiocytoma	Midthigh	178	NC	Marginal excision	Dubious	>90	Yes	12 living NED
7	M	50	Mixoid liposarcoma	Upper thigh	185	NC	Wide excision	Yes	<50	No	11 living NED
8	M	24	Synovial sarcoma	Upper thigh	173	<50%	Marginal excision	Dubious	>90	Refused	12 living M+ (lung)
9	F	55	Rhabdomyosarcoma	Upper thigh	184	NC	Wide excision	Yes	>50	No	9 living M+ (lung)
10	M	15	Clear cell sarcoma	Upper thigh	165	>50%	Wide excision	Yes	100	No	7 living NED
11	M	13	Malignant schwannoma	Shoulder	128	<50%	Marginal excision	Dubious	<50	Yes	3 living NED
12	F	56	Malignant fibrous histiocytoma	Upper thigh	166[a]	NC	Waiting for surgery				3 M+ (lung) synchronous
13	F	57	Mixoid liposarcoma	Upper thigh	180	NC	Marginal disarticulation	Dubious	None	Yes	2 living NED

[a] See text

NC, no change; NED, no evidence of disease; M+, with metastases; RT, radiotherapy; ADM, adriamycin between the numbers of men and women afflicted. All patients were given the infusion drug at the proposed dose: mean total dose 164.7 mg adriamycin, range 116–185 mg.

Our data are summarized in Table 1. No complications occurred during the infusion treatment, with the exception of a reduction in pulse and a peculiar reddish color to the homolateral hand of a 13-year-old boy who had been given chemotherapy via the branchial artery; however, no vascular deficit occurred. Toxicity from adriamycin was typical and acceptable in all cases; all patients experienced alopoecia, and the range of WBC was 700–2,500, with a mean low of 1,950. There was no cardiotoxicity. It is noteworthy that there were also no complications after surgery, even when the operation was performed in the presence of leukopenia. Wound healing was normal in all patients.

The time between infusion treatment and surgery is too short to achieve a significant clinical evaluation of a possible response. Nevertheless, five patients showed clinical improvement in the dimension or consistency of the tumor, but in only one case was it judged to be more than 50%. On the other hand, response was proven histologically in ten of 12 evaluated specimens, and in seven of these it was more than 90%: in one case no residual neoplastic tissue was found in the necrotic areas.

All patients underwent radical surgery. In no case was macroscopic residual neoplastic tissue left in the surgical bed, but in five cases the operation was marginal, according to Enneking's classification (Enneking et al. 1980). In three cases clinical improvement made it possible to perform conservative surgery rather than disarticulation.

The first patient entered this study in January 1981 and the follow-up period has not been very long (see Table 2): seven patients are now in the second year of follow-up. No patient has died; no relapses have been documented, but four have developed lung metastases. In one patient a synchronous solitary lung metastasis was detected during the infusion treatment (case no. 12, Table 1); after the first intra-arterial dose of adriamycin two more doses were delivered intravenously at 21-day intervals; local radiotherapy was also employed, and the patient is waiting for surgical treatment of primary and secondary lesions. This high incidence of metastases is probably due to an unfortunate and spontaneous selection of highly malignant histotypes which included four malignant fibrous histiocytomas (two now have metastases), one synovialsarcoma, one rhabdomyosarcoma, and one undifferentiated sarcoma (the last three all with metastases). The onset of metastases occured after a mean interval of 7.3 months (range 4–10).

In our opinion this study is distinctive for the strict selection of operable, similar cases, and for the administration of adriamycin as a single high dose, higher than others reported in the literature (Didolkar et al. 1978; Di Pietro et al. 1973; Karakousis et al. 1980; Kraybill et

Table 2. Follow-up data

	No. of cases	Mean follow-up (months)
Living NED	7	11.4
Living with metastases	4	11.3
Dead	0	–
Lost to follow-up	0	–
Still not evaluated	2	–
Total	13	11.4

NED, no evidence of disease

al. 1977; Maree et al. 1980; Weisenburger et al. 1981). The number of patients who entered the study is limited, but new cases of soft tissue sarcomas are not very frequent and, except for the analysis by Weisenburger et al. (1981), no author has presented a larger series of selected cases.

Conclusions

Based on this pilot study, and in view of our stated aims, we can conclude that:

1. Preoperative intra-arterial chemotherapy is feasible and leads to no complications or unexpected side effects.
2. Clinical improvement sometimes makes it possible to perform conservative surgery rather than amputation or disarticulation.
3. The early metastatic spread seen in our series suggests the presence of latent metastases at the beginning of therapy; in any case, this multimodal treatment schedule does not seem to prevent metastatic onset.
4. Tumor chemosensitivity to adriamycin was well documented in almost all the patients. The response rate (ten in 12 cases) is remarkably high, if we consider that previous analysis of adriamycin for advanced sarcomas revealed objective response in less than 30% of treated cases (Gottlieb et al. 1976).

We now intend to modify the schedule, administering adriamycin over 4 rather than 8 days (at the same total dose) for two or three cycles at 21-day intervals in order to achieve a better clinical evaluation and to improve conservative surgery; should the response to chemotherapy be good, postoperative systemic treatment with the same drug is planned.

References

Didolkar MS, Kanter PM, Baffi RR, Schwartz HS, Lopez R, Baez N (1978) Comparison of regional systemic chemotherapy with adriamycin. Ann Surg 187: 332–336

Di Pietro S, De Palo GM, Gennari L, Molinari R, Damascelli B (1973) Cancer chemotherapy by intraarterial infusion with adriamycin. J Surg Oncol 5: 421–430

Enneking WF, Spanier SS, Goodman MA (1980) A system for the surgical staging of musculoskeletal sarcoma. Clin Orthop 153: 106–120

Gottlieb JA, Baker LH, O'Bryan RM, Sinkovics JG, Hoogstraten B, Quagliana JM, Rivkin SE, Bodey GP, Rodriguez VT, Blumenschein GR, Saiki JH, Coltman C Jr, Burgees MA, Sullivan P, Thigpen T, Bottomley R, Balcerzak S, Moon TE (1976) Adriamycin (NSC-123127) used alone and in combination for soft tissue and bone sarcomas. Cancer Treat Rep 60: 199–203

Karakousis CP, Lopez R, Catane R, Rao U, Moore R, Holyoke ED (1980) Intraarterial adriamycin in the treatment of soft tissue sarcomas. J Surg Oncol 13: 21–27

Kraybill WM, Harrison M, Sasaki T, Fletcher WS (1977) Regional intraarterial infusion of adriamycin in the treatment of cancer. Surg Gynecol Obstet 144: 335–338

Marée D, Bui NB, Chauvergne J, Avril A, Richaud P (1980) Traitment des sarcomes des tissus mous localement évoluées. Intérêt de la chimiothérapie d'induction par voie intra-artérielle. Bull Cancer (Paris) 67: 175–182

Weisenburger TH, Eilber FR, Grant TT, Morton DL, Mirra JJ, Steinberg M, Rickles D (1981) Multidisciplinary 'limb salvage' treatment of soft tissue and skeletal sarcomas. Int J Radiat Oncol Biol Phys 7: 1495–1499

Discussion

Leakage in isolated estremity perfusions seems to range between 5% and 12%. Most surgeons measure leakage, and stop perfusing when it exceeds 20%. Bone-marrow depression resulting from melphalan perfusion occurs very rarely incidence is generally below 1%.

Isolated extremity perfusions for primary melanomas are performed at Clark level III−IV, with a tumor thickness of at least 1.5 mm. In cases of acrolentiginous or nodular melanomas, perfusion is repeated 4 or 6 weeks later.

In recurrent melanomas there is a therapeutic indication for isolated perfusion. To determine adjuvant indication in stage-I patients a controlled randomized trial was requested by several speakers.

Hyperthermic Regional Perfusion in High-Risk Stage-I Malignant Melanomas of the Extremities

H. Schraffordt Koops and J. Oldhoff

Division of Surgical Oncology, University Hospital Groningen, Groningen, The Netherlands

Malignant melanoma of the skin is an erratic tumor of rather unpredictable behavior. The prognosis is influenced by the presence or absence of metastases. In recent years studies by Clark et al. (1969) and Breslow (1975) have revealed several additional clinical and histologic characteristics of the primary tumor to which prognostic significance can be ascribed. Tumor size, depth of invasion, ulceration, vascular invasion, and lymphoid reaction along the under side of the tumor have been reported to be of importance in this respect. Olsen (1966), Bodenham (1968), Davis (1976), Milton (1977), and Shaw et al. (1978) reported that the location of the primary tumor and the patient's sex are also factors influencing survival.

Materials and Methods

During the period from 1965 to 1976, 158 patients with malignant melanoma Clark level IV or V and a tumor thickness of more than 1.5 mm located on one of the extremities, without demonstrable metastases, were treated in our department. Treatment was comprehensive and consisted in all cases of a combination of surgery and chemotherapy: wide local excision and regional perfusion.

In order to study survival and local recurrence in our patients, all sections from tumors were reassessed. Because our analysis is based primarily on reexamination of representative sections through the lesions rather than of the entire melanoma, it is possible that thicker areas may have existed in unsampled portions of the specimens.

Regional Perfusion

The treatment of cancer by regional perfusion with cytostatic agents resulted from a study by Klopp et al. (1950), who found that pain was alleviated and tumor size reduced when small doses of nitrogen mustard (chlormethine) were injected into the supplying arteries. The best results were obtained when venous return from the area involved was blocked.

In 1959 Creech et al. combined this procedure with extracorporeal circulation, using a pump oxygenator which made it possible to administer large doses of nitrogen mustard continuously.

In 1960 Stehlin et al. reported on 116 regional perfusions carried out in the M.D. Anderson Hospital, Houston. The majority of patients had tumors on the extremities; the remainder had tumors of the pelvic region and the head and neck area. Luck (1956) established in animal experiments that melphalan (L-phenylalanine mustard) was the most active agent to inhibit the growth of malignant melanoma in mice; this cytostatic drug has since been the agent of choice in perfusions.

In 1967 Cavaliere et al. laid the foundations for perfusions under hyperthermia. In a biochemical and clinical study they described the susceptibility of cancer cells to high temperatures.

The literature (Krementz et al. 1979; McBride et al. 1975; Schraffordt Koops et al. 1977, 1981; Stehlin et al. 1979; Sugarbaker and McBride 1976) of the past few years shows that regional perfusion is really practicable only in the extremities, where adequate vascular occlusion can be achieved. In other parts of the body this is difficult because leakage to the systemic circulation becomes excessive; the advantage of regional perfusion − high local doses of the cytostatic agents without systemic toxic reactions − is consequently lost.

Technique of Perfusion

For perfusion of a lower extremity the external iliac artery and vein were exposed just above the inguinal ligament. The vessels were cannulated and occluded above the catheter with vascular clamps and a tourniquet. The extremity was perfused with the aid of a pump oxygenator containing a heat exchanger in the circuit.

The drug dosage was determined on the basis of local tissue tolerance and leakage to the systemic circulation (1−1.5 mg phenylalanine mustard per kg body wt. for the lower extremity and 0.5−0.7 mg/kg for the upper). Leakage was measured using a radioactive tracer in the external circulation and an NaI scintillation detector placed over the heart (Schraffordt Koops et al. 1981).

Until 1969 the perfusate was introduced at a temperature of approximately 37.5° C and the perfusion time was 45 min. In subsequent years the temperature and the perfusion time have been increased to 40° C and 60 min.

For perfusion of the upper extremity the axillary vessels were cannulated high in the axilla and the perfusion procedure was carried out as for the lower extremity, but with a smaller dose of phenylalanine mustard.

In patients with melanomas of the upper extremity, a single axillary perfusion was performed. Patients with a melanoma on the lower extremity located above the level of the ankle underwent an external iliac perfusion. Since melanomas of the lower extremity below the level of the ankle have a higher tendency to local recurrence, patients with the primary tumor at this level had the limb perfused twice, with the external iliac perfusion followed by a popliteal perfusion 6 weeks later.

Results

Complications After Perfusion

The relevant literature describes a variety of post-perfusion complications. In our patients postoperative complications were relatively rare (Table 1). Two patients died as a result of the operation. There were some lasting postoperative complications which occurred mainly

Table 1. Major complications in 158 patients after 201 perfusions for primary melanomas

	No. of patients	(%)
Mortality	2	1.3
Amputation	2	1.3
Impaired leg/hand function	5	3.2
Pulmonary embolism	2	1.3

during the first years of our perfusion treatment: two patients had late pulmonary embolism after 7 and 8 months; in two others amputation of the lower extremity was necessary because of serious burns following hyperthermic perfusion.

Status and Determinate Survival

Of the 158 patients who have undergone perfusion and excision, 112 are alive with no evidence of disease. Four died of documented intercurrent disease without evidence of melanoma 1 or more years after perfusion. One patient developed a second primary tumor 6 years after perfusion and died of this tumor 3 years later. Two patients died as the result of an operative complication: diffuse intravascular coagulation of unknown origin a few hours after perfusion. No patient has been lost to follow-up. Determinate survival for 5 years or more is 112 of 151 patients, or 74%.

Survival in Relation to Histologic Features

There was a marked correlation between tumor thickness and survival. In tumors over 5 mm thick, the survival rate fell from 82% to 50% (Table 2). In our patients the different levels of invasion were also associated with evident differences in survival. The Clark levels (Table 3) show that the prognosis is evidently more unfavorable as tumor invasion is deeper (78% survival at level IV, 33% at level V).

Recurrence in the Extremity After Perfusion

Recurrent melanomas are defined here as tumors developing in or adjacent to the scar of the excision of the primary lesion, or cutaneous or subcutaneous lymphatic metastases (in-transit metastases) between the site of the primary lesion and the regional lymph nodes.

Of the 151 patients, 14 had a recurrence in the extremity during the follow-up of 5–16 years. In nine patients the recurrence became manifest in the perfused extremity after systemic metastases were detected at 8, 12, 21, 36, 43, 72, 80, 80, and 84 months after treatment (mean: 48 months). Five had recurrence without distant metastases at 21, 37, 65, 72, and 77 months (mean: 54) after therapy.

So far, this series of patients has shown no statistically significant difference in local recurrence after normothermic and hyperthermic perfusion, two of 19 (11%) and 12 of 132

Table 2. Observed survival in relation to tumor thickness (follow-up 5−16 years)

Thickness (mm)	No. of patients	No evidence of disease	
		Patients (n)	Percent (%)
1.5 −3.00	65	58	89
3.01−4.00	16	12	75
4.01−5.00	22	18	82
> 5.01	48	24	50

Table 3. Observed survival in relation to Clark staging

Level of invasion	No. of patients	No evidence of disease	
		(n)	(%)
IV	139	108	78
V	12	4	33

(9%) respectively. However, mean tumor thickness in the patients treated by hyperthermic perfusion proved to exceed that in the normothermically perfused patients.

In this series it was possible to determine the timing of the first recurrence in the perfused extremity. Stehlin and Clark (1965) stated that the first 24 months after definitive therapy are critical as far as regional recurrences are concerned; if recurrences develop, they do so within this period in 80% of patients. In our group, however, recurrence came much later than two years after perfusion. It seems that perfusion at least delays local recurrence, if it does not prevent it. The five patients with local recurrence and without distant metastases are all alive and show no evidence of disease 91, 35, 43, 2, and 36 months after retreatment. Amputation for uncontrolled in-transit metastases was not necessary.

Regional Lymph Node Metastases

Lymph node metastases occurred during the follow-up of 5−16 years in 30 of 151 patients (20%). This proved to be an unfavorable prognostic sign.

Summary

Local recurrence after conventional surgical treatment of malignant melanomas of the extremities has frequently been observed in our department in the past. As at other centers, this sometimes necessitated amputation, and on a few occasions amputations were performed exclusively for palliative reasons.

In an effort to improve this situation, regional perfusion as local regional treatment was added to conventional therapy in 1965. We have since observed no further instances of massive local tumor growth, and since that time no amputations have had to be performed for this reason.

Of course this complicated therapy caused new problems, particularly in the early years, but we have learned to reduce these to what we believe to be an acceptable minimum. In the last 2 years we have done nearly 100 perfusions and have had no major complications.

A comparison of the results of regional perfusion plus local excision in the treatment of stage-I melanoma with those of other reported series (Cascinelli et al. 1978; Elder et al. 1979; Fortner et al. 1977; Goldsmith et al. 1970; Lee 1979; McCarthy et al. 1974; Veronesi et al. 1977; Wanebo et al. 1975) treated only by local excision is difficult, owing to the complexity of the known variables relating to survival and local recurrence. The 5–16 year determinate survival rate for our perfusion patients was 74%.

The local recurrence rate in the perfused extremities was 9%, 14 patients, and nine of these 14 had distant metastases as well. The other five patients still show no evidence of disease after retreatment. It is of interest that when a recurrence developed after perfusion it appeared more than 5 years after initial treatment in seven of 14 patients.

The latest local recurrence developed after 84 months, which means that perfused patients should have a follow-up period of at least 10 years. It seems likely that perfusion delays the appearance of recurrence; it may also be that retreatment of local recurrence has a very high success rate. This is illustrated by the five patients with local recurrence and without distant metastases, who are all alive with no evidence of disease.

So far, our series of patients has shown no statistically significant difference in local recurrence rate after normo- and hyperthermic perfusion. However, mean tumor thickness in the patients treated by hyperthermic perfusion proved to exceed that in the normothermically perfused patients.

Lymph node metastases occurred during the follow-up period of 5–16 years in 20% of patients.

The most important achievement of regional perfusion is that amputation – a procedure widely used in the treatment of malignant melanoma 20 years ago – is now seldom, if ever, necessary.

References

Bodenham DC (1968) A study of 650 observed malignant melanomas in the South-West Region. Ann R Coll Surg Engl 43: 218

Breslow A (1975) Tumor thickness, level of invasion, and node dissection in stage I cutaneous melanoma. Ann Surg 182: 572

Cascinelli N, Van der Esch EP, Morabito A (1978) Stage I melanoma of the limbs: assessment of prognosis by levels of invasion and maximum thickness. Tumori 64: 273

Cavaliere R, Ciocatto EC, Giovanella BC et al. (1967) Selective heat sensitivity of cancer cells. Biochemical and clinical studies. Cancer 20: 351

Clark WH, From L, Bernardino EA, Mihm MC (1969) The histogenesis and biological behaviour of primary human malignant melanomas of the skin. Cancer Res 29: 705

Creech O, Ryan RF, Krementz ET (1959) Treatment of malignant melanoma by isolation perfusion technique. JAMA 169: 339

Davis NC (1976) Cutaneous melanoma; the Queensland experience. Curr Probl Surg 13: 5

Elder DE, Ainsworth AM, Clark WH Jr (1979) The surgical pathology of cutaneous malignant melanoma. In: Clark WH, Goldman LJ, Mastrangelo MJ (eds) Human malignant melanoma. Grune and Stratton, New York, p 55

Fortner JG, Woodruff J, Schottenfeld D, MacLean B (1977) Biostatistical basis of elective node dissection for malignant melanoma. Ann Surg 186: 101

Goldsmith HS, Shah JP, Kim DH (1970) Prognostic significance of lymph node dissection in the treatment of malignant melanoma. Cancer 26: 606

Klopp CF, Alford TC, Bateman J, Berry GN, Winship T (1950) Fractionated intra-arterial cancer chemotherapy with methyl bis amine hydrochloride: a preliminary report. Ann Surg 132: 811

Krementz ET, Carter RD, Sutherland CM, Campbell M (1979) The use of regional chemotherapy in the management of malignant melanoma. World J Surg 3: 289

Lee YTN (1979) Diagnosis, treatment and prognosis of early melanoma. Ann Surg 191: 87

Luck JM (1956) Action of p-[di(2-chloroethyl)]-amino-L-phenylalanine on Harding-Passey mouse melanoma. Science 123: 984

McBride CM, Sugarbaker EV, Hickey RC (1975) Prophylactic isolation-perfusion as the primary therapy for invasive malignant melanoma of the limbs. Ann Surg 182: 316

McCarthy JC, Haagensen CD, Herter FP (1974) The role of groin dissection in the management of melanoma of the lower extremity. Ann Surg 179: 156

Milton GW (1977) Malignant melanoma of the skin and muccous membranes. Churchill Livingstone, Edinburgh, p 26

Olsen G (1966) The malignant melanoma of the skin. Thesis, Finsen Institute and Radium Center, Aarhuus Stiftsbogtrykkerie

Schraffordt Koops H, Oldhoff J, Van der Ploeg E, Vermey A, Eibergen R (1977) Regional perfusion for recurrent malignant melanoma of the extremities. Am J Surg 133: 221

Schraffordt Koops H, Beekhuis H, Oldhoff J, Oosterhuis JW, Van der Ploeg E, Vermey A (1981) Local recurrence and survival in patients with (Clark level IV/V and over 1.5 mm thickness) stage I malignant melanoma of the extremities after regional perfusion. Cancer 48: 1952

Shaw HM, Milton GW, Farago G, McCarthy WH (1978) Endocrine influences on survival from malignant melanoma. Cancer 42: 669

Stehlin JS Jr, Clark RL (1965) Melanoma of the etremities. Experiences with conventional treatment and perfusion in 339 cases. Am J Surg 110: 336

Stehlin JS, Clark RL, White EC et al. (1960) Regional chemotherapy for cancer: experiences with 116 perfusions. Ann Surg 151: 605

Stehlin JS, Giovanella BS, De Ipolyi PD, Anderson RF (1979) Eleven years' experience with hyperthermic perfusion for melanoma of the extremities. World J Surg 3: 305

Sugarbaker EV, McBride CM (1976) Survival and regional disease control after isolation-perfusion for invasive stage I melanoma of the extremities. Cancer 37: 188

Veronesi U, Adamus J, Bandiera DC et al. (1977) Inefficacy of immediate node dissection in stage I melanoma of the limbs. N Engl J Med 297: 627

Wanebo HF, Fortner JG, Woodruff J, MacLean B, Binkowski E (1975) Selection of the optimum surgical treatment of stage I melanoma by depth of microinvasion. Ann Surg 182: 302

Hyperthermic Perfusion in Malignant Melanoma: 5-Year Results

J. Tonak[1], W. Hohenberger[1], F. Weidner[2], and H. Göhl[1]

1 Chirurgische Universitätsklinik Erlangen, Maximilliansplatz, 8520 Erlangen, FRG
2 Dermatologische Abteilung der Chirurgischen Universitätsklinik Erlangen,
Maximilliansplatz, 8520 Erlangen, FRG

Introduction

A special problem in the treatment of malignant melanomas is the management of occult regional metastases. The incidence of these metastases is directly related to the depth of invasion of the primary tumor (Breslow 1970; Fortner et al. 1977; Tonak et al. 1981; Wanebo et al. 1975).

Melanomas have the special characteristic of not only leading to lymph node and distant metastases, but also to so-called in-transit metastases. These are tumor cells which are deposited in tissue or lymph vessels somewhere between the primary melanoma and the regional lymph nodes, and which finally develop into clinically manifest tumors. In advanced melanomas of the limbs we have to reckon with the presence of in-transit metastases in 20%−30% of cases (Sugarbaker and McBride 1976).

One can assume that the treatment of advanced malignant melanomas would be especially successful if not only the primary tumor and the regional lymph nodes were removed, but also the occult tumor cells present between the primary tumor and the lymph nodes were distroyed. This goal can be achieved for melanomas of the limbs by perfusion, with the simultaneous use of cytotoxic drugs and hyperthermia (Ghussen et al. 1981; Illig and Aigner 1980; Krementz et al. 1979; Schraffordt Koops et al. 1977; Stehlin et al. 1975, 1979; Tonak et al. 1981).

Material and Methods

Since 1969 all patients with malignant melanoma treated at Erlangen University have been registered in a special cancer file. Up to December 31, 1981 a total of 784 cases of malignant melanomas were included in this register. Clinical and pathological findings on all patients are documented in a standardized manner. The pathohistological examination of all tumor specimens is carried out according to the same principle by two independent pathologists. For the purpose of this study, 154 patients with potentially curable melanomas of the extremities who had undergone curative operations between December 1, 1975 and December 31, 1980 were selected from this register.

The basic treatment for primary malignant melanoma consisted in wide local excision, elective dissection, and hyperthermic perfusion of the extremity. In patients with regional

Table 1. pTNM classification and clinical data on 154 cases of melanomas of the extremities treated by perfusion

Stage	n	%	Female	Male	Upper extremities	Lower extremities
Ia	13	8				
Ib	90	59	110	44	47	107
II	51	39	(71%)	(29%)	(31%)	(69%)

metastases we performed a wide local excision of the primary tumor, a therapeutic lymph-node dissection, and hyperthermic perfusion.

In cases of patients with numerous in-transit metastases which were not surgically removable, or with satellitosis, we carried out hyperthermic perfusion without further surgical treatment.

The follow-up of all patients covers at least 1 year, but the average follow-up has been 39 months. None of the patients has been lost to follow-up.

The TNM classification of the Union Internationale Contra le Cancer (1978) is used (Table 1). In 107 patients a lower extremity was perfused, and in 47 patients an upper; 110 patients were female and 44 male.

Of our 154 patients, 61 (40%) had a superficial spreading melanoma, 42 (27%) a nodular melanoma, nine (6%) a lentigo maligna melanoma, and 19 (12%) an acral-lentiginous melanoma. Of the remaining 15% (23 patients) one patient had a malignant melanoma arising from a blue nevus, one a malignant melanoma from a giant cellular nevus, and one an unclassified melanoma. In 20 patients with stage-II disease the diagnosis was first established through already existing regional metastases.

Indications

We see an indication for perfusion at the present time in primary malignant melanomas with a tumor diameter of more than 1.5 mm, or in those at microstages 4 and 5. In terms of the pT classification of the UICC, this is to say that we consider pT 1 and pT 2 melanomas of the extremities low-risk tumors, for which wide local excision is sufficient. Numerous in-transit metastases or satellitosis which cannot be removed surgically are a special indication for perfusion.

Elective dissection and adjuvant perfusion are now performed only for pT 3 and pT 4 melanomas. However, until 2 years ago we also used adjuvant perfusion and elective lymph-node dissection for patients with melanomas at microstage 3 and with tumors between 0.76 and 1.5 mm in diameter, which correspond to pT 2 tumors. Among 21 patients so treated, there were no lymph node metastases in the specimens examined histologically, and no metastases have since occurred; no patients have died. The 5-year survival rate was 100%, irrespective of whether adjuvant perfusion was carried out in addition to the excision and dissection (Fig. 1). We therefore believe that in such tumors local excision with a wide margin of safety is sufficient, and that no further measures are required.

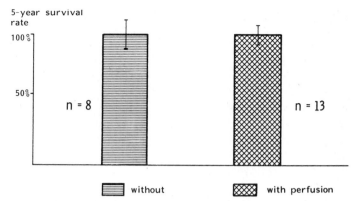

Fig. 1. Five-year survival rates (corrected for age − Berkson-Gage, Erlangen) for 21 patients with stage-I, pT 2 melanomas of the extremities, treated by excision and dissection, *with* or *without* perfusion

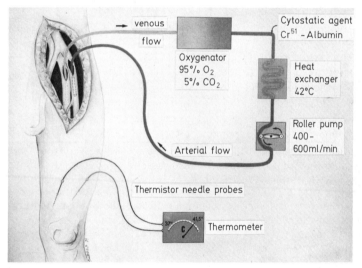

Fig. 2. Hyperthermic perfusion system and procedure

Operative Procedures

Figure 2 illustrates the procedure of hyperthermic perfusion. We have followed the method recommended by Creech and Krementz (1966) and Schraffordt-Koops et al. (1977, 1981). The vessels of a lower or upper extremity are cannulated and connected to an oxygenator; the isolated extremity is perfused with a pump oxygenator containing a heat exchanger in the circuit. The limb temperature is continuously monitored during the procedure by subcutaneous thermist or needle probes. The chemotherapeutic agents are added to the perfusate; we use melphalan at an average dose of 1.2 mg/kg body wt. In case of regional metastases we employ a combination of melphalan and actinomycin-D (average dose 0.01 mg/kg body wt.). Perfusion time is 1 h. During perfusion the limb temperature usually reaches 41.5−42° C. The elective axillary or inguinal lymph-node dissection is performed synchronously. Normally, the primary tumor is removed several days earlier, and histologically examined.

Results

The 4-year-survival rate for our 103 patients with stage I disease is 90% ± 9% following perfusion. The 5-year-survival rate is 80% ± 17%. These survival rates are higher than those of a historic group of patients, who between 1969 and 1975 received the same type of surgical treatment, with excision and dissection, but no perfusion. However the difference is not statistically significant after the third year of follow-up (Fig. 3).

For 90 patients with stage-I disease and prognostically unfavorable pT 3 and pT 4 melanomas who received perfusion the 4- and 5-year survival rates are 89% ± 11% and 78% ± 16% respectively (Fig. 4).

Comparison with another historical group of 51 patients with pT 3 and pT 4 melanomas who were treated at our hospital in the same manner by surgical excision and dissection but

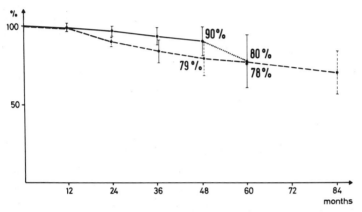

Fig. 3. Five-year age-corrected survival rates (Berkson-Gage) for 169 patients with stage-I, pT 2−pT 4 melanomas of the extremities. *Solid line*, 103 treated by excision and dissection with perfusion; *dotted line*, less than ten patients, follow-up not statistically relevant; *broken line*, 66 patients treated by excision and dissection and without perfusion

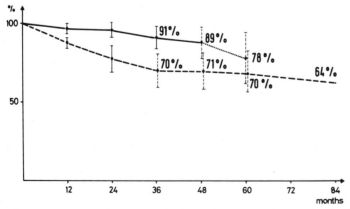

Fig. 4. Age-corrected 5-year survival rates for same patients as in Fig. 3, excluding those with pT 2 melanomas. *Solid line*, 90 treated by excision, dissection, and perfusion; *dotted line*, less than ten patients followed up in the 5th year; *broken line*, 51 treated by excision and dissection without perfusion

without perfusion shows that the patient group with perfusion had statistically significant ($p < 0.05$) higher survival rates up to 5 years' follow-up.

Less than ten patients of the groups represented in Figs. 3 and 4 were followed up for 6 years, so a statistically relevant comparison for this time period is not possible.

The survival rates of 51 patients with stage-II disease, i.e., with regional metastases, who received perfusion were on average 30% higher than those for 23 patients who were treated before 1975 with excision and dissection only (Fig. 5).

Recurrences

Among our 103 patients with stage-I disease, 19 developed metastases during the observation period. The incidence of local recurrence after adjuvant perfusion in our patients is low, at 3%. Seven of 103 perfused patients developed distant metastases within 2 years. In these seven patients no local recurrence or regional metastases occurred in the area of the perfused limb. In two cases satellitosis on the treated limb could be observed in

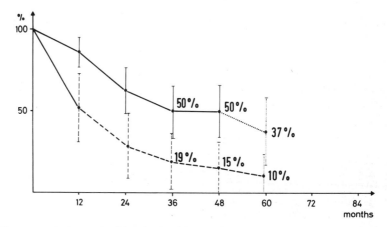

Fig. 5. Age-corrected 5-year survival rates for 74 patients with stage-II melanomas of the extremities. *Solid line,* 51 treated by excision, dissection, and perfusion; *dotted line,* less than ten patients in follow-up; *broken line,* 23 treated by excision and dissection only

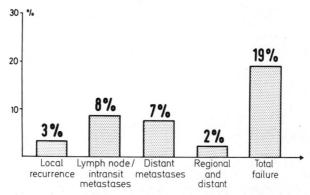

Fig. 6. Observed incidence of first recurrence in 103 patients with stage-I melanomas of the extremities, treated by excision, dissection, and perfusion (only pT 2−pT 4 tumors) (compare Table 2)

Table 2. Comparison of reports in the literature on first recurrence in patients treated by perfusion

Report	Patients treated (n)	Tumor type	Adjuvant dissection	Local recurrence, n (%)	Lymph node metastases, n (%)	Distant metastases, n (%)	Regional and distant metastases, n (%)	Total treatment failures n (%)
Schraffordt-Koops 1981	104	pT3 and pT4	None	9 (9)	18 (17)	None	4 (4)	27 (26)
Krementz 1979	286	pT2–pT4	Usually	8 (3)	17 (6)	27 (9)	9 (3)	61 (21)
Sugarbaker 1976	197	pT2–pT4	Usually none	4 (2)	30 (15)	15 (8)	None	49 (25)
Erlangen 1982	103	pT2–pT4	Always	3 (3)	8 (8)	7 (7)	2 (2)	19 (19)

incidence of patients who later developed in-transit or lymph node metastases was 8% (Fig. 6).

A comparison of these results with reports from the literature shows that all physicians who do not perform elective dissection report a higher frequency of late-developing lymph node metastases (Table 2).

Side Effects

Hyperthermic perfusion is fraught with a number of characteristic side effects, the severity of which depends on the duration of perfusion, the tissue temperature, the dose of cytostatic drug administered, and individual circumstances. With increasing experience on the part of the surgeon, these complications can be minimized. The following severe side effects occurred in our group of 154 patients:

1. One had rebleeding with reoperation (1%).
2. Three developed arterial thromboses (2%).
3. Six experienced permanent swelling [postthrombotic syndrome (4%)].
4. Four exhibited neurologic disturbances [permanent paralysis of the femoral or peroneal nerves (3%)].
5. One had extensive necrosis which led to amputation (1%).

The amputation was of a right leg 12 weeks after perfusion, and took place 4 years ago; we have not seen any permanent damage following perfusion during the past $2^1/_2$ years.

There have been three deaths as a result of the operation, owing to (a) rebleeding 14 days later, (b) pulmonary embolism 10 days later, and (c) pulmonary embolism 14 days later.

Discussion

The use of hyperthermic limb perfusion as a prophylactic measure for high-risk melanomas of the extremities is still under discussion. Opponents of this method (Davis 1979) argue that its efficiency has not yet been proven in prospective randomized trials. To our knowledge there is only one investigation under way in the world, which is being conducted by the Southwest Oncology Group in Kansas, United States, to compare wide excision with and without adjuvant hyperthermic perfusion (National Institutes of Health 1980) using melphalan.

We have not conducted such a prospective trial, nor have other physicians in Germany who in the meantime use hyperthermic perfusion as a routine method. Other authors have shown in a large number of cases (Ariel 1980; Weidner 1981) that in pT 3 and pT 4 melanomas of the extremities 8- to 10-year survival rates between 45% and 60% can be achieved using surgical methods only. Well-documented studies (Krementz et al. 1979; Schraffordt-Koops and Oldhoff 1980; Stehlin et al. 1979) have shown that survival rates for patients with these high-risk melanomas can be increased by an average of 20% if adjuvant perfusion is applied.

In addition, many authors have shown (Lejeune et al. 1977; Nachbur 1980; Tonak et al. 1981; Stehlin et al. 1975) perfusion to be effective in primary tumors or metastases which were not surgically removed. In more then half of these cases tumors disappeared completely after the treatment, at least on a temporary base. These data have convinced us that a prospective randomized trial is no longer justified. In our own study the 4-year survival rate for patients with pT 4 and pT 3 melanomas of the limbs is 89% at present. This leads us to expect that 8−10 year survival rates of about 80% can also be achieved for our patients.

Putting this in relation to the total number of perfused patients, one can conclude that in two thirds of cases malignant melanomas and their occult metastases respond to the treatment. It remains to be seen whether the use of other chemotherapeutic agents will further increase the response rate. Of special interest in this connection are investigations which are aimed at determining the sensitivity of tumors to individual cytostatic drugs. In limb perfusion not only the type of cytostatic drug but also the type of hyperthermia used is of special importance (Martijn et al. 1981; Tonak et al. 1981).

Stehlin et al. (1975) for example were able to prove that only the concomitant use of hyperthermia makes perfusion clinically effective. Therefore, we are of the opinion that a more intensive degree of hyperthermia should be used than that described by some authors (Krementz et al. 1979; Schraffordt-Koops and Oldhoff 1981, Sugarbaker and McBride 1976).

By increasing the temperature in perfused tissue to above 41.5° C we hope that not only the increased action of the cytostatic drug caused by an increase in metabolic activity and increased uptake into the melanoma cells, but also the hyperthermia itself will have a significant cytotoxic effect. Experiments with animals and clinical investigations have shown that hyperthermia alone, provided it is above 41.5° C, will destroy malignant tumors, and especially malignant melanomas (Cavaliere et al. 1967). A significant increase in undesirable side effects was not observed in our own clinical series up to a temperature of 42° C (Tonak et al. 1981). Despite the high temperature the only damage we have seen in the past 2 years was one transient peroneal paralysis. Extensive damage to healthy tissue can be prevented when our modern knowledge of the physiology of perfusion is properly applied (Wieberdink and van Slooten 1976).

Death following the procedure was caused in two of three cases by lethal pulmonary embolisms. A certain risk of venous thrombosis is always present in operations in the groin and in those involving large veins. We limit this danger by early mobilization of the patients and the administration of high-dose heparin (4 × 5,000 U) for the duration of the hospital stay. The morbidity and mortality associated with the method seem to us acceptable, as they are limited to a small percentage of patients, and in view of the malignancy of the basic disease and the improved survival rates.

Perfusion causes disappearance of regional metastases in almost 50% of cases, at least on a temporary basis. This is clearly reflected in the survival rates of patients with stage-II disease, which are almost 30% better than those with conventional surgical therapy.

In conclusion, we are able to confirm the good results of other investigators in handling these advanced metastasizing melanomas (Krementz et al. 1979; Lejeune et al 1977; Martijn et al. 1981; Stehlin et al. 1979). In patients who have numerous skin or in-transit metastases which cannot be removed surgically, hyperthermic perfusion is the treatment of choice at the present time.

Summary

Between December 1975 and December 1980 a total of 154 patients with potentially curable malignant melanoma were treated by adjuvant hyperthermic perfusion. The basic therapy consisted in local excision of the primary tumor with elective dissection of the regional lymph nodes.

The 4- and 5-year survival rates for our 103 patients with stage-I disease who were perfused are 90% ± 9% and 80% ± 17%. The 4- and 5-year survival rates for 51 patients with stage-II disease are 50% ± 16% and 37% ± 28%.

Compared with historic control groups of patients who were treated at our hospital with the same surgical methods but without perfusion, essentially better results were achieved with adjuvant hyperthermic perfusion.

It is concluded from our results that hyperthermic perfusion can further improve the prognosis for patients with malignant melanomas of the limbs.

References

Ariel M (1980) Malignant melanoma of the lower extremity: Evaluation of 453 patients. J Surg Oncol 15: 147

Breslow A (1970) Thickness, cross-sectional areas and depth of invasion in the prognosis of cutaneous melanoma. Ann Surg 172: 902

Cavaliere R, Ciocatto EC, Giovanella BC, Heidelberger C, Johnson RO, Margottini M, Mondovi B, Moricca G, Rossi-Fanelli A (1967) Selective heat sensivity of cancer cells. Cancer 20: 1351

Creech O Jr, Krementz ET (1966) Techniques of regional perfusion. Surgery 60: 938

Davis NC (1979) Comment regarding hyperthermic perfusion. World J Surg 3: 308

Fortner JG, McLean BJ, Woodruff J, Schottenfeld D (1977) Biostatistical basis of elective node dissection for malignant melanoma. Ann Surg 186: 101

Ghussen F, Nagel K, Groth W (1981) Regionale hypertherme Zytostatikaperfusion bei malignen Melanomen der Extremitäten. Dtsch Med Wochenschr 106: 1612

Illig L, Aigner K (1980) Therapie des malignen Melanoms unter besonderer Berücksichtigung der isolierten Extremitätenperfusion. Dtsch Ärzteblatt 49: 2911

Krementz ET, Carter RD, Sutherland CM, Campbell M (1979) The use of regional chemotherapy in the management of malignant melanoma. World J Surg 3: 289

Lejeune FJ, Mathieu M, Kenis Y (1977) Hyperthermic isolation-perfusion with melphalan. A preliminary appraisal of local and general effects in malignant melanoma. Tumor 63: 289

Martijn H, Oldhoff J, Schraffordt-Koops H (1981) Regional perfusion in the treatment of patients with a locally metastasized malignant melanoma of the limbs. Eur J Cancer 17: 471

Nachbur B (1980) Regionale Chemotherapie in der Behandlung des malignen Melanoms. 16th annual meeting of the Swiss society for plastic and reconstructure surgery, Basel 18–20 Sept, 1980

National Institutes of Health (1980) Compilation of cancer therapy, protocol summaries, 4th edn. Publication Nr. 80–1116, Protocol Nr. SWOG 7737, p 438

Schraffordt-Koops H, Oldhoff J (1981) Survival and local recurrence after regional perfusion in patients with a deep growing primary malignant melanoma of the extremities. In: Weidner F, Tonak J (eds) Das maligne Melanom der Haut. Perimed, Erlangen

Schraffordt-Koops H, Oldhoff J, van der Ploeg E, Vermey A, Eibergen R, Beekhuis H (1977) Some aspects of the treatment of primary malignant melanoma of the extremities by isolated regional perfusion. Cancer 39: 27

Sugarbaker EV, McBride CM (1976) Survival and regional disease control after isolation perfusion for invasive stage I melanoma of the extremities. Cancer 37: 188

Stehlin JS, Giovanella BC, de Ipolyi PD, Muenz LR, Anderson RF (1975) Results of hyperthermic perfusion for melanoma of the extremities. Surg Gynecol Obstet 140: 339

Stehlin JS, Giovanella BC, de Ipolyi PD, Anderson RF (1979) Eleven year's experience with hyperthermic perfusion for melanoma of the extremities. World J Surg 3: 305

Tonak J, Gall FP, Hermanek P (1980) Die prophylaktische Lymphknotendissektion beim malignen Melanom. Dtsch Med Wochenschr 105: 1782

Tonak J, Weidner F, Hoferichter S, Altendorf A (1981) Erlanger Therapieschema. Grundlagen, Ergebnisse und Behandlung von Rezidiven. In: Weidner F, Tonak J (eds) Das maligne Melanom der Haut. Perimed, Erlangen

Union Internationale Contre le Cancer (UICC) (1978) TNM Classification of malignant tumors, 3rd ed. UICC, Geneva

Wanebo HJ, Woodruff J, Fortner JG (1975) Malignant melanoma of the extremities: a clinicopathologic study using levels of invasion (microstage). Cancer 35: 666

Weidner F (1981) Eight-year-survival in malignant melanoma related to sex and tumor location. Dermatologica 162: 51

Wieberdink J, van Slooten EA (1976) Regional perfusion with chemotherapeuticals. Paper given at meeting of the EORTC Melanoma Group, Moscow, September 1976

Regional Perfusion with cis-Platinum and Dacarbazine

K. Aigner, P. Hild, K. Henneking, E. Paul, and M. Hundeiker

Allgemeinchirurgische Klinik des Zentrums für Chirurgie, Justus-Liebig-Universität, Klinikstrasse 29, 6300 Giessen, FRG

In October 1979, the isolated extremity perfusion for treatment of malignant melanomas and sarcomas was introduced in Giessen. Improvements in perfusion technique have been incorporated in the method continuously. Within the first $2^1/_2$ years 190 extremity perfusions were performed. The drug combination most commonly used was melphalan with dactinomycin. Besides this we started using nitrogen mustard, and after having worked out the dosage schedules in animal experiments we introduced dacarbazine and cis-platinum for isolation perfusion.

Materials and Methods

In primary perfusions the external iliac artery and vein are exposed above the inguinal ligament. In this area collateral vessels are ligated. While cannulating the iliac vessels, attention is focused on placing the tip of the arterial catheter proximal to the bifurcation of the femoral vessels so that the perfusate will enter both vessels. Thus a homogeneous distribution of the drug and hyperthermia in the upper and lower limb can be achieved. The cannulas are connected to an extracorporeal circuit, consisting of a roller pump and an oxygenator with a heat exchanger. The oxygenator is filled with 500 ml blood and 500 ml 5% glucose. A tourniquet is placed around the root of the limb in order to avoid leakage of the perfusate into the systemic circulation. The flow rate of 300–600 ml/min for the lower limb and hyperthermia of 40° C, measured with four thermistor probes in the muscular tissue of the upper and lower leg as well as subcutaneously near the tumor-bearing area, are maintained during the 60-min perfusion period. The extremities are usually wrapped in a metal sheet. In axillary perfusions the flow rate is 150–300 ml/min.

When performing a second perfusion we use a similar approach to the vessels. Proximal to the bifurcation the two branches of a Y-catheter are introduced – one into the deeper, one into the superficial femoral artery. Again, this procedure is likely to allow a homogeneous perfusion of the limb (Aigner and Schwemmle, to be published).

Dacarbazine (DTIC) or cis-platinum was usually administered in cases of histologically verified disseminated tumors 2 weeks prior to tumor excision, in order that we could observe regression rates. The dosage of the drugs used was based on the volume of the perfused limb, measured by water displacement (Fig. 1). We usually give 20 mg cis-platinum per liter extremity at a temperature not exceeding 40° C (Aigner and Schwemmle, to be published). Otherwise severe nerve damage may occur. DTIC is well

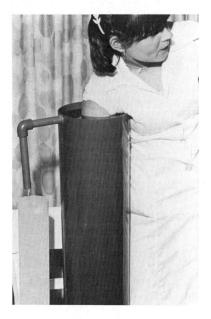

Fig. 1. Volumetry by water displacement

tolerated up to 130 mg/l at a maximum temperature of 40° C, a dosage schedule that has been worked out in animal experiments (Aigner et al. 1980, to be published). In five patients DTIC was added to the perfusate. One of the five had a primary melanoma, three had in-transit metastases, and one suffered from a soft tissue sarcoma in the upper arm.

Isolated perfusions with *cis*-platinum have been performed in a total of 12 patients, five of whom had in-transit metastases and seven, local disease, satellitosis, or cutaneous metastases. A combination treatment with *cis*-platinum and dactinomycin was carried out in six patients, in two of whom the tumors had already been excised, following a primary perfusion with melphalan and dactinomycin.

Results

In the five patients treated with DTIC in perfusion there were no signs of systemic or local toxicity after the operation, despite a slight edema of the perfused extremity for a few days and redness of the skin in the perfused area. No signs of vascular damage or neurotoxicity were observed. Tumor regression of at least 30% was noted in each patient. In the widely excised tumor tissue, regression was confirmed histologically as described elsewhere (Aigner et al., to be published). One DTIC patient had very impressive macroscopic regressions of about 80%–90%; however, the tumors recurred. In three patients the outcome of the DTIC perfusion was troubled by local recurrences between 1.5 and 4 months later. These were cases with multiple in-transit metastases, some of which had no longer been palpable 3 weeks postoperatively.

Of six patients perfused with *cis*-platinum and dactinomycin, two had in-transit metastases; in two cases a tumor excision had been carried out before the perfusion; one patient had a primary tumor; one had satellitosis (Table 1). Since this combination therapy did not produce superior short-term results, we eliminated dactinomycin and started a mono-

Table 1. Dosage, temperature, and percentage of tumor regression in isolated perfusions with *cis*-platinum and dactinomycin (1 mg)

Diagnosis	Dosage of *cis*-Pt (mg/l extremity)	Temperature (° C)	Regression (%)
Satellitosis	16	38.5	20
In-transit disease	17.5	39.6	80
Local disease	16	39.7	50−60
Second perfusion	19	39.4	−
Second perfusion	18	39.4	−
In-transit disease	22	39.8	40−50

Table 2. Isolated perfusion with *cis*-platinum in local disease, satellitosis, and cutaneous epidermotrophic metastases

Diagnosis	Dosage (mg/l extremity)	Temperature ° C	Regression (%)
Cutaneous metastases	28	39.5	50
Local disease	28	38.5	30
Local disease	28	39.5	50
Local disease	20	39	70
Satellitosis	20	40	50
Cutaneous metastases	20	37.5	50
Cutaneous metastases	20	40	50

Table 3. Isolated perfusion with *cis*-platinum in in-transit metastases in subcutaneous or muscular tissue

Diagnosis	Dosage (mg/l extremity)	Temperature (° C)	Regression (%)
In-transit	24	39.7	70
In-transit, LN	16	40	70−90
In-transit	25	39.9	100
In-transit	20	39.6	80
In-transit	25	39.7	100

LN, lymph node

therapy series with *cis*-platinum. This collective, which was divided into two groups − one with primary lesions or cutaneous metastases (Table 2), the other with in-transit metastases in deeper layers such as subcutaneous or muscular tissue (Table 3) − showed better short-term results. Judging clinically, regressions in deeper tissue layers were obviously more impressive. Tumor regression within 2 weeks following *cis*-platinum perfusion at 20 mg/l extremity at approximately 40° C is illustrated by Figs. 2 and 3. A quite similar result can be observed in Figs. 4 and 5, the latter also taken 2 weeks after perfusion. The superficial tumors developed crusts that could be peeled off within several days. In the excised palpable material, however, tumor tissue could be verified histologically, while

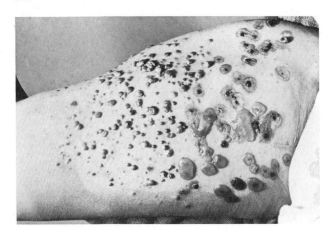

Fig. 2. Multiple cutaneous metastases on the upper thigh of a patient prior to perfusion, some having been treated by cryosurgery

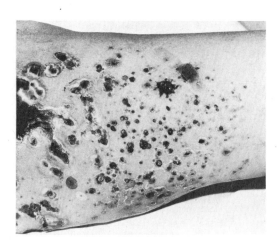

Fig. 3. Multiple cutaneous metastases of same patient as represented in Fig. 2, 2 weeks after *cis*-platinum perfusion

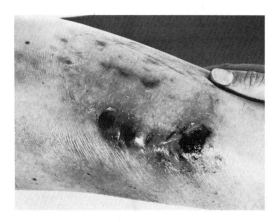

Fig. 4. In-transit metastases in the lower leg before perfusion

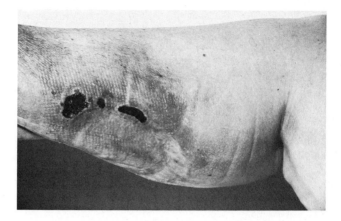

Fig. 5. Same patient as in Fig. 4, 14 days after *cis*-platinum perfusion (20 mg/liter extremity)

Table 4. Disease-free interval from perfusion with *cis*-platinum to tumor recurrence

Interval (months)	No. of patients	Clinical staging
3	4	III AB ($n = 3$) III A ($n = 1$)
4	2	III AB
5	1	III AB
8	1	III A
9	1	II

Table 5. Current follow-up of 13 patients with malignant melanomas and differing clinical staging, after isolated extremity perfusion with *cis*-platinum; at preparation of data all patients were free of disease

Time since perfusion (months)	No. of patients	Clinical staging
4	1	III A
5	2	III A
6	1	III A
7	1	III A
14	2	Acral-lentiginous ($n = 2$)
17	1	III A
18	3	III B ($n = 1$) I ($n = 2$)
19	1	I
20	1	II

subcutaneous metastases generally showed faster shrinkage and often were not palpable after 14 days.

Separated into two groups, representing patients with and without local recurrences, the first group (Table 4) consisting of patients who were mainly stage III AB of disease showed tumor recurrences within 4 months. In the second group (Table 5) with no evidence of disease, about 50% of the patients have had no local recurrences for between 14 and 20 months now. Two patients suffering from acral-lentiginous melanomas died after 14 months due to distant metastases.

Complications

Edema is generally mild after a *cis*-platinum perfusion under mild hyperthermia at 39.5°–40° C. When this temperature limit was exceeded, as in three patients, extensive edema occurred and peridural anesthesia was required for treatment of pain (Aigner and Schwemmle, to be published; Biscoping et al. 1982). All patients, even those with slightly overheated extremities, developed footdrop, a sign of peroneal nerve damage. Renal toxicity was not observed since the leakage rate did not exceed 10%, as measured after radioiodinated serum-albumin injection into the extracorporeal circuit. Bone marrow depletion never occurred.

Discussion

Although complete, or at least partial, remissions can generally be expected after *cis*-platinum perfusions, recurrences may occur within 3 or 4 months, predominantly in stage-III AB cases (Table 4). This requires either a second perfusion or intra-arterial treatment. Two of our stage-III AB patients had no evidence of local recurrence but died of distant metastases. It appears to us that in advanced cases or acral-lentiginous melanomas isolated perfusion is very efficient as far as the regional metastases are concerned, but it obviously cannot prevent the growth of distant metastases if they have already been disseminated. Thus, in such cases, the survival rate cannot be influenced to a significant extent. Many stage-III melanomas which have invaded the regional lymph nodes, have apparently already disseminated distant metastases as well. This supports our opinion that there will be no greater advantage in amputation of the limb as compared with regional perfusion combined with local tumor resection and lymph node dissection (Schraffordt Koops et al. 1981). Though immunological stimulation after isolated perfusion has been considered (McBride 1970; Stehlin et al. 1975), in our follow-up there is no striking evidence that such reactions generally occur.
Our response rates achieved with isolated DTIC perfusion (Aigner et al; to be published) were significantly higher than those achieved with systemic chemotherapy using DTIC in combination or as monotherapy (Lejeune et al. 1978; Luce 1972).
Perfusions with *cis*-platinum carry the risk of neurotoxicity as soon as the tissue temperature exceeds 40° C. In two of our first patients perfused with *cis*-platinum the tissue temperature temporarily reached 41° and 41.5° C. This resulted in severe damage to the peroneal nerve which is normally seen starting on the second postoperative day (Aigner and Schwemmle, to be published). It must be emphasized that short-term hyperthermia at between 40° and 42° C in cytostatic perfusion obviously leads to complications rather than to significantly better results — especially when *cis*-platinum is used.
In 13 of 22 patients having no evidence of disease the longest follow-up period has now been of a stage-II patient for 20 months. However, there are no stage-III AB cases in this group. One III A and one III B have now been disease free for 17 and 18 months respectively, the latter perhaps due to immunological stimulation with an effect on distant micrometastases. The two patients with acral-lentiginous melanoma, having no evidence of local disease in the limb, died of distant metastases 14 months after perfusion (Table 5).
The duration of remission in the group with no evidence of disease cannot yet be foreseen but might be in agreement with observations by other authors (Martijn et al. 1981; Stehlin et al. 1975, 1979). Only one of our patients was perfused between normothermic and

hyperthermic conditions at a temperature of 38.5° C. In this patient tumor regression did not exceed 30%. This again supports the theory that hyperthermic perfusion enhances the efficacy of drugs (Krementz and Ryan 1972).

It may be that in advanced cases better long-term results could be obtained by regional perfusion and resection of the tumor-bearing area and adjuvant systemic or intra-arterial chemotherapy. This can only be answered by means of a controlled prospective trial.

Summary

In 22 patients isolated extremity perfusion with *cis*-platinum for treatment of malignant melanoma was performed; 18 had local metastatic disease (M. D. Anderson stages II and III A, B, AB) and four were stage I. A further five patients were submitted to isolated DTIC perfusion. DTIC-perfused tumors showed regression rates of 30%−80%, followed by recurrences within 4 months. After *cis*-platinum perfusion stage-III AB cases tended to show tumor recurrence within 4 months, while to date stage-III A and stage-II cases have reached disease-free survival times of 17 and 20 months respectively. While in DTIC perfusion the tissue temperature may range between 40° and 41° C, in *cis*-platinum perfusions 40° C should not be exceeded; otherwise neural damage will occur.

References

Aigner K, Schwemmle K (to be published) Technik der isolierten Extremitätenperfusion. Langenbecks Arch Chir

Aigner K, Hild P, Henneking K, Paul E, Hundeiker M, Breithaupt H, Merker G, Jungbluth A (1980) DTIC − Studies in isolated perfusion of the leg and the liver in dogs. EORTC Melanoma Meeting, Lausanne 24/25 April 1980

Aigner K, Hild P, Breithaupt H, Hundeiker M, Schwemmle K, Henneking K, Illig L, Merker G, Paul E, Brodkorb J, Jungbuth A (to be published) The isolated extremity perfusion with DTIC − an experimental and clinical study. Anticancer Res

Biscoping J, Aigner K, Hempelmann G (1982) Erfahrungen mit einer kontinuierlichen Plexus-Anaesthesie des Armes nach Melanomperfusion. Region Anaesth 5: 62−63

Krementz ET, Ryan RF (1972) Chemotherapy of melanoma of the extremities by perfusion: fourteen years' clinical experience. Ann Surg 175: 900

Lejeune FJ, DeWasch G (1978) Malignant melanoma. In: Staquet MJ (ed) Randomized trials in cancer: a critical review by sites. Raven, New York, p 339

Luce JK (1972) Chemotherapy of malignant melanoma. Cancer 30: 1604

Martijn H, Oldhoff J, Schraffordt Koops H (1981) Regional perfusion in the treatment of patients with a locally metastasized malignant melanoma of the limb. Eur J Cancer 17: 471

McBride CM (1970) Advanced melanoma of the extremities. Treatment by isolation perfusion with a triple drug combination. Arch Surg 101: 122

Schraffordt Koops H, Beekhuis H, Oldhoff J, Oosterhius JW, van der Ploeg E, Vermey A (1981) Local recurrence and survival in patients with (Clark level IV/V and over 1.5 mm thickness) stage I malignant melanoma of the extremities after regional perfusion. Cancer 48: 1952

Stehlin JS, Giovanella BC, de Ipolye PD, Muenz LR, Anderson RF (1975) Results of hyperthermic perfusion for melanoma of the extremities. Surg Gynecol Obstet 140: 338

Stehlin JS, Giovanella BC, de Ipolyi PD, Anderson RF (1979) Results of eleven years' experience with heated perfusion for melanoma of the extremities. Cancer Res 39: 2255

Fluorescence-Histochemical and Electron-Microscopical Investigations in Melanoma Patients After Isolated Cytostatic Perfusion

E. Paul[1], M. Ishii[2], K. Aigner[3], P. Hild[3], and L. Illig[1]*

1 Zentrum für Dermatologie, Andrologie und Venerologie, Justus-Liebig-Universität, Gaffkystrasse 14, 6300 Giessen, FRG
2 Department of Dermatology, Osaka City University, Medical School, Osaka, Japan
3 Abteilung für Chirurgie, Justus-Liebig-Universität, Klinikstrasse 29, 6300 Giessen, FRG

Introduction

In the light-microscopic examination of melanoma metastases with heavily damaged tumor cells after isolated cytostatic perfusion it is often difficult to decide whether the therapy has completely destroyed all tumor cells or has only partly affected them. It must be assumed that viable tumor cells resistant to therapy may be the source of repeated tumor growth, i.e., relapse of further spreading of tumor cells.

However, there is a method of "illuminating" vital pigment cells described by Rorsman (1974), the formalin-induced fluorescence method (FIF method after Falck et al. 1962), in which a yellow-green fluorophore results from the histochemical reaction between 5-S-cysteinyldopa, an intermediate product of melanin, and formaldehyde.

In addition, electron-microscopic investigations give a direct insight into the subcellular structures, and the extent of cellular damage can be determined by the structural changes.

Material and Methods

A total of 62 in-transit metastases from 30 patients with malignant melanomas of the extremities were examined after isolated cytostatic perfusion (method see Schraffordt Koops et al. 1977; Illig and Aigner 1980). The following cytostatics were used: melphalan, cis-platinum, or nitrogen mustard, alone or in combination with actinomycin-D, and dacarbazine alone (for details see Aigner et al. "Regional Perfusion with cis-Platinum and Dacarbazine," this volume).

In cases of multiple in-transit metastases, tissue specimens were taken prior to perfusion, and 4 and 14 days thereafter. In some cases, additional specimens were taken at other times. Immediately after excision the tissue was cooled to the temperature of liquid nitrogen. After being freeze-dried the specimens were treated with formaldehyde vapor

* The authors are grateful to Dr. S. Syed Ali, at the Center of Anatomy and Cytobiology for assistance in ultrastructural studies, and to Mrs. G. Thiele, at the Department of Clinical and Experimental Dermatology, for skilled technical assistance. We are indebted to Prof. Dr. Dr. h.c. A. Oksche and Prof. Dr. R. Lange, at the Center of Anatomy and Cytobiology, for the provision of a work place

according to the method of Håkanson and Sundler (1974), then embedded in paraffin in 10-μm thick sections and mounted in liquid paraffin. Fluorescence-microscopic examination with an epi-illuminator (Ploem-Opak) followed using a filter combination of BG 12 and K 510 and Ilford HP 5 film material.

For electron-microscopic examination the tissue was fixed in glutaraldehyde and embedded in Durcupan. Semithin and ultrathin sections were done on the LKB Ultrotom III with the use of a diamond knife. Contrasting: Uranylacetate and lead citrate were used for contrast, and the electron microscope was a Philips 201, the film material Kodak fine grain.

Results

Of the 62 metastases examined under the fluorescence microscope, only eight (13%) were completely negative after the perfusion. In ten metastases (16%) some fluorescent tumor cells (0%−5%) were found only focally or regionally, while 17 (27%) showed approximately 50% of their cells to be still fluorescent, and 27 (44%) (from 19 patients) had been only slightly or not at all affected by therapy. In these cases the fluorescence-microscopically positive cells were clearly predominant (> 50%).

In some cases in which several second-look biopsies were examined at varying intervals after perfusion, the lowest percentage of fluorescent cells was observed some days after the operation, while the number of FIF-positive cells significantly increased again within 1 or 2 weeks thereafter.

The arrangement of the tumor cells within the metastases seemed to be of great importance for the effect of perfusion. Clusters of tumor cells, loosely distributed in the connective tissue, were more resistant to therapy than melanoma cells in compact tumor nodes. In compact metastases we often observed what we have called the "central-peripheral phenomenon." This means that the central part of the tumor node is completely necrotic, while the periphery of the metastases shows a more-or-less broad zone of viable and fluorescent cells (Fig. 1).

Also, the localization of the metastases within the various dermal layers seemed to have an influence on the therapeutic response to perfusion: In general, it appeared that subcutaneous metastases responded more favorably to perfusion than did cutaneous nodes.

Tumor cells in the papillary body of the dermis, in the epidermis, or around hair follicles are most likely to resist therapy (Fig. 2).

Under the electron microscope all degrees of cell damage up to complete disintegration could be observed.

The ultrastructural studies have shown that the tumor cells of a circumscribed area are not always damaged to the same degree. We have frequently seen that some tumor cells with intact structures and virtually no signs of cell damage were surrounded by highly damaged cells with pyknotic nuclei and vacuolated cytoplasm (Fig. 3).

Minor damage to the cytoplasm was manifested by a swelling of the mitochondria and by the occurrence of vacuoles and autophagosomes, which were frequently found in deep invaginations of the nucleus. The nuclear changes were even more impressive: invagination, lobulation, and deformation of the nucleus extending to complete destruction of the nuclear membrane.

In necrotic areas we found complete destruction of all cytoplasmic organelles and of the cell membrane. The nucleus and nuclear membrane, too, were almost completely dissolved. Only the nucleoli showed relatively normal structure and electron density (Fig. 4).

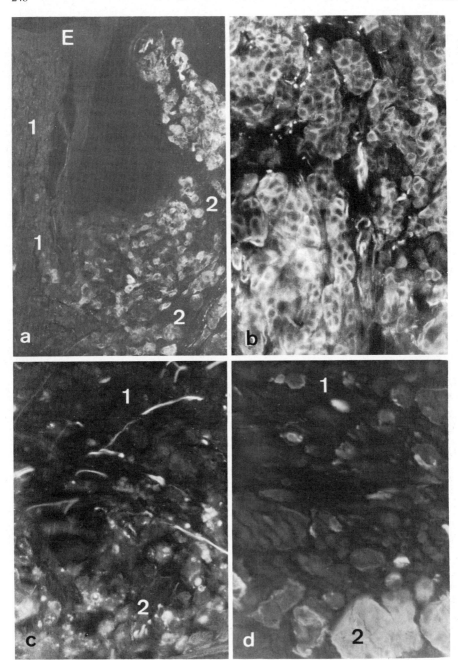

Fig. 1a–d. "Central-peripheral phenomenon" in melanoma metastases after isolated cytostatic perfusion. **a** General view. *1*, Fluorescence-histochemically negative center with necrotic cells; *2*, periphery of the metastasis with intact, fluorescent tumor cells; E epidermis at the surface of the metastasis. **b** Section from the periphery. Tumor cell complexes show typical FIF fluorescence. **c** and **d** Sections from the transitional zone center and periphery in two other patients. *1*, center; *2*, periphery, in between a transitional zone with sporadically occurring fluorescent cells. **a** × 110; **b–d** × 250

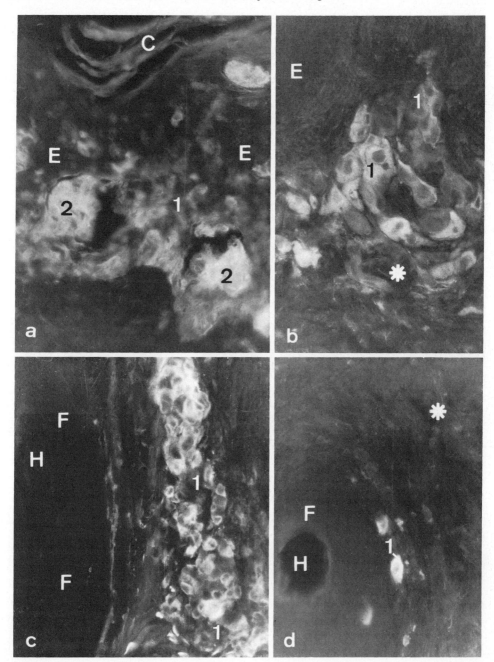

Fig. 2a—d. Remains of fluorescent tumor cells in melanoma metastases after isolated cytostatic perfusion at typical localization. **a** Intraepidermal tumor cells (*1*) and nests (*2*) of an epidermotropic metastasis. *C*, corneal layer (nonspecific fluorescence); *E*, epidermis. **b** Fluorescent tumor cells (*1*) in the upper papillary body. The deeper protions (*) are fluorescence-histochemically negative. *E*, epidermis. **c** and **d** Fluorescent tumor cells (*1*) in close vicinity to a hair follicle (*F*); *H*, hair shaft; (*) shadowed fluorescence-microscopically negative tumor cells

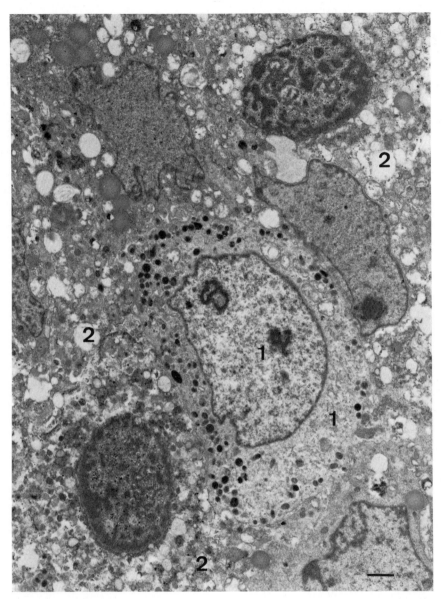

Fig. 3. Patient E.K., 2 days after perfusion with 140 mg *cis*-platinum and 1 mg actinomycin-D. × 7200; bar 1 μm. Normal-looking tumor cells (*1*) surrounded by damaged cells (*2*) showing cytoplasmic vacuolization, extensive loss of cell membrane, and nuclear changes

Discussion

We have repeatedly used the FIF method to demonstrate vital melanoma cells (Paul et al. 1975b; Illig and Paul 1976). It can be safely assumed that tumor cells with positive and specific formalin-induced fluorescence have intact membranes and are therefore viable. On the other hand, 5-*S*-cysteinyldopa would certainly diffuse from a dead cell, as has been shown, with delayed freezing in liquid nitrogen (compare Björklund et al. 1972).

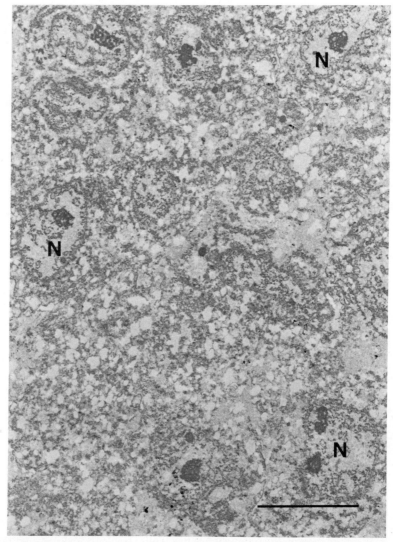

Fig. 4. Patient E.K., 2 days after perfusion with 140 mg *cis*-platinum and 1 mg actinomycin-D. × 2800; bar 10 μm. Nearly complete cellular destruction in the center of a compact metastasis; only shadowy appearance of the nuclei (*N*)

Therefore, the demonstration of fluorescent tumor cells seems to be of high diagnostic value. In our opinion, it is more probable that FIF-positive cells would indicate an insufficient therapeutic effect than that negative cells would indicate a therapeutic success, because in both primary tumors and metastases FIF-negative cell areas may sometimes be observed in the absence of therapy (Paul et al. 1975a).

After isolated perfusion with dacarbazine, the loss of fluorescence might also be due to the immediate cytostatic effect on pigment synthesis, without the vitality of the cells necessarily being reduced (cf. Morgan et al. 1976).

Further statistics are required to clarify whether complete loss of fluorescence of all tumor cells after perfusion does in fact correlate with a better prognosis. Within our follow-up period of 2 weeks it is not possible to clearly determine the definite effect of perfusion on the tumor cells. Earlier authors (Krementz and Creech 1970; Stehlin et al. 1975) reported that complete clinical regression of the tumor had sometimes been observed only after months.

Multiple biopsies taken from the same patient at varying intervals showed the lowest percentage of fluorescent cells immediately after the perfusion and on the following days. Thereafter, the number of fluorescence-microscopically positive cells often increased again.

While this "restoration" of metastases may be explained by the formation of new cells through cell division, it is also possible that some tumor cells were only temporarily affected, and recovered after some days. An increased membrane permeability (cf. Strom et al. 1973) might have caused a transitory loss of fluorophores by diffusion. At 2 weeks after perfusion the transient membrane damage is likely to have compensated, so that second-look biopsies at this time are probably most suitable for assessing the therapeutic effect.

We suppose that the regionally different response of the tumor cells within the metastases, which leads to the so-called central-peripheral phenomenon, and the less favorable response of intra- and subepidermal tumor parts are due to a common factor, the vascular supply. For example, it is possible that tumor cells in the upper papillary body or around a hair shaft have a lower blood supply than cell complexes which are loosely distributed within the connective tissue. Intraepidermal tumor cells are possibly not reached by the required cytostatic effect.

On the other hand, in an apparent contradiction, the peripheral parts of solid metastases, which are better supplied with blood, seemed to remain unaffected, while the center of the metastases became necrotic. In such cases it must be assumed that the cytostatic drug alone was not able to destroy all tumor cells in the periphery of the metastasis. However, in the poorly supplied center of the metastasis, the additive effect of cytostatic agent, hypoxia, and hyperthermia caused necrosis, resulting in the "central-peripheral phenomenon" (compare Dietzel 1975; Harisiadis et al. 1975; Tonak 1981). Thus, the spontaneous tendency to central necrosis observed in some metastases might be intensified by perfusion therapy.

The structural changes observed in our material under the electron microscope several days after perfusion are so-called late changes, which are probably not due to the immediate effect of temperature because only 24 h after hyperthermia David et al. (1971) could not find any changes in the organelles of liver cells. While the cytoplasmic alterations are likely to be reversible, the severe nuclear changes are probably expressive of irreversible damage. However, typical nuclear changes such as apoptosis, as observed by Kerr and Searle (1980) in irradiated tumors, were not seen in our patients.

The damage observed in tumor cells after isolated cytostatic perfusion seems to be multifactorial. It appears that in only some of the cases is the cytostatic effect sufficient to destroy all tumor cells. In other cases there are indications that the cytostatic effect is supported by the effect of hyperthermia, and possibly that of hypoxia.

Summary

The effect of isolated cytostatic perfusion was determined in in-transit metastases from malignant melanomas at various times after therapy. Fluorescence-microscopically positive tumor cells (formalin-induced fluorescence) were regarded as viable and possibly capable of dividing. Most of the metastases examined showed fluorescent cells even after perfusion, and these were often found at characteristic sites within the metastases.

Under the electron microscope, the cell damage was seen mainly in the nucleus, but also in the organelles of the cytoplasm. The source of cell damage might be multifactorial, and the cytostatic effect could not be clearly separated from the effect of hyperthermia or hypoxia.

References

Björklund A, Falck B, Owman C (1972) Fluorescence-microscopic and microspectrofluorometric techniques for the cellular localization and characterization of biogenic amines. In: Kopin J (ed) Methods of investigative and diagnostic endocrinology. North Holland, Amsterdam

David H, Uerlinge J, Grupe M (1971) Strukturveränderungen von Leberzellen bei supranormalen Temperaturen. Exp Pathol 5: 2−10

Dietzel F (1975) Tumor und Temperatur. Urban and Schwarzenberg, München

Falck B, Hillarp N-Å, Thieme G, Torp A (1962) Fluorescence of catecholamines and related compounds condensed with formaldehyde. J Histochem Cytochem 10: 348−354

Håkanson R, Sundler F (1974) Formaldehyde condensation at reduced temperature. Increased sensitivity and specificity of the fluorescence-microscopic method for demonstrating primary catecholamines. J Histochem 22: 887−894

Harisiadis L, Hall EJ, Kraljevic U, Borek C (1975) Hyperthermia: biological studies at the cellular level. Radiation Biology 117: 447−452

Illig L, Aigner K (1980) Therapie des malignen Melanoms unter besonderer Berücksichtigung der isolierten Extremitätenperfusion. Dtsch Ärzteblatt 77: 2911−2925

Illig L, Paul E (1976) Unspezifische Immuntherapie des malignen Melanoms der Haut mit DNCB nach Malek-Mansour. Hautarzt 27: 579−587

Kerr JFR, Searle J (1980) Apoptosis: its nature and kinetic role. In: Meyn RE, Withers HR (eds) Radiation biology in cancer research, Raven, New York pp 367−384

Krementz ET, Creach O Jr (1970) Advances in the treatment of malignant melanoma. Proc Natl Canc Conf 6: 529−542

Morgan LR Jr, Samuels MS, Carter RD, Krementz ET (1976) Effects of dimethyltriazeno imidazole carboxamide (DTIC; NSC 45, 388) on melanoma metabolites and enzymes. Pigment cell 2. Karger, Basel, 327−338

Paul E, Hartwig H-G, Möller W, Illig L (1975a) Fluoreszenzhistochemische Untersuchungen und mikrofluorometrische Analysen an pigmentbildenden Tumoren der Haut (unter besonderer Berücksichtigung der Melanom-Theorie von Mishima). Arch Dermatol Res 253: 125−144

Paul E, Illig L, Möller W (1975b) Vitalitätsbeurteilung von Metastasen eines malignen Melanoms nach endolymphatischer Radionuklidtherapie mit der Falck-Hillarp-Methode. Hautarzt 26: 317−320

Rorsman H (1974) The melanocyte illuminated. Trans St John's Hosp Derm Soc 60: 135−141

Schraffordt Koops H, Oldhoff J, van der Ploeg E, Vermey A, Eibergen R, Beekhuis H (1977) Some aspects of the treatment of primary malignant melanoma of the extremities by isolated regional perfusion. Cancer 39: 27−33

Stehlin JS Jr, Giovanelly BC, de Ipolyi RD, Muenz LR, Anderson RF (1975) Results of hyperthermic perfusion for melanoma of the extremities. Surg Gynecol Obstet 140: 338−349

Strom R, Santoro AS, Crifo C, Bozzi A, Mondovi B, Rossi-Fanelli A (1973) The biochemical mechanism of selective heat sensitivity of cancer cells. Inhibition of RNA synthesis. Eur J Cancer 9: 103−112

Tonak J (1981) Die hypertherme Zytostatikaperfusion beim malignen Melanom. Eine experimentelle und klinische Untersuchung. In: Nagel G, Sauer R, Schreiber HW (eds) Zuckschwerdt, München

Tissue Toxicity in Experimental Isolated Perfusion with Adriamycin

K. Henneking, K. Aigner, C. Deeg, G. Merker, H. W. Spelz, and M. Hundeiker

Abteilung für Chirurgie, Justus-Liebig-Universität, Klinikstrasse 29, 6300 Giessen, FRG

Since the introduction of isolated regional perfusion in 1958 by Creech et al. this method has been employed for the treatment of various tumors of the extremities.

During the period from October, 1979 to March, 1982 we perfused 183 melanomas and seven soft tissue sarcomas with various cytostatic drugs by this method (Aigner and Schwemmle, to be published).

In 1976 Schraffordt Koops et al. reported successful treatment of soft tissue sarcomas of the extremities by adjuvant isolated regional perfusion. In all cases the cytostatic agent was melphalan, in some cases combined with dactinomycin.

For about 10 years adriamycin, an antitumor antibiotic obtained from *Streptomyces* fermentation, has been used in chemotherapy (Fig. 1). It is an antineoplastic agent with a broad spectrum of activity for human malignancies (Carter 1980; O'Bryan et al. 1977). In order to be able to use this effective cytostatic agent in isolated perfusion we determined its tissue toxicity and its highest tolerable concentration.

Material and Methods

Twelve dogs with an average weight of 32 kg received isolated perfusion in the right hind leg for 1 h under normothermic conditions between 36° C and 37° C. Operations were performed with the animals under halothane nitrous oxide inhalation anesthesia.

After cannulation of the femoral vessels the hind leg was isolated to an extracorporeal circuit consisting of a roller pump and a Bentley Bos 5 oxygenator. The flow rate ranged between 150 and 250 ml/min, arterial pressure between 80 and 140 mm Hg.

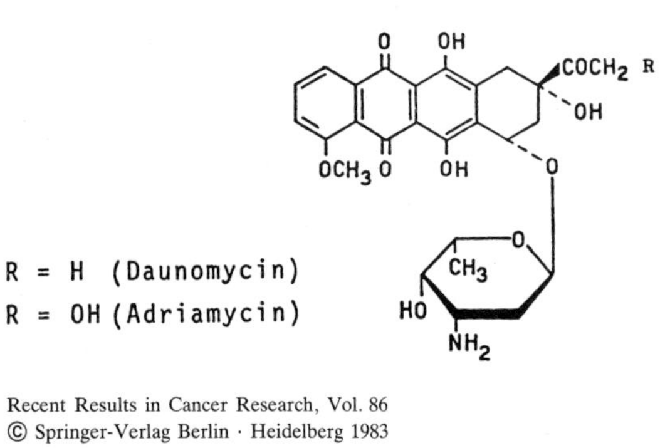

R = H (Daunomycin)
R = OH (Adriamycin)

Fig. 1. Structure of adriamycin — polycyclic aglycone and amino sugar — which differs from daunomycin in the substitution of a hydroxyl for a hydrogen atom at C-14

During the perfusion blood gas analyses were performed and acidosis was normalized with sodium bicarbonate. The range of pO_2 in the perfusion solution was between 100 and 400 mm Hg.

The volume of the perfused hind legs was determined by measurement of water displacement, the average volume amounting to 1.6 l. Dosage of adriamycin was steadily increased; we started with a dose of 6.5 mg adriamycin/l extremity volume and increased up to 15.0 mg/l extremity volume.

The dogs were killed on the 18th postoperative day and the perfused hind legs were examined histologically.

Results

Reversible edema was the most common toxicity observed. There is a direct relationship between dosage and postoperative edema (Table 1), vascular damage, and necrosis of muscular tissue (Table 2).

Dogs perfused with up to 10 mg adriamycin/l extremity showed slight and reversible edema only. They used the perfused hind leg on the 4th postoperative day at the latest.

Neither macroscopic impression of the perfused leg nor histological examination of artery, vein, nerve, and muscle showed any pathological signs after perfusion with 10 mg adriamycin/l extremity. Examination with the electron microscope revealed no structural changes of the muscular tissue (Fig. 2).

Table 1. Intensity of edema according to dose of adriamycin

Group of dogs (n = 2/group)	Dosage of adriamycin (mg/l extremity)	Edema, 3 days postoperative	Edema, 8 days postoperative
I	6.5	−	−
II	8.5	+	−
III	10.0	−	−
IV	12.5	+++	++
V	13.5	++	+
VI	15.0	+++	+++

Table 2. Relation of dose to vascular damage and necrosis of muscular tissue

Group of dogs (n = 2/group)	Dosage of adriamycin (mg/l extremity)	Vascular damage	Necrosis of muscular tissue
I	6.5	−	−
II	8.5	−	−
III	10.0	−	−
IV	12.5	+	−
V	13.5	++	+
VI	15.0	+++	+++

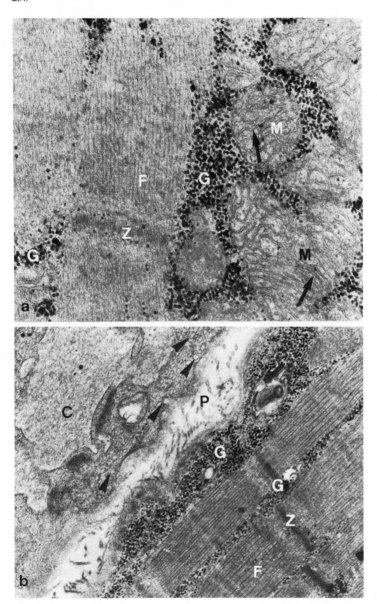

Fig. 2a, b. Musculus tibialis anterior of a dog, 18 days after perfusion with 10 mg adriamycin per liter extremity. No structural changes are observed. Note the numerous vesicles in the endothelial cells of a capillary (*arrowheads,* **b**), possibly indicating increased micropinocytosis. *C,* capillary; *F,* muscle filaments; *G,* glycogen stores; *P,* perivascular space; *Z,* Z line; *arrows,* mitochondrial christae. Durcupan (Fluka); **a** × 62,600; **b** × 28,200

Mitochondria and the membranes of the sarcoplasmic reticulum were intact; glycogen was deposited in close proximity to the sarcoplasmic reticulum and between the myofilaments. In the capillary wall, however, numerous endothelial micropinocytosis vesicles occurred, possibly indicating increased exchange across the capillary wall.

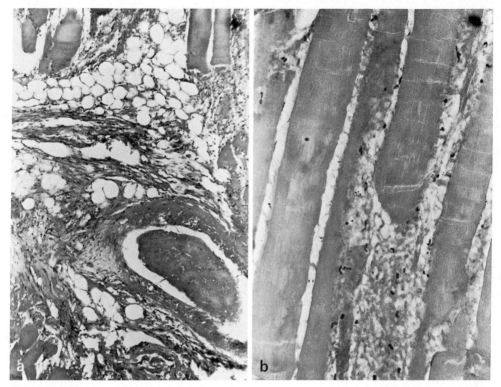

Fig. 3. Histological presentation of (**a**) a small vein and (**b**) musculature, after perfusion with 15 mg adriamycin

After perfusion with 13 mg/l adriamycin the arteries showed no morphological changes, but the veins exhibited severe intima lesions with thrombosis.

Doses of between 14 and 15 mg adriamycine resulted in skin ulcerations, necrosis of muscular tissue and damage of the vessels. Figure 3a shows thrombosis and necrosis of the wall in a small vein and loss of nuclear staining within the striated muscle cells 10 days after perfusion with 15 mg adriamycin. Striated muscle cells with nearly total loss of nuclear staining and partial loss of striation can be observed in Fig. 3b. These animals were killed as early as the 10th postoperative day because of severe edema and pain in the perfused leg.

After perfusion with adriamycin no structural changes could be noted in liver tissue or samples of kidney tissue. Even after high doses the structure of the cell organelles in liver and kidney seemed to be unaffected.

In all cases blood tests were always within normal limits. Only the dogs that received doses higher than 14 mg/l extremity showed an increase in transaminases, which normalized on the 8th postoperative day (Figs. 4 and 5). Since the liver was not exposed to adriamycin in our experiments this transitory dose-dependent increase of liver enzymes might be an effect of transfer from the extracellular to the intracellular compartment during perfusion.

Our experiments show that dosages of about 10 mg/l perfused extremity were well tolerated by the animals. Lower concentrations did not result in any side effects. In most cases, dosages higher than 10 mg/l extremity induced severe edema, pain, and histological changes.

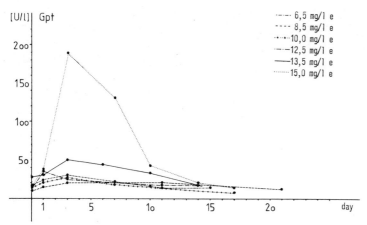

Fig. 4. Range of glutamic-pyruvic transaminase (*GPT*) after perfusion with various doses of adriamycin per liter extremity (*e*)

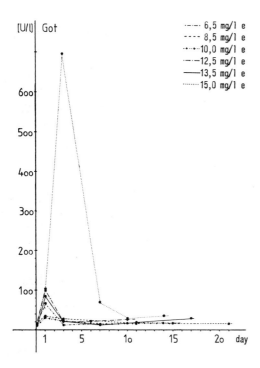

Fig. 5. Range of glutamic-oxaloacetic transaminase (*GOT*) after perfusion with various doses of adriamycin per liter extremity (*e*)

Discussion

Isolated perfusion allows the use of high concentrations of cytotoxic drugs in the extremity without the risk of high toxicity in the entire organism.

To date we have employed melphalan, dactinomycin, dacarbazine, *cis*-platinum, and nitrogen mustard as cytostatic agents for isolated extremity perfusion (Aigner and Schwemmle, to be published). By our experiments we wanted to enlarge this spectrum, using another drug which appears to be effective in a large variety of tumors, for instance, soft tissue sarcomas and osteosarcomas (Gottlieb et al. 1975).

The systemic toxicity of intra-arterial adriamycin appears to be equivalent to that seen in intravenous administration (Haskel et al. 1975), whereas isolated extremity perfusion reduced the systemic side effects of adriamycin to a minimum.

We used heparin in our isolated perfusion, as did the group from the National Cancer Institute in Milan, Italy (Di Petro et al. 1973), and never observed precipitations in the extracorporeal circuit as reported by the UCLA group (Haskel et al. 1974).

Braat et al. (1981) reported on regional perfusion with adriamycin from 1975 to 1981 in 14 patients suffering from soft tissue sarcomas. A severe, non-dose-related toxicity was observed in three cases.

Our experimental isolated perfusion in twelve dogs showed dose-related occurrence and increase of edema, and vascular and muscular damage.

Histological and ultrastructural sections verified irreversible tissue damage after perfusion with 15 mg adriamycin/l extremity volume, but isolated perfusion under normothermic conditions with 10 mg adriamycin/l did not result in severe tissue toxicity and was well tolerated by the animals.

Summary

Adriamycin is known as an antineoplastic agent with a broad spectrum of activity for human malignancies. To determine the highest tolerable concentrations of adriamycin in isolated perfusion of the extremities the hind legs of 12 dogs were isolated in an extracorporeal circuit and perfused under normothermic conditions.

Dosages of about 10 mg/l perfused extremity were well tolerated by the animals, and lower concentrations did not result in any side effects. However, in most cases, dosages higher than 10 mg adriamycin/l extremity volume induced severe edema, pain, and histological changes.

References

Aigner K, Schwemmle K (to be published) Technik der isolierten Extremitätenperfusion – Erfahrungen an 171 Fällen. Langenbecks Arch Chir

Braat RP, van Slooten E, Wieberdink K, Olthuis J (1981) Regional perfusion with adriamycin in soft tissue sarcomas. EORTC Melanoma Meeting, 26–28 Oct 1981, Lausanne

Carter SK (1980) The clinical evaluation of analogs. III. Anthracyclines. Cancer Chemother Pharmacol 4: 5–10

Creech O, Krementz ET, Ryan RF, Winblad JM (1958) Chemotherapy of cancer: Regional perfusion utilizing an extracorporal circuit. Ann Surg 148: 616–632

DiPietro S, DePalo G, Gennari L (1973) Cancer chemotherapy by intra-arterial infusion with adriamycin. J Surg Oncol 5: 421–430

Gottlieb JA, Baker LH, O'Bryan RM, Sinkovics JG, Hoogstraten B, Quagliana JM, Rivkin SE, Bodey GP, Rodriguez VT, Blumenschein GR, Saiki JH, Coltman C, Burgess MA, Sullivan P, Thigpen T, Bottomley R, Balcerzak S, Moon TE (1975) Adriamycin (NSC-123127) used alone and in combination for soft tissue and bony sarcomas. Cancer Chemother Rep 6: 271–283

Haskel CM, Silverstein MJ, Rangel DM (1974) Multimodality cancer therapy in man: a pilot study of adriamycin by arterial infusion. Cancer 33: 1485–1490

Haskel CM, Eilber FR, Morton DL (1975) Adriamycin (NSC-123127) by arterial infusion. Cancer Chemother Rep 6: 187–189

O'Bryan RM, Baker LH, Gottlieb JE, Rivkin SE, Balcerzak SP, Grumet GN, Salmon SE, Moon TE, Hoogstraten B (1977) Dose-response evaluation of adriamycin in human neoplasia. Cancer 39: 1940–1948

Schraffordt Koops H, Eibergen R, Oldhoff J, van der Ploeg E, Vermey A (1976) Isolated regional perfusion in the treatment of soft tissue sarcomas of the extremities. Clin Oncol 2: 245–252

Regional Perfusion with Adriamycin in Soft Tissue Sarcomas

R. P. Braat, J. Wieberdink, E. van Slooten, and G. Olthuis

Daniel Den Hoech Kliniek, Rotterdamsch Radio-Therapeutich Instituut,
Groene Hilledijk 301, P.O. 5201, 3075 EA Rotterdam, The Netherlands

Since 1973 isolation perfusion of the extremities has been performed at the Rotterdam Radiotherapeutic Institute, and since 1975 perfusions have been done at the Antoni van Leeuwenhoekhuis in Amsterdam. Since 1977 they have been done at both cancer institutes by the same team using identical techniques and, for melanoma, identical indications.

In Amsterdam from the start, perfusions have been performed for sarcoma and sarcoma-like tumors. Adriamycin (doxorubicin) was chosen as the cytotoxic drug because of promising results obtained with systemic adriamycin therapy in sarcoma patients. At the beginning melphalan was used as well.

Table 1. Data on 14 patients who received isolated perfusion with adriamycin

Diagnosis	Patient		Year perfused	Clinical staging
	Sex	Age (years)		
Low-grade fibrosarcoma	F	50	1975	II B
	M	15	1976	I B
	M	10	1976	I B
	F	11	1977	II B
	F	16	1980	II B
Synovial sarcoma	M	14	1975	I B
	M	11	1976	II B
	M	25	1977	I B
	F	24	1981	III A
Liposarcoma	M[a]	51	1980	III B
	M	56	1980	III A
Aggressive lipomatosis	F	11	1976	II B
Postmastectomy lymphangiosarcoma	F	69	1976	I B
Malignant fibrous histiocytoma	M	51	1981	II B

[a] Received two perfusions

Perfusion was considered for a sarcoma patient when the only alternative treatment was amputation, and when the chance of distant metastases was believed to be rather low.

We have perfused a total of 14 patients, one of them twice (Table 1). Five had nonresectable primary tumors, six had nonresectable local recurrences, two had local recurrences with (resected) positive lymph glands, and one had local recurrence with distant metastases at the time of perfusion.

Treatment

Of the 14 patients, one was treated palliatively by perfusion alone. Of the 13 treated curatively, five received only perfusion, six a combination of perfusion with surgery, one perfusion and radiotherapy, and one, all three procedures.

Six patients were treated for lesions of the upper extremities — four perfused via the axillary artery and two via the brachial — and eight for lesions of the lower extremities (one leg was perfused twice); four of these nine perfusions were via the iliac artery, three via the femoral, and two via the popliteal.

During the early series (1975–1977) dosage was calculated in mg/kg body wt. Expressed as mg/l perfused tissue, this led to a considerable range of doses: 5–40 mg adriamycin per liter, with or without 4–25 mg melphalan per liter. In the new series (since 1980) the dose is standardized at 10 mg adriamycin per liter of perfused tissue.

Results

Perfusion alone, or perfusion with other treatment modalities resulted in only one case of local recurrence; eight patients are free of disease and five, three of whom died, developed distant metastases. The important point here is that there was only one patient with local recurrence, this being the one with aggressive lipomatosis. However, the local spread of this disease seems to have stopped at this time.

Eight patients have been followed up for more than 5 years; six of these may be cured (Table 2). Table 3 details the tumor response to perfusion in nine patients; four with more

Table 2. Data on eight patients followed up for 5 years or more

Diagnosis	Treatment	Duration of follow-up (years)
Low-grade fibrosarcoma	Perfusion only	6.5
Lymphangiosarcoma[a]		5.5
Low-grade fibrosarcoma		5.0
Synovial sarcoma	Perfusion and local resection	6.5
Low-grade fibrosarcoma		5.0
Aggressive lipomatosis[a]	Perfusion and local resection	6.0
Low-grade fibrosarcoma		5.0
Synovial sarcoma		5.0

[a] Patient not free of disease

Table 3. Tumor response to perfusion measured in nine cases

	Diagnosis	No. of cases	Method of examination
Complete remission	Low-grade fibrosarcoma	2	C
	Lymphangiosarcoma	1	C
	Low-grade fibrosarcoma	1	H
Partial or no remission	Low-grade fibrosarcoma	1	C
	Aggressive lipomatosis	1	H
	Liposarcoma	1	H
	Malignant fibrous histiocytoma	1	H
	Synovial sarcoma	1	H

C, clinical; *H*, histological

than 5 years' follow-up show complete remission, so that adriamycin and melphalan perfusion, as the only form of treatment, seems to have cured three low-grade fibrosarcomas and one lymphangiosarcoma.

Although most of the perfusions were done to avoid amputations, five did have to be performed. In two cases local resection was not possible, and in the other three cases severe reaction of the tissues to the perfusion necessitated the amputation; the specific doses administered were 15 mg adriamycin with 10 mg melphalan, 7 mg adriamycin with 4 mg melphalan, and 10 mg adriamycin given twice, all expressed as mg per liter of perfused tissue.

Side Effects

Of the four children in the early series, two had a shorter leg after perfusion and one a shorter arm, most likely due to a toxic effect on the epiphyseal growth plates of the long bones, which probably fused too early. There was one case of general toxicity without isotope leakage. One patient developed skin ulcers where radiotherapy had previously been administered. Metastases of one desmoid tumor to the subclavian scar were detected 2 years after perfusion. Neither results nor local toxicity seem to be dose related.

From our clinical material, and from the work done on the rat model by Dr. Benckhuijsen in Amsterdam since 1977, we have derived some recommendations for relatively safe perfusion with adriamycin:

1. Dose should not exceed 10 mg/l.
2. Perfusion with adriamycin should not be repeated too early.
3. Peak levels of the drug in the perfusate should be avoided.
4. High pO_2 in the perfusate should be avoided.
5. There may be a danger if radiotherapy is administered within several months before or after perfusion.

Conclusions

Regional perfusion with adriamycin and melphalan may cure some soft tissue sarcomas, and perfusion can be a valuable adjuvant therapy to the surgical treatment of soft tissue sarcomas of the extremities.

References

Benckhuijsen C, van Dijk WJ, van 't Hoff SC (1982) High-flow isolation perfusion of the rat hind limb in vivo. J Surg Oncol 21: 249−257
McBride CM (1974) Sarcomas of the limbs − Results of adjuvant chemotherapy using isolation perfusion. Arch Surg 109: 304−308

Peripheral Nerve Damage
Following Isolated Extremity Perfusion with cis-Platinum

O. Busse[1], K. Aigner[2], and H. Wilimzig[2]

1 Neurologische Universitätsklinik, Am Steg, 6300 Giessen, FRG
2 Allgemeinchirurgische Klinik des Zentrums für Chirurgie, Justus-Liebig-Universität, Klinikstrasse 29, 6300 Giessen, FRG

Introduction

Temporary or permanent nerve injuries have been observed in 0.5%−7% of patients following isolated hyperthermic extremity perfusion with cytostatic agents (Krementz and Ryan 1972; McBride et al. 1975; Schraffordt Koops et al. 1977; Stehlin 1960; Tonak 1981). The cytostatic agent administered was usually melphalan, either alone or in combination with others. The peroneal nerve was the most affected after lower limb perfusion; this is believed to be due to postoperative edematous swelling in the anterior lateral compartment of the lower leg. The tourniquet and neurotoxicity of high cytostatic doses have also been discussed as causes (Krementz and Ryan 1972).

Material, Methods and Results

At the University Hospital of Surgery in Giessen 22 patients received extremity perfusions with *cis*-platinum over a period of 18 months. No patient showed any peripheral nerve lesion in the extremity to be perfused prior to the operation.

Arm perfusions were carried out in only three patients, one of whom suffered a plexus injury caused by the tourniquet. Of the 19 patients who received lower limb perfusion, 16 could be examined neurologically and neurophysiologically, some at regular intervals. All patients showed postoperative peripheral nerve lesions, two thirds with severe pareses. Sometimes the neurological symptoms appeared within a few hours after perfusion, but it usually developed within 2 days, rarely after 3 or 4 days. The more severe the injury the earlier it was manifested. In most cases the pareses were distributed equally between the extensor and felxor muscles of the lower leg and foot, in severe cases also involving the thigh muscles. They were always combined with a stocking shaped diminution of sensibility. Almost all patients complained of severe causalgia in the foot and lower leg for several months.

The extent of the neurological deficit correlated with the *cis*-platinum dose (Fig. 1). The severity of the pareses was graded according to the remaining strength of the muscles of the lower leg and foot. On this scale "0" stood for total paralysis of muscles, while "20" was assigned to their normal function. While there is indeed a parallel between the extent of the neurological deficit and the *cis*-platinum dose, it is not statistically significant.

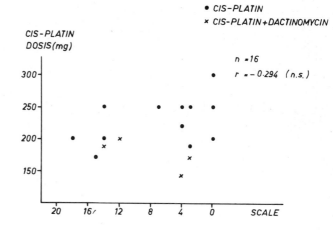

Fig. 1. Correlation between severity of peripheral nerve lesion and *cis*-platinum dose level

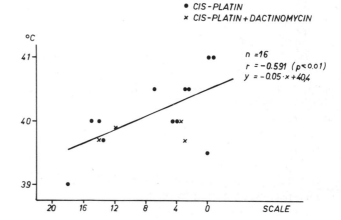

Fig. 2. Correlation between severity of peripheral nerve lesion and perfusion temperature

Figure 2 shows the relationship between peripheral paresis and perfusion temperature which is statistically significant; the severity of nerve injury increases with increased temperature of the perfusate. Figure 3 also illustrates this relationship. All lesions were severe when temperatures above 40° C were used. At temperatures of 40° C and below the incidence of severe and moderate or slight pareses was about equally distributed.

The influence of edema on the extent of the peripheral nerve lesion was also examined (Fig. 4). More than half of the severe pareses were accompanied by extensive edema, while moderate and slight pareses never were. This shows that the swelling in the lower leg compartments may influence the severity of the neurological deficit. On the other hand, nerve lesions also occur in the complete absence of edema.

Unfortunately, not all patients could be observed over longer time spans. Only seven patients were available for 3−14 months. Proximal pareses were always reversible. The tendency for distal pareses to improve was generally small but always present, with the exception of one case. In one case only there was complete remission of slight paresis, but diminished sensibility remained. The improvement was in inverse proportion to the severity of the neurological deficit, the dose of *cis*-platinum, and the perfusion temperature.

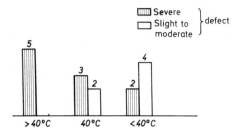

Fig. 3. Results of Fig. 2 as a block diagram

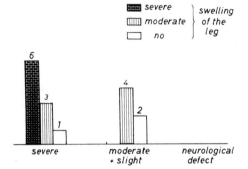

Fig. 4. Relationship between edematous swelling of the leg and severity of neurological deficit

Discussion

Isolated hyperthermic extremity perfusion with *cis*-platinum has a very high rate of complications. Because of the relationship between severity of the nerve damage and perfusion temperature we have ceased to use temperatures above 40° C. In view of the − less pronounced − relationship between the *cis*-platinum dose and the extent of paresis we now use doses of 2.5−2.7 mg/kg body wt., or 20 mg/l perfused extremity. Peripheral nerve lesions are probably not avoided by this treatment, but can nevertheless be reduced in severity.

The incidence of complications with administration of *cis*-platinum is far higher than that for other cytostatic agents. Our patients, perfused with melphalan alone or in combination with dactinomycin, developed lesions in no more than 5% of peripheral nerves. This correlates with reports in the literature. In our opinon the neurotoxicity of *cis*-platinum plays a major role in the development of the nerve damage, even though the toxic effect is viewed as relatively small in systemic administration (Becher et al. 1980; Kedar et al. 1980; Lokich 1980; Ostrow et al. 1980; Von Hoff et al. 1979). The postoperative edematous swelling potentiates the peripheral nerve damage, but we feel that it cannot be the only cause. Without the assumption of the neurotoxicity of *cis*-platinum which increases with application of heat, it would be difficult to explain why melphalan and other cystostatic agents are relatively much less injurious than *cis*-platinum, in spite of edema development. The neurophysiological examinations also indicate that a neurotoxic nerve lesion must be the major factor. Electromyographic changes typical for ischemic lesions following edematous compartment syndrome were observed in only three patients who had complete paralysis of the lower leg muscles.

Summary

Of 16 patients treated, all who could be examined after isolated hyperthermic lower limb perfusion with cis-platinum showed peripheral nerve damage, particularly of the lower leg and foot. We found a close correlation between the severity of neurological deficit and the perfusion temperature. The dose of cytostatic agent also plays a role in development of the nerve lesion. The major cause of the nerve damage seems to be the neurotoxicity of cis-platinum. The edematous swelling in the compartments in the lower leg have an influence. The reversibility of the pareses was generally very small.

References

Becher R, Schütt P, Osieka R, Schmidt CG (1980) Peripheral neuropathy and ophthalmologic toxicity after treatment with cis-Diamminedichloroplatinum II. J Cancer Res Clin Oncol 96: 219–221

Kedar A, Cohen ME, Freeman AI (1980) Peripheral neuropathy as a complication of cis-diamminedichloroplatinum (II) treatment: A case report. Cancer Treat Rep 62: 819–821

Krementz ET, Ryan RF (1972) Chemotherapy of melanoma of the extremities by perfusion: fourteen years' clinical experience. Ann Surg 175: 900–917

Lokich JJ (1980) Phase I study of cis-damminedichloroplatinum (II) administered as a constant 5-day infusion. Cancer Treat Rep 64: 905–908

McBride ChM, Sugarbaker EV, Hickey RC (1975) Prophylactic isolation perfusion as the primary therapy for invasive malignant melanoma of the limbs. Ann Surg 1982: 316–324

Ostrow S, Egorin MJ, Hahn D, Markus S, Leroy A, Chang P, Klein M, Bachur NR, Wiernik PH (1980) cis-Diamminedichloroplatinum and adriamycin therapy for advanced gynecological and genitourinary neoplasms. Cancer 46: 1715–1721

Schraffordt-Koops HJ, Oldhoff E, van der Pleog A, Vermey R, Eibergen P, Beekhius H (1977) Some aspects of the treatment of primary malignant melanoma of the extremities by isolated regional perfusion. Cancer 39: 27–33

Stehlin JS (1960) Hyperthermic perfusion with chemotherapy for cancer of the extremities. Surg Gynecol Obstet 129: 305–308

Tonak J (1981) Die hypertherme Zytostatikaperfusion beim malignen Melanom. Zuckschwerdt, München

von Hoff DD, Schlisky R, Reichert CM, Reddick RL, Rosencweig M, Young RC, Muggia FM (1979) Toxic effects of cis-diamminedichloroplatinum (II) in man. Cancer Treat Rep 63: 1527–1531

Objective Regression of Unexcised Melanoma in-Transit Metastases After Hyperthermic Isolation Perfusion of the Limbs with Melphalan

F. J. Lejeune, T. Deloof, P. Ewalenko, J. Fruhling,
M. Jabri, M. Mathieu, J.-M. Nogaret, and A. Verhest*

Institut Jules Bordet, Centre des Tumeurs de l'Université Libre de Bruxelles,
Rue Héger Bordet 1, 1000 Bruxelles, Belgium

Introduction

In-transit metastases of melanoma of the limbs represent a challenging problem to the surgeon. Before the introduction of isolation perfusion, the only treatment available was major amputation, without there being evidence, however, of increased patient survival (McPeak et al. 1963; Miller 1977). Complete remissions after hyperthermic isolation perfusion with melphalan (HIPM) were reported by Stehlin et al. (1975) on some unexcised primaries and regional metastases of melanoma. However most authors (Au and Goldman 1979; Creech and Krementz 1964; Krementz and Ryan 1972; Martijn et al. 1981; Stehlin et al. 1975) have favored the policy of metastasis excision, followed or preceded by isolation perfusion. The rate of cure is between 50% and 75%, but it seems difficult to ascertain the value of adjuvant isolation perfusion because it is administered simultaneously with surgery.

The addition of heat in isolation perfusion seems to have consistently increased the cytotoxicity of the procedure. Although experimental studies indicate that heat at 43° C is selectively cytotoxic to melanoma cells (Giovanella et al. 1976), Stehlin et al. (1975) advocated that mild hyperthermia at 39° to 41° C reduces the toxicity to normal tissue, without obviously impairing the efficacy of HIPM. A 5-year survival rate of 74% was reported (Stehlin et al. 1979) for patients with in-transit metastases treated according to this procedure.

In 1977 we reported (Lejeune et al. 1977) on a pilot study of HIPM, with regressions of some unexcised regional metastases.

In order to objectively appraise the regional efficacy of HIPM we initiated a prospective study on stage IIa disease (in-transit metastases) and stage IIa b (with additional involvement of regional lymph nodes) where metastases were left unexcised after the procedure.

We report here on a series of 23 stages IIa and IIa b patients, prospectively treated according to a protocol, and all operated upon by the same surgeon within a 5-year period.

---

* We are grateful to A. Gerard, head of the Department of Surgery, for his support. M. C. Hennaut, R.N., and E. Pataschnik are acknowledged for their skillful assistance

Patients and Methods

Eligibility of Patients

Patients with in-transit metastasis of the limbs, stage IIa, and with additional regional lymph node metastases, stage IIa b, with no sign of distant metastases, no other malignancy, and no severe arterial insufficiency were admitted to the study. There were four men and 19 women, ranging in age from 40 to 79 years (mean: 59). For 16 patients the disease was classified as stage IIa, for seven as stage IIa b. Two patients had melanoma of an upper limb and 21 of a lower limb. Previous treatment consisted of chemotherapy for one, immunotherapy for four, and radiotherapy for three patients.

Workup for Staging of the Disease

After physical examination, all patients were subjected to complete blood tests, including haematology, coagulation screening, and biological functions. The technical workup consisted of lung X-rays including tomography, liver scintigraphy, or echography and/or a CAT scan, bone scintigraphy, EEG, brain scintigraphy, and a brain CAT scan. Some patients underwent laparoscopy with a liver biopsy at the time of the operation, according to a method already published (Bleiberg et al. 1980). No patient in this series had to be withdrawn because of the detection of distant metastases. Histological and/or cytological analysis of at least one in-transit metastasis was obtained in each patient.

Technique of HIPM

Our perfusion technique has already been described in part (Lejeune et al. 1977). It is essentially the technique of Stehlin (1963, 1975) with some minor modifications. The temperature of proximal/distal muscle and skin was recorded every 5 min with thermistor probes. Hyperthermia was induced both by heating the blood to 43° C with a temptrol "Infant" oxygenator and by heating the skin with a heating blanket. To ensure the stability of the tourniquet we inserted two Steinman pins in the iliac and the Esmark bandage was fastened to a Sandow fixed on the table close to the patient's opposite shoulder. Leakage was measured by isotopic dilution in the peripheral plasma 5 min after injecting radioiodinated serum albumin (RISA) into the extracorporeal circuit. Melphalan (Alkeran in freshly made solution was injected in to the arterial line when the skin temperature in the major tumor area reached 39° C. The maximal temperature allowed was 41° C. The maximum dosage of melphalan was 100 mg for iliac and femoral (1.3−1.5 mg/kg), 75 mg for popliteal, and 50−75 mg for axillary HIPM. Duration of perfusion was exactly 60 min.

For stage IIa b disease we always performed a radical inguinoiliac dissection. For stage IIa we did so for the first ten patients, and then abandoned this procedure because of increased complications with wound healing delay and edema.

We performed 22 perfusions via the iliac artery, three via the femoral, one via the popliteal, and two via the axillary. Of the 23 patients 18 recived one perfusion each and five received two. Four metastases were excised and 24 were left unexcised. Isotope leakage during the first 5 min averaged 7.95% (0%−30%).

Assessment of Response

Tumor diameters were assessed before HIPM and each week thereafter. The major diameter and the one perpendicular to it were measured with a micrometric caliper. Photographs were taken at a constant distance at weekly or biweekly intervals. For patients with numerous in-transit metastases, response was assessed by comparing consecutive slides.

Complete remission represents complete disappearance of the tumors. For some patients this was studied with xeroradiography. Partial remission means that the multiplication product of the two recorded diameters was reduced by at least 50%.

When residual tumor or pigmentation was found during the follow-up biopsies were done.

Results

Objective Response to Isolation Perfusion

The in-transit metastases were left unexcised in 24 of 28 perfusions. In one case evaluation was not possible because an amputation had to be performed on the 6th postoperative day due to severe destruction of tissue. As seen in Table 1, 65% of the perfusions produced complete remission (CR), 26% partial remission (PR), and only 9% had no effect. The two failures occurred in the stage-II-a b group.

Time to response was compared between CR, PR, and parameters of tumor burden such as number of nodules and average nodule diameter (Table 2). The mean times to response ranged between 46 and 53 days. No significant difference could be detected.

However, significant differences in remission durations were found. Mean duration was 23.7 weeks (6 months) and 81.34 weeks (20 months) for PR and CR respectively. Patients with no more than five nodules also had more than twice the remission duration of the patients with more than five. No significant differences were found between patients with tumor diameter of less than or equal to 1 cm and those with tumors of more than 1 cm, nor between those with stage IIa and those with IIa b.

The five cases with two perfusions are analysed for response in Table 3. There seems to be no predictive value for the second perfusion in the type of response to the first perfusion, nor in the disease free interval. Case 2 hat bony involvement with ulceration in the tibial diaphysis. The patient experienced PR after iliac perfusion and CR 7 months later, after a popliteal perfusion.

Table 1. Objective response to isolation perfusion of 23 patients

Stage	No. of patients	No. of perfusions	Unexcised metastases	Response		
				CR	PR	O
IIa	16	21	17	11 of 16	5 of 16	0 of 16
IIab	7	7	7	4 of 7	1 of 7	2 of 7
Total	23	28	24	15 of 23 (65%)	6 of 23 (26%)	2 of 23 (9%)

CR, complete remission; PR, partial remission

Table 2. Time to response and duration of remission after isolation perfusion

	Number of patients	Mean time to response in days (range)	Mean remission duration in weeks (range)	
Response				
PR	6	50.67 (21−120)	23.70 (4.3−67)	} $p < 0.05$
CR	15	49.33 (8−120)	81.34 (8.6−260)	
No remission	2	−	− (2−13)	
Tumor burden				
≤ 5 nodules	14	53.07 (8−120) } NS	65.61 (8.6−260)	} $p < 0.05$
> 5 nodules	5	46.20 (21−60)	27.65 (4.3−52)	
≤ 1 cm diameter	15	49.86 (9−120)	66.60 (8.6−260)	} NS
> 1 cm diameter	5	49.20 (8−120)	82.77 (26−173)	
Stage				
IIa	19	−	65.25 (4.3−260)	} NS
IIa b	7	−	37.44 (2−104)	

Table 3. Response to first and second perfusion in five cases

Case no.	Response to first perfusion (weeks)	Interval (months)	Response to second perfusion
1	PR 4.3	24	PR 5
2	PR 67	7	CR 173
3	CR 67	17	Postoperative death
4	Excision 52	14	PR 13
5	CR 52	12	Excision 22

PR, partial remission; *CR*, complete remission

Complete healing was achieved, allowing the patient to go back to bicycling and walking.

Survival After Isolation Perfusion

The median follow-up time has been 42 months. Since most patients died within the first 3 years, the median survival has been 20 months. A trend in favor of stage IIa over IIa b was found (Table 4). However no difference was detected between complete and partial remissions.

Types of Progression After Isolation Perfusion

Only 7 of 20 patients who survived and did not undergo amputation (35%) had recurrence in the perfused limb. Of 22, 11 (50%) developed distant metastases: two in skin and soft tissues, two in bones, eight in viscera, one in brain, and two in other organs.

Table 4. Survival after first isolation perfusion

	Median survival (months)	No. of patients
All patients	18.2	23
Evaluable patients	20	20
Stage IIa	24	15
Stage IIa b	9.6	5
Complete remission	21.6	15
Partial remission	18.3	6
No response	(4 and 10)	2

Further Treatment

Following perfusion, two patients with PR were submitted to local radiotherapy which resulted in CR in one case and had no effect in the other. Intralesional bacille Calmette Guérin (BCG) was given to two patients with recurrence after perfusion. Complete regression of the inoculated lesion was temporarily seen, followed by BCG-resistant new nodules. Various chemotherapeutic regimens were given systemically to 11 patients after isolation perfusion. Two received adjuvant chemotherapy with dacarbazine (DTIC), alternating with lomustine (CCNU)-vincristine (VCR)-bleomycin (BLM); these treatments did not prevent dissemination. Nine patients who developed disseminated disease were treated with one of the following drugs: DTIC alone; a combination of CCNU, VCR, and BLM; vindesine alone; phosphoroacetyl-L-aspartate (PALA); or a combination of *cis*-platinum and vindesine.

Only one patient receiving the last schedule experienced PR, with distant lung and muscular metastases.

Complications

All patients developed erythema as expected, with a peak on day 10. Complications due to isolation perfusion were classified as mild, medium, or severe (Table 5). Edema was the most common side effect and it was accompanied by a drop in protein concentration during the first operative week. In recent cases edema has been successfully prevented by prophylactic administration of plasma cryoprecipitate and human albumin during the first 10 postoperative days.

Extensive necrosis due to accidental overheating required amputation in one case. Arterial thrombosis of the thumb required a later amputation of the second phalanx. The two cases of hemorrhage occured in patients who had previously been subjected to radiotherapy of the iliac region. The first required an arterioplasty and the second, arterial ligation; this was followed by good circulation and limb function. Reversible neuropathy was seen in 11 patients, consisting mainly in footdrop.

During the first 5 min after RISA injection into the extracorporeal circuit, mean leakage was 7.95%.

Two patients had severe bone marrow depletion. Both were obese (95 and 102 kg) and the leakage averaged 30%. One died of complete agranulocytosis while the other completely recovered. One 75-year-old woman died of cardic failure after a second perfusion. A

Table 5. Major complications observed following isolation perfusion

Complication	No. of patients, according to degree		
	Mild	Medium	Severe
Regional			
Edema	4	4	1
Necrosis		2	1 (Amputation)
Thrombosis		1	
Hemorrhage			2
Neuropathy	5	3	3
Wound infection	1	4	
General			
Bone marrow depletion	4		2 (One death)
Cardiac failure			1 (Death)
Liver hemorrhage			1

55-year-old woman was submitted for liver biopsy immediately prior to perfusion; she developed severe liver hemorrhaging as a result of full heparinization, which was required for the subsequent perfusion, but recovered completely after hepatic artery ligation.

Discussion

This prospective study on the effects of HIPM on unexcised, in-transit metastases of melanoma allows the objective appraisal of its direct effect on measurable tumors.

Regression of Metastases After HIPM

Melphalan at a lethal concentration — 4–6 times higher than the maximum tolerable concentration when injected intravenously — produced, with the addition of heat, a response rate of 81% (CR + PR), which is about 8 times the response rate that can be reached after systemic administration (Lejeune and de Wasch 1978). In addition, to the best of our knowledge, no systemic chemotherapy has ever been shown to be so effective on skin and soft tissue melanoma metastases. Nitrosourea derivatives, DTIC used as monotherapy or in combination (Luce 1972), and *cis*-platinum in combination with vindesine were usually shown to provide response rates of 20%–25% (Mulder et al., to be published).

The median remission duration was 6 months for PR and 19 months for CR: this is also superior to the several months expected after systemic chemotherapy (Luce 1972; Lejeune and de Wasch 1978; Mulder et al., to be published).

Our results, however, are in agreement with the findings of others (Martijn et al. 1981; Stehlin et al. 1975, 1979) after separate analysis of cases with unexcised metastases subjected to HIPM. Stehlin et al. (1975) mentioned a few cases of tumor eradication after HIPM. Of nine patients who failed to regress after intralesional BCG, Storm et al. 1979 found local disease control in seven, with 10 months' median duration, which is somewhat shorter than the median duration reached in this study.

Other studies did not use the addition of heat to melphalan. The early report by Stehlin et al. (1963) mentions approximately 33% response in unexcised metastases. A 48% PR rate was achieved for 7 months in a recent series, with 50% after perfusion with three drugs (McBride 1970) − melphalan, actinomycin-D, and mechlorethamine hydrochloride − also under normothermic conditions.

The earlier claim (Krementz and Ryan 1972; Stehlin 1969) that hyperthermia − 39°−41° C − increases the efficiency of melphalan is supported by our results.

Survival After HIPM for Stage IIa and IIa b Melanomas

Our patients experienced a rather short survival after HIPM, averaging 18.2−20 months, despite the high response rate in terms of complete and partial remission. Moreover, it seems that CR patients did not do significantly better than PR patients; the two no-response patients had very short survival times of 4 and 10 months. The same survival times were observed by others (Bulman and Jamieson 1980; Storm et al. 1979; Weaver et al. 1975) who also had good regional response after HIPM. In contrast, Stehlin et al. (1979) found an unexpected 74% 5-year survival rate. We do not have any explanation for this discrepancy but it might be a selection factor. Although some authors (McBride 1970; Stehlin et al. 1975) have suggested that HIPM may have an indirect effect, through immunological stimulation it seems difficult to believe that regional chemotherapy and hyperthermia could have a favorable systemic effect on distant micrometastases.

It is worth pointing out that in our study, leaving the regional metastases does not seem to have been detrimental to our patients' survival, when we compare with the work done on excision following HIPM (Martijn et al. 1981).

Prognostic Factors after HIPM

Time to response did not vary significantly according to either the response itself or the tumor burden (Table 2). In contrast, remission duration was significantly longer for CR (Table 2) than for PR, and the tumor burden was inversely proportional to the remission time. Neither the average tumor diameter nor the stage of disease influenced remission. In addition, there was no obvious difference in terms of response between stages IIa and IIa b (Table 1), despite the great difference in survival time.

The magnitude of response to the first HIPM did not seem predictive of the second HIPM response in the five available patients (Table 3). It is worth pointing out that there was a long period of CR after the second HIPM, though only PR was induced by the first (case no. 2, Table 3).

Recurrence and Further Treatment

The rate of recurrence (35%) in the perfused limb in our study is identical to the results obtained by Martijn et al. (1981) who perfused twice, sometimes with two drugs, and widely excised after the second HIPM.

Therefore, it may be suggested that the major effect can be obtained by HIPM alone and that wide excision of the in-transit metastases sites is not useful, except in isolated individual cases, e.g., for debulking and in case of local hemorrhage. Salvage of the limb is the ultimate reasonable aim in such cases, and our results confirm this, as do others (Krementz and Ryan 1972; Stehlin et al. 1975; Storm et al. 1979; Weaver et al. 1975).

Distant metastases have been recorded in 50% of our cases and their distribution does not seem to differ from what is reported in the literature (Sacre and Lejeune 1982).

The response rate to systemic chemotherapy after HIPM in cases of distant metastases and/or limb recurrences in our series was extremely poor: one response in 11 cases. The patient received *cis*-platinum-vindesine according to the EORTC protocol no. 18802 which reports a total response rate of approximately 21% (Mulder et al., to be published). These poor results obtained with systemic chemotherapy after HIPM suggest the possibility of the occurrence of a selective drug-resistance phenomenon.

In contrast, radiotherapy and intralesional BCG produced objective response in four cases after HIPM. These therapies might be worth investigating further as combination therapy in conjunction with HIPM (Krementz and Ryan 1972; Stehlin 1969; Storm et al. 1979).

Complications After HIPM

The main complication has been edema of the perfused leg. It seems to be due, in our cases, to the addition of radical lymph node dissection, which we used to perform, either prophylactically or therapeutically, in the first half of our patients. It was indeed claimed (Creech and Krementz 1964; Krementz and Ryan 1972; McBride 1970) that complications, including necrosis, infections, and accumulation of serum were common, as in our cases, after regional node dissection. Our remaining cases were treated in two steps; when a lymph node dissection had to be performed therapeutically, it was done 4–6 weeks after HIPM, with no complications.

In conclusion, HIPM – using the alkalating agent melphalan with medium heat – seems to be a valuable method for treating regional melanoma spreading on the limb, as it provides a 91% objective response rate, resulting in limb salvage for most patients. However, survival does not seem to be affected by this treatment when it is applied to stage IIa and IIa b melanomas.

References

Au FC, Goldman LI (1979) Isolation perfusion in limb melanoma: A critical assessment and literature review. In: Clark WH, Goldman LI, Mastrangelo MJ (eds) Human malignant melanoma. Clinical oncology. Grune and Stratton, New York, p 295

Bleiberg H, La Meir E, Lejeune F (1980) Laparoscopy in the diagnosis of liver metastases in 80 cases of malignant melanoma. Endoscopy 12: 215

Bulman AS, Jamieson CW (1980) Isolated limb perfusion with melphalan in the treatment of malignant melanoma. Br J Surg 67: 660

Creech O, Krementz ET (1964) Regional perfusion in melanoma of limbs. JAMA 188: 855

Giovanella BC, Stehlin JS, Morgan AC (1976) Selective lethal effect of supranormal temperatures on human neoplastic cells. Cancer Res 36: 3944

Krementz ET, Ryan RF (1972) Chemotherapy of melanoma of the extremities by perfusion: fourteen years clinical experience. Ann Surg 175: 900

Lejeune FJ, De Wasch G (1978) Malignant melanoma. In: Staquet MJ (ed) Randomized trials in cancer: a critical review by sites. Raven, New York, p 339

Lejeune FJ, Mathieu M, Kenis Y (1977) Hyperthermic isolation perfusion with melphalan. A preliminary appraisal of local and general effects in malignant melanoma. Tumori 63: 289

Luce JK (1972) Chemotherapy of malignant melanoma. Cancer 30: 1604

Martijn H, Oldhoff J, Schraffordt Koops H (1981) Regional perfusion in the treatment of patients with a locally metastasized malignant melanoma of the limbs. Eur J Cancer 17: 471

McBride CM (1970) Advanced melanoma of the extremities. Treatment by isolation perfusion with a triple drug combination. Arch Surg 101: 122

McPeak CJ, McNeer GP, Whiteley HW, Booker RJ (1963) Amputation for melanoma of the extremity. Surgery 54: 427

Miller TR (1977) Hemipelvectomy in lower extremity tumors. Orthop Clin North Am 8: 903

Mulder JH, Dodion P, Cavalli F, Czarnetzki B, Clavel M, Thomas D, Suciu S, Rozencweig M (to be published) Cisplatin and vindesine combination chemotherapy in advanced malignant melanoma: an EORTC phase II study

Sacre R, Lejeune FJ (1982) Pattern of metastases distribution in 173 stage I or II melanoma patients. Anticancer Res 2: 47

Stehlin JS (1969) Hyperthermic perfusion with chemotherapy for cancers of the extremities. Surg Gynecol Obstet 129: 305

Stehlin JS, Clark RL, Vickers WE, Monges A (1963) Perfusion for malignant melanoma of the extremities. Am J Surg 105: 607

Stehlin JS, Giovanella BC, de Ipolyi PD, Muenz LR, Anderson RF (1975) Results of hyperthermic perfusion for melanoma of the extremities. Surg Gynecol Obstet 140: 338

Stehlin JS, Giovanella BC, de Ipolyi PD, Anderson RF (1979) Results of eleven years' experience with heated perfusion for melanoma of the extremities. Cancer Res 39: 2255

Storm FK, Sparks FC, Morton DL (1979) Treatment for melanoma of the lower extremity with intralesional injection oif bacille Calmette Guérin and hyperthermic perfusion. Surg Gynecol Obstet 149: 17

Weaver PC, Wright J, Brander WL, Wesbury G (1975) Salvage procedures for locally advanced malignant melanoma of the lower limb (with special reference to the role of isolated limb perfusion and radical lymph adenectomy). Clin Oncol 1: 45

Results of Regional Hyperthermic Perfusion for Primary and Recurrent Melanomas of the Extremities

P.-E. Jönsson, L. Hafström, and A. Hugander

Department of Surgery, University of Lund, 22185 Lund, Sweden

Introduction

The technique for regional isolated perfusion has remained essentially the same since it was introduced in 1957, with the exception that heat was added in 1967 (Creech et al. 1958; Stehlin 1969). The anticancer drug most consistently used since 1957 is melphalan (Alkeran). The aim of isolation perfusion is to subject the tumor-bearing region to the influence of a high concentration of anticancer drugs in such a way that contamination of other parts of the body does not occur to any significant extent (Stehlin 1969). Malignant melanoma of the extremities seems especially suitable for this treatment, because local and regional metastases occur in up to 20% of patients (McBride et al. 1975). Reports of prolonged survival and local control of tumor growth have also encouraged many centers to perform this kind of treatment, not only for palliative (therapeutic) but also for curative (adjuvant) purposes (McBride et al. 1975; Stehlin et al. 1975; Martijn et al. 1982).

In this report the experience with, and results of, hyperthermic melphalan perfusion for primary and recurrent melanoma in Lund since 1976 are presented.

Material and Methods

From 1976 to 1979 32 patients (nine males, 23 females; age range 25−75 years, median age 55 years) with primary melanoma on the extremities, and from 1976 to 1981 36 patients (11 males, 25 females; age range 32−80 years, median age 66 years) with recurrent melanoma on the extremities were perfused. In the group with primary, the tumor site was on the upper extremity in four patients and on the lower extremity in 28. According to the Clark classification, the primary melanoma was level III in one patient, level IV in 25, and level V in six. After lymph node dissection eight patients were found to have micrometastases and were therefore considered clinical stage IIIB while the remaining 24 were still stage I.

In all 36 patients with recurrent melanoma, the diagnosis was verified by excision or fine-needle biopsy. This patient group included 12 with stage II, eight with stage IIIA, eight with IIIB, seven with IIIAB, and one with IV. The total of 68 patients underwent 80 perfusions; four patients with primary were reperfused and eight with recurrent disease.

Recent Results in Cancer Research, Vol. 86
© Springer-Verlag Berlin · Heidelberg 1983

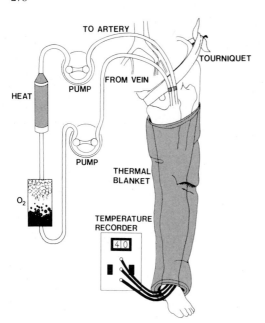

Fig. 1. Illustration of technique for regional perfusion of lower extremity with cytostatics and controlled hyperthermia

Checkups included physical examination, laboratory tests, chest X-rays, and liver scans on a regular basis. Whenever neurological symptoms appeared, a brain scan or computed tomography of the brain was performed.

Technique of Hyperthermic Perfusion

Our technique is the same as that described by Stehlin et al. (1975); Fig. 1 illustrates the setup. For lower extremity perfusion the femoral artery and vein were cannulated, and for upper extremity the axillary vessels. The perfusion circuit consisted of a pediatric heart-lung machine with a membrane oxygenator and a heat exchanger. The perfusion fluid consisted of blood and Ringer solution, and its temperature was maintained at 41.5°−42° C. Perfusion pressure was kept just below the mean systemic arterial blood pressure. The flow rate was 400−600 ml/min. The temperature was monitored continuously by thermistor probes placed intramuscularly, subcutaneously, and cutaneously at different levels of the extremity.

The dosage of melphalan was 0.9 mg/kg body wt. for the lower extremity and half that amount for the upper extremity. Half the amount of the drug was added to the perfusate when the intramuscular temperature had reached 38°−39° C, and the other half when half of the perfusion time had passed. The perfusion time was 1 h for adjuvant and 2 h for therapeutic perfusions. When the perfusion time was over the extremity was rinsed with Ringer solution.

For staging purposes an inguinal lymph node dissection was performed when the femoral vessels were isolated. The lymphatic tissue around the common iliac vessel was also dissected through a separate incision above and parallel with the inguinal ligament. For upper extremity perfusions a staging axillary node dissection was made.

Results

Perfusion for Primary

The follow-up time for patients perfused for primary melanoma was 3−6.5 years, with a median time of 4.5 years. The first sign of tumor progress was local in six patients (19%) and systemic in two (6%). Relapse of disease occurred after 11−37 months with a median time of 24 months (Fig. 2). Recurrence of disease in relation to Clark level and clinical stage is shown in Table 1. The crude 3-year survival was 94%.

Perfusion for Recurrent Disease

The follow-up time for patients with recurrent melanoma was 6 months to 7 years, median time 3.5 years. Fifteen patients with manifest tumor at the time of perfusion had tumor

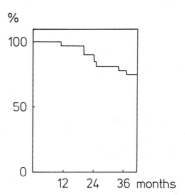

Fig. 2. Percentage of patients free of recurrence from start of therapy

Table 1. The first recurrence site in relation to Clark level and clinical stage after adjuvant perfusion

Clarc level	Recurrence site		Stage	Recurrence site	
	Local	Systemic		Local	Systemic
IV	5 of 25	1 of 25	I	4 of 24	1 of 24
V	1 of 6	1 of 6	IIIB	2 of 8	1 of 8

Table 2. Evaluation of treatment effect on manifest tumor in 15 patients

Regression of local tumor (%)	No. of patients
100	1
> 50	10
< 50	3
0	1

Table 3. Complications in 68 patients who underwent 80 perfusions

	Adjuvant perfusion	Therapeutic perfusion
Seroma	12	6
Wound infection	4	5
Hematoma	2	1
Arterial bleeding	–	1
Venous thrombosis	1	–
Skin necrosis	–	1
Compartment syndrome	1	–

response evaluated (Table 2). One patient with a tumor 3 cm in diameter at the elbow had complete regression. After removal of the tumor histopathological examination did not reveal any signs of viable tumor cells.

After treatment seven patients had local recurrence on the extremity as the first manifestation of tumor progress; in four of these patients it was the only manifestation of the disease. Eight patients had systemic metastases as the first sign of recurrence. The median time for new recurrences on the extremity was eight months (1–20 months) and for systemic metastases seven months (5–30 months). Twenty-two patients are still alive; 14 have died of progressive disease, after a median time of 17 months.

Complications

The distribution of complications in adjuvant and therapeutic perfusions are shown in Table 3. Three major complications were registered, skin necrosis, thrombosis in the lower leg, and compartment syndrome. There was no toxic effect on the bone marrow observed in any patient.

Discussion

Partial tumor response has been reported by several authors when perfusion was performed for manifest melanoma (Stehlin et al. 1975; Martijn et al. 1982; Sugarbaker and McBride 1976; Lejeune et al. 1977). The results concerning survival in different series are impossible to analyze properly because or the lack of uniformity in classification, and in performance of the perfusion treatment. In a comprehensive study of melanoma patients with in-transit metastases (IIIA) improved survival figures are reported specifically after hyperthermic perfusion (Stehlin et al. 1975). Other reports, even if not comparable, indicate a somewhat lower survival rate (Lejeune et al. 1977; Schraffordt Koops et al. 1977). Compared with surgical excision or amputation, the gain by regional hyperthermic perfusion is convincing (Krementz et al. 1979; Fortner et al. 1974; Cox 1974).

The clinical course after therapeutic perfusion is related to the extension of local and regional tumor growth (Schraffordt Koops et al. 1977; Hafström and Jönsson 1980). Patients with regional lymph node metastases usually developed distant metastases as the first sign of tumor progress.

When regional perfusion has been performed in stage I patients as an adjuvant therapy to standard surgical treatment, a 5-year survival rate of 80%–85% is reported (Stehlin et al.

1975; Schraffordt Koops et al. 1977). The local recurrence rate within 5 years in many of these series is approximately 5%. For comparison there are now reports of the same 5-year disease-free survival and a local recurrence rate below 10% in series treated by surgery alone (Day et al. 1981). It is difficult to interpret our results as compared with others because of differences in tumor staging, in the primary standard surgical treatment, and histopathological classification. The 3-year survival in the present series is comparable to previous reports, but the local recurrence rate is significantly higher. Unfortunately, the tumor thickness in our patients is unknown. This has to be evaluated before definitive conclusions can be drawn. The immediate result, however, does not indicate any decrease with adjuvant perfusion in the local recurrence rate.

The incidence of complications from regional hyperthermic perfusion must be considered low. In 13 cases of 2,000 perfusions reported in the literature, amputation of the perfused extremity was performed due to tissue necrosis (less than 0.1%) (Hafström and Jönsson 1979). The myelosuppressive effect is limited, as well, to approximately 4% of patients. To conclude, the complication rate is not of such a magnitude that the procedure is contraindicated in other than exceptional cases.

Opinions as to the value of regional hyperthermic perfusion range from enthusiastic to maximally negative. All authors who have employed the technique are pleased with the results. Our negative experience with adjuvant hyperthermic perfusion in high-risk primary melanoma does not mean that there is no benefit from this treatment. There may be a subgroup of patients, e.g., primary melanoma thicker than 3−4 mm, who might benefit from the procedure. Although good tumor response is seen in perfusion for recurrent melanoma evaluation of the definitive value of this type of treatment as compared with surgery is mandatory. Such a clinical trial is now underway in the Swedish Melanoma Study Group. A similar study would also be most welcome for in primary melanoma (e.g., thicker than 3−4 mm), but the approach should be limited to those individuals and institutions equipped to perform the procedure and follow-up in a controlled manner. There are also many other factors which have to be further evaluated, e.g., the rationale for using hyperthermia, the proper drugs, the importance of oxygenation and leakage, many questions which have to be solved by experiments. Recent results of Karakousis et al. (1979) indicating that tourniquet infusion with anticancer drugs give tissue levels comparable to those after hyperthermic perfusion is of great interest. This underlines the importance of further evaluation of anticancer drugs to determine which is the most suitable for hyperthermic perfusion.

References

Cox KR (1974) Survival after amputation for recurrent melanoma. Surg Gynecol Obstet 139: 720

Creech O Jr, Krementz ET, Ryan RF, Winblad JN (1958) Regional perfusion utilizing an extracorporeal circuit. Ann Surg 148: 616

Day CL, Sober AJ, Kopf A, Lew RA, Mihm MC (1981) A prognostic model for clinical stage I melanoma of the lower extremity. Surgery 89: 599

Fortner JG, Strong EW, Mulcare RJ, Schottenfield D, Maclean BJ (1974) The surgical treatment of recurrent melanoma. Surg Clin North Am 54: 865

Hafström L, Jönsson P-E (1979) Regional perfusion with anticancer drugs for treatment of malignant tumors. In: Pettersson HI (ed) Tumor blood circulation CRC, Florida, p 217

Hafström L, Jönsson P-E (1980) Hyperthermic perfusion of recurrent melanoma on the extremities. Acta Chir Scand 146: 313

Karakousis CP, Kanter PM, Lopez RE, Moore R, Holyoke ED (1979) Modes of regional chemotherapy. J Surg Res 26: 134

Krementz ET, Carter RD, Sutherland CM, Campell M (1979) The use of regional chemotherapy in the management of malignant melanoma. World J Surg 3: 289

Lejeune FJ, Mathieu M, Kenis Y (1977) Hyperthermic isolation perfusion with melphalan. A preliminary appraisal of local and general effects in malignant melanoma. Tumori 63: 289

Martijn H, Oldhoff J, Schraffordt-Koops H (1982) Hyperthermic regional perfusion with melphalan and a combination of melphalan and actinomycin D in the treatment of locally metastasized malignant melanomas of the extremities. J Surg Oncol 20: 9

McBride CM, Sugarbaker EV, Hickey RC (1975) Prophylactic isolation perfusion as the primary therapy for massive malignant melanoma of the limbs. Ann Surg 182: 316

Schraffordt-Koops H, Oldhoff J, van der Ploeg E, Vermey A, Eiberger R (1977) Regional perfusion for recurrent melanoma of the extremities. Am J Surg 133: 221

Stehlin JS Jr (1969) Hyperthermic perfusion with chemotherapy for cancer of the extremities. Surg Gynecol Obstet 129: 305

Stehlin JS Jr, Giovanella BC, de Ipolyi PP, Muenez LR, Anderson RF (1975) Results of hyperthermic perfusion for melanoma of the extremities. Surg Gynecol Obstet 140: 338

Sugarbaker EV, McBride CM (1976) Survival and regional disease control after isolation perfusion for massive stage I melanoma of the extremities. Cancer 37: 188

First Histologic Findings in Metastases of Colorectal Carcinoma Following Isolated Liver Perfusion with Cytostatics

A. Schulz and J. Kracht

Zentrum für Pathologie, Universitätsklinikum, Langhansstrasse 10, 6300 Giessen, FRG

Introduction

The development of different forms of tumor therapy specific for individual tumor forms or tumor groups has increased the demands made on clinical pathology. One of the major tasks is precise morphological tumor diagnosis. This requires the use of immunological and electron microscopic techniques in addition to conventional histology (Kuzela et al. 1982; Themann 1980). For a number of epithelial and mesenchymal tumors, highly effective oncological therapy regimens based on precise diagnosis have been developed. Tumor sensitivity to treatment is mainly controlled by means of clinical parameters, such as tumor markers in serum, sonography, and computerized tomography (Clark 1982), but modern clinical pathology has also been assigned new tasks in connection with therapeutic effectiveness control. The pathologist is asked the following questions:

1. Which signs of tumor regression resulting from oncological therapy can be demonstrated?
2. Can a definite therapeutic effect be verified on the basis of the tumor regression signs?
3. Is the treatment employed effective, and therefore the right one for the respective tumor?

To determine a therapeutic effect a "second-look" biopsy is performed in the course of treatment (Alken et al. 1975), or a tumor resection specimen is histologically examined after chemotherapy (Rosen et al. 1982). Experience gathered so far has resulted in the establishment of various morphological regression grades. In this context the tendency of

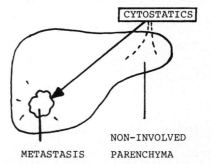

Fig. 1. Effect of perfusion with cytostatics on tumor and liver

tumors to spontaneous regression in the form of necrosis must also be kept in mind (Mavligit et al. 1981).

This study is concerned with the regression of liver metastases of colorectal carcinomas after liver perfusion with cytostatic substances. In addition to evaluating the extent of tumor regression, we also wanted to determine whether high levels of the cytostatic substance cause damage to the noninvolved liver parenchyma (Fig. 1).

Material and Methods

In two patients who had undergone surgery for colorectal carcinoma, liver metastases occurred after intervals of 1 and 12 months. Since there were no other metastases, isolated liver perfusion with 5-fluorouracil (300 mg and 450 mg) was performed using a newly

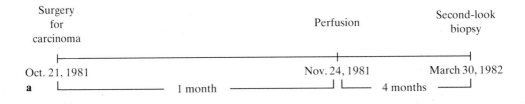

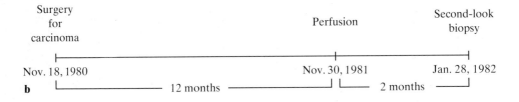

Fig. 2. Time tables for **a** case 1 and **b** case 2. Case 1 is a 58-year-old woman, A. H., with well-differentiated rectal adenocarcinoma and metastases to the liver; Duke's stage C. Case 2 is a 61-year-old man, W. W., with moderately differentiated rectal adenocarcinoma and metastases to the liver; Duke's stage C. Both were perfused with 5-FU

Table 1. Histologic regression of liver metastases after perfusion with 5-FU

Therapeutic effect	Grade of regression			Case
None	No regression	NR	I	
Possible	Stable tumor	ST	II	
				A.H.
Probable	Partial regression (40−60%)	PR −	III	
				W.W.
Definite	Partial regression	PR +	IV	
	Complete regression	CR	V	

developed method (Aigner et al. "First Experimental Results of Isolated Liver Perfusion with Cytostatics in Metastases from Colorectal Primary", this volume). At the time of perfusion, biopsies of liver tissue and metastatic tumor tissue were taken to serve as a basis for further evaluation. After intervals of 2 and 4 months second-look surgery was performed, during which liver tissue and metastatic tumor tissue were again obtained to monitor the effectiveness of treatment (Fig. 2a and b). The tissue was processed according to conventional histologic technique by paraffin embedding. To assess tumor regression and therapeutic effect a five-grade regression grading system based on that of Mavligit et al. (1981) was used (Table 1).

Results

In both patients the primary tumor was rectal adenocarcinoma with regional lymph node metastases. Accordingly, a Duke's stage-C tumor was diagnosed at the time of surgery. The tumor was highly differentiated in one patient and moderately differentiated in the other. Tumor differentiation was also identical in the liver metastases. The interval between initial surgery and second-look surgery was between 2 and 4 months in the two patients. The post-perfusion findings also differed in these two patients. One exhibited a relatively strong regression of tumor tissue, exceeding 60% of the metastastic tissue examined, whereas tumor regression in the other patient was maximal at 40%. On the basis of the regression grading employed the therapeutic effects, as measured against the quantitative changes, must be assessed with caution.

Patient 1 (A. H.) with 40% tumor regression was classified between grades II and III (therapeutic effect, possible to probable) whereas patient 2 (W. W.) with tumor regression between 60% and 90% was rated as a case between grades III and IV (therapeutic effect, probable to definite) (Table 1).

A qualitative assessment of the effect of treatment gives results that are a little better: the tumor tissue showed areas of stromal fibrosis in both patients. The tumor cell complexes in the fibrotic areas exhibited distinct cytological regression phenomena, consisting of regressive nuclear polymorphy due to nuclear pyknosis and chromatin condensation, as well as cytoplasmic changes in the form of hydropic swelling, vacuolization, and loss of the glandular pattern (Figs. 3 and 4).

The liver parenchyma of both patients was also thoroughly studied histologically before and after perfusion. Morphologically, neither of them showed any liver damage. Before perfusion one of them was found to have merely a slight focal fatty degeneration of the liver parenchyma (under 10%) which was still present to the same extent after perfusion.

Discussion

Isolated liver perfusion is used to bring high doses of a cytostatic substance to the liver metastases. The blood containing the cytostatic agent is supplied via a second circulatory system which is isolated from the other circulation, with separate oxygenation of the blood of the hepatic artery and the portal vein by a heart-lung machine (Aigner et al. "First experimental Results of Isolated Liver Perfusion with Cytostatics in Metastases from Colorectal Primary"). In this manner the remaining organism is not affected by the cytostatic substance.

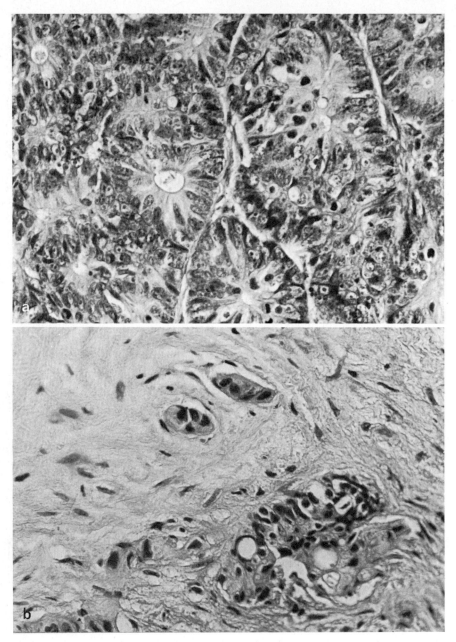

Fig. 3. a Liver metastases in patient no. 1 before perfusion therapy; highly differentiated adenocarcinoma. **b** Regressive changes of liver metastases following perfusion therapy. Loss of glandular pattern, nuclear pyknosis, stromal fibrosis. H and E, × 240

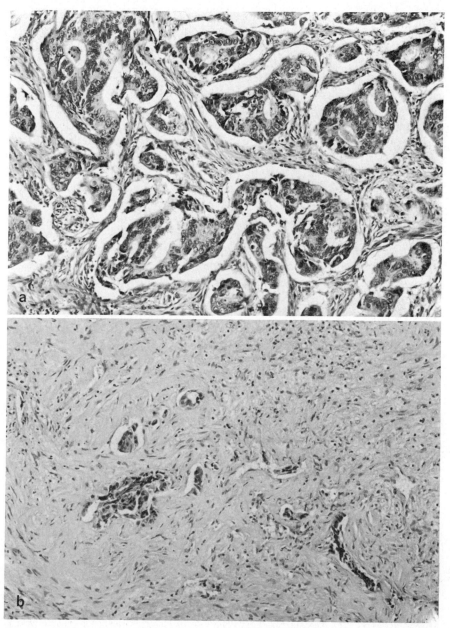

Fig. 4. a Liver metastases of colorectal carcinoma in patient no. 2 before liver perfusion therapy; moderately differentiated adenocarcinoma. **b** Regressive changes following perfusion therapy as described for patient no. 1. H and E, × 120

During this isolated high loading with 5-fluorouracil the liver parenchyma must be regarded as being particularly endangered. However, no morphological indication of liver damage was found in the two patients after 2 and 4 months. Despite the relatively high doses of 300 mg and 450 mg no hepatotoxic effect had been reached in the patients we examined. The therapeutic tolerance range does not even seem to have been fully exhausted, since in experiments with dogs nearly double the dosage (10 mg/kg) resulted in no signs of a hepatotoxic effect (Daly et al. 1982).

Even without therapy, metastatic tumors show regression signs in the form of tumor necroses. In most cases they are to be interpreted as being the result of circulatory disturbances arising from insufficient vascularization of the tumor tissue. The tendency to spontaneous necrosis differs quantitatively in different tumors and must be taken into account in the assessment of therapeutic effects. Differentiation between spontaneous and therapy-induced involution of tumor tissue is facilitated by cellular regression phenomena, which have already been established by Alken et al. (1975) during the biopsy examination and therapy control of prostatic carcinoma. According to these authors regressive nuclear polymorphy and vacuolization of the cytoplasm constitute definite regression signs on a cellular basis. An additional histological finding is fibrosis of the tumor, which we were able to demonstrate to some extent in the two cases we investigated (Figs. 3b and 4b).

In the quantitative assessment of therapy-induced tumor regression not only the extent of necrosis but also the typical cytologic and histologic criteria must therefore be considered. As a measure for assessing the effectiveness of therapy a five-grade regression grading analogous to that of Mavligit et al. (1981) was used. According to this grading system, a therapeutic effect is probable only if partial tumor regression exceeds 60%. If regression is less than 40%, a therapeutic effect is merely possible. The changes found in the metastatic tumor tissue of the two investigated patients after perfusion therapy were assigned to these two regression grades. This critical assessment of the examination results is necessary because the present observations are based on analogous conclusions which as yet do not permit of generalization. Further experimental and clinical studies on the results of perfusion therapy are needed. The optimal dose of the cytostatic substance and the most favorable time for biopsy control must be ascertained.

References

Alken CE, Dhom G, Strauber W, Braun JS, Kopper B, Rehker H (1975) Therapie des Prostatacarcinoms und Verlaufskontrolle. Urologe A 14: 112

Clark RL (1982) Cancer 1980: Achievements, challanges and prospects. Cancer 49: 1739−1745

Daly JM, Smith G, Frazier H, Stanley JD, Copeland E (1982) Effects of systemic hyperthermia and intrahepatic infusion with 5-fluorouracil. Cancer 49: 1112−1115

Kuzela DC, True LD, Eiseman B (1982) The role of electron microscopy in the management of surgical patients. Ann Surg 195: 1

Mavligit GM, Benjamin R, Patt YZ, Jaffe N, Chuang V, Wallace S, Murray J, Ayala A, Johnston S, Hersh EM, Calvo DB (1981) Intraarterial cis-platinum for patients with inoperable skeletal tumors. Cancer 48: 1−4

Rosen G, Caparros B, Huvos AG, Kosloff C, Nirenberg A, Cacavio A, Marcove RC, Lane JM, Mehta B, Urban C (1982) Preoperative chemotherapy for osteogenic sarcoma: Selection of postoperative adjuvant chemotherapy based on the response of the primary tumor to preoperative chemotherapy. Cancer 49: 1221−1230

Themann H (1980) Möglichkeiten und Grenzen der Transmissionselektronenmikroskopie (TEM) in der Diagnostik. Mikroskopie 36: 274−318

Subject Index

abscess, hepatic 70, 72
actinomycin D 182, 196, 231, 246, 254
adenosine triphosphate (ATP) 95
adriamycin 3, 14, 38, 133, 152, 160, 182, 197, 218, 220, 254, 260
agranulocytosis 84, 85
alcohol 180
alkaline phosphatase 64
alopezia 39
amphothericin B 180
amputation 124, 127, 204, 206, 218, 221, 225, 244, 261, 270, 281
analgesic therapy 26, 37
analgesics 33
anesthesia in isolated liver perfusion 110
angiography 51, 72, 83, 128, 205
−, pelvic 27
angiomas 42
anorexia 126
antimetabolite 49
aortic, bifurcation 33
−, therapy 27
−, wall necrosis 133
arterial pressure 94, 95
− access 130, 134
arteriosklerosis 128
arteritis 197
artery, axillary 126, 194, 224, 261, 269, 278
−, brachial 50, 94, 126, 215, 218, 261
−, bronchial 129, 134
−, coeliac 52, 126
−, common, carotid 169, 174
−, −, iliac 43
−, deeper femoral 239
−, epigastric 126, 196

−, external carotid 10, 142, 149, 152, 162, 165, 169, 206
−, − iliac 194, 218, 224, 239, 261, 269
−, femoral 26, 52, 194, 215, 218, 261, 269, 278
−, gastroduodenal 69, 70, 87
−, hepatic 1, 50, 70, 83, 87, 94, 99
−, −, aneurysmn 70
−, −, ligation 76
−, −, occlusion 91
−, hypogastric 31
−, intercostal 130
−, internal, carotid 41
−, −, iliac 16, 38
−, −, thoracic 130
−, mammary 126
−, maxillary 153
−, morphology in perfusion, adriamycin 257
−, perforation 30
−, popliteal 261, 269
−, pulmonary 128, 134
−, regeneration 70
−, renal 44
−, splenic 52
−, subclavian 126
−, superficial, femoral 205, 215, 239
−, −, temporal 142, 149, 153, 162, 165
−, transverse facial 142, 149
ascites 80

bacille Calmette Guerin (BCG) 273
bile duct 13, 94
biopsies, liver tissue 285
−, metastases 285
bleeding 23, 35, 84
bleomycin 3, 23, 149, 152, 160, 167, 171

Recent Results in Cancer Research

Sponsored by the Swiss League against Cancer. Editor in Chief: P. Rentchnick, Genève

D